# Experimental Design and Statistical Analysis for Pharmacology and the Biomedical Sciences

Wilcoxon
Hypothesis
freedom
chi-square
descriptive
Tukey SNK
mode
ANOVA
statistic
paired variance
standard
Mann-Whitney mean
confidence degrees
Friedman independ

z-score
Dunnett
deviation family
error
Type

# Experimental Design and Statistical Analysis for Pharmacology and the Biomedical Sciences

Paul J. Mitchell
Department of Pharmacy and Pharmacology
University of Bath
Bath, UK

Department of Pharmacology and Therapeutics
National University of Ireland (NUI)
Galway, Ireland

WILEY Blackwell

*Registered Offices*

John Wiley & Sons, Inc., 111 River Street, Hoboken, NJ 07030, USA

John Wiley & Sons Ltd, The Atrium, Southern Gate, Chichester, West Sussex, PO19 8SQ, UK

*Editorial Office*

9600 Garsington Road, Oxford, OX4 2DQ, UK

For details of our global editorial offices, customer services, and more information about Wiley products visit us at www.wiley.com.

Wiley also publishes its books in a variety of electronic formats and by print-on-demand. Some content that appears in standard print versions of this book may not be available in other formats.

*Library of Congress Cataloging-in-Publication Data*

Names: Mitchell, Paul J. (Senior lecturer and Associate Professor in pharmacology) author.
Title: Experimental design and statistical analysis for pharmacology and
 the biomedical sciences / Paul J. Mitchell.
Description: Hoboken, NJ : John Wiley & Sons, Inc., 2022. | Includes
 bibliographical references and index.
Identifiers: LCCN 2021034578 (print) | LCCN 2021034579 (ebook) | ISBN
 9781119437635 (paperback) | ISBN 9781119437673 (adobe pdf) | ISBN
 9781119437666 (epub)
Subjects: MESH: Research Design | Pharmacology | Data Interpretation,
 Statistical
Classification: LCC RM301.12  (print) | LCC RM301.12  (ebook) | NLM QV 20.5
 | DDC 615.1–dc23
LC record available at https://lccn.loc.gov/2021034578
LC ebook record available at https://lccn.loc.gov/2021034579

Cover design: Wiley
Cover image: © RomanOkopny/Getty Images

Set in 9.5/11.5pt Minion by Straive, Pondicherry, India

*This book is dedicated to my parents Alec and Jean, long gone but never, ever, forgotten, and to my wife, Angela, and our children Matthew and Samantha of whom I am immensely proud.*

# Biography

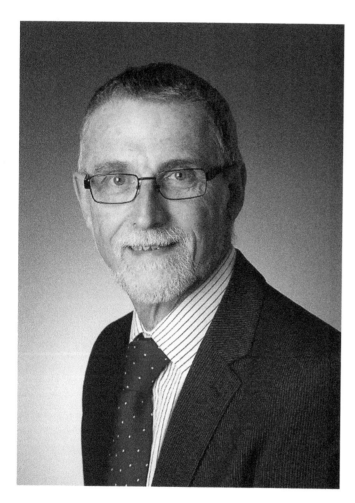

**D**r Paul J Mitchell is a Senior Lecturer and an Associate Professor in the Department of Pharmacy and Pharmacology, University of Bath, United Kingdom, and Adjunct Lecturer in the Department of Pharmacology and Therapeutics, National University of Ireland (NUI), Galway, Ireland.

His career in pharmacology started in 1975 when he joined the cardiovascular group led by Dr Bob Poyser at Beecham Pharmaceuticals, Harlow, United Kingdom. After five years, during which he also graduated with an Upper Second BSc in Applied Biology (Pharmacology) from North East London Polytechnic under Prof Geof B West, he transferred to the CNS disorders group led by Dr Mike Clarke. Dr Mitchell left Beecham in 1985 to start post-graduate studies with Dr (now emeritus Prof) Peter Redfern in the School of Pharmacy and Pharmacology, University of Bath, United Kingdom. After successfully defending his PhD thesis on the *Effect of Antidepressant Treatment on Social Behaviour and Circadian Rhythms of Locomotor Activity in the Rat* in 1989, he joined the research laboratories of Wyeth-Ayerst, Taplow, principally to examine the potential antidepressant activity of novel psychotropic compounds in the rodent models of social behaviour that were developed during his postgraduate studies. The results of these behavioural studies were pivotal in the company's decision to fully develop venlafaxine (known in-house as Wy 45030) to the clinic. Subsequently, Dr Mitchell became heavily involved in the further pre-clinical development of venlafaxine (Effexor®, Efexor®), the world's first SNRI antidepressant drug, which was approved by the U.S.FDA in 1993 and by the MHRA in the United Kingdom in 1994.

In 1995, Dr Mitchell returned to the University of Bath to set up his own lab to continue examining the effect of antidepressant drugs on rodent social behaviour (Resident-Intruder test and Social Hierarchy model of social behaviour), while working very closely with the pharmaceutical industry (principally colleagues at Wyeth-Ayerst in the USA, Lundbeck in Denmark, and Organon in the United Kingdom).

Over the last 25 years, Dr Mitchell has collaborated with colleagues at the University of Bath and NUIGalway to develop a coherent strategy to teach experimental design and statistical analysis to undergraduate and postgraduate students across subject areas in the Life and Biomedical sciences.

Dr Mitchell has been a member of the British Pharmacological Society since 1985. He is currently working closely with the society on a residential training workshop on the topic of this book covering the principles of robust, rigorous, experimental design, and statistical analysis. This course is ideal for early career researchers working in drug discovery or academia.

# Contents

# Acknowledgements

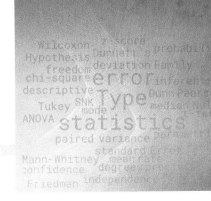

## Homo Sapiens – Part 1

Looking back over copious notes and draft versions of this book, I've come to realise that this project has taken me far longer than my initial 12-month plan envisaged. But let me take you back to the beginning of the 2016–2017 academic year when I confronted a group of pharmacology undergraduate students who had just returned from a year's placement and were about to embark on the final year of their degree programme. My question 'So, how're your stats skills coming along now you've been in the big wide world?' was met with a mixture of dismay and disdain, not to say contempt for mentioning the S word! The ensuing conversation quickly dispelled any thoughts on my part regarding their progress and so I quickly put together an intense four-week package, which covered all my statistics lectures and hands-on data analysis workshops to get them up to speed. The feedback I received suggested that delivering such material in such a short period was successful, but one important component was missing; they had no access to a suitable concise textbook covering descriptive and inferential statistics suitable for undergraduate pharmacology students. Indeed their major complaint was that currently available textbooks were either focused on statistical theory (suitable only for highly competent students of mathematics) or were simply user guides for statistical software packages; both of which were totally inappropriate for students who simply wanted to know which statistical tests they had to use to analyse different types of experimental data. In short, they needed a concise 'textbook' book, which showed them how to use statistics as a *tool* with which they could analyse their experimental data and arrive at appropriate conclusions, thereby revealing the relationship of their data to the real world. So, it seems obvious to me that the first group of individuals that I should thank, and you, dear reader, should blame for kick-starting this project which has resulted in the contents of this book, are the infamous seven final year pharmacology students from 2016: Charlotte Bell, Charlotte Day, Sam Groom, James Miles (yes, that cocky bugger), Katy Murrell, Gemma Wilkinson, and Alex Williams – according to my latest information most if not all have now completed (or nearly so) their subsequent PhD studies and are now forging research careers on their own (and most notably without my help!). If this book is in any way successful, then clearly you seven should be held totally accountable!

Of course, when you embark on a project that is clearly not your day job, then you need a lot of support to help you to find the time in the working day that enables you to turn that germ of an idea into fruition. My sincere thanks to all my colleagues in the Department of Pharmacy and Pharmacology at the University of Bath that in many, diverse, ways have enabled me to focus on putting this manuscript together, that have humoured me while I've ranted on regarding the statistical inadequacies in the scientific press or listened quietly while I've bombarded them with different ideas on how to describe quite complex statistical issues that an inexperienced undergraduate student may (hopefully) understand. Most importantly, my thanks to Profs Steve Ward and Roland Jones who agreed for me to move my teaching duties around that created gaps in my teaching load, which allowed me to concentrate on writing. This book is full of data examples, which, I hope, will enable the reader to understand more-fully descriptive and inferential statistics and to envisage statistics in action. Most of the data examples are my own, and for all other examples I am very grateful to Dr Malcolm Watson. I must also thank Prof Steve Husbands and Dr Christine Edmead for their helpful comments, encouragement, and suggestions after reading the first completed draft version of the manuscript; of course, considering Steve is a medicinal/organic chemist, who (by his own admission) failed to understand anything described in the book, his comments were totally ignored!

For the last 15–20 years or so, I have worked very closely with Prof John Kelly, Department of Pharmacology and Therapeutics, NUIGalway, during which we have tried, successfully it must be said, to develop a fully integrated series of lectures and workshops to teach undergraduate and postgraduate students in pharmacology, neuropharmacology, toxicology, and drug discovery the vagaries of robust experimental design and statistical analysis. I still travel to Galway every year to expose John's postgraduate students to an English sense of humour in my attempt to run hands-on statistical workshops – I must be doing OK as John keeps inviting me back! My sincere thanks to John for all the support and encouragement he has given me during that time and to other colleagues in Galway, notably Ambrose O'Halloran and Sandra O'Brien, who were instrumental in preparing the initial versions of the lectures, which I now subject my own students to back in Bath and which are closely aligned to the contents and flavour of this book.

During the life of this project, I have worked closely at various times with the management team for the British Pharmacological Society and I would like to convey my thanks to David James (Executive Director, Business Development) for his initial help and advice to get this project off the ground, and latterly to Katherine Wilson (Director, Research Dissemination) and Lee Page (Head of Education and Engagement) for their help and advice on 'what to do next'!

I am also very grateful to everybody at Wiley from Alison Oliver, who as Publications Manager and Commissioning Editor back in 2016 took a risk and encouraged me to put my ideas into a proposal, which subsequently became a formal agreement between myself and Wiley, to James Watson (Publications Manager), Kimberly Monroe-Hill (Managing Editor), and Tom Marriott (Assistant Editor, Health and Life Sciences) who have guided me through all the steps following formal submission of the final manuscript through to publication. My thanks also to the reviewers of my initial proposal to Wiley who thought this project was a good idea, who have encouraged me to complete the project ever since (hi John and Steve, you know who you are) and who also opened my eyes that this work may be not only useful within the realm of pharmacology but also throughout the biomedical and life sciences!

My career in pharmacology has taken me from the pharmaceutical industry with Beecham Pharmaceuticals in the 1970s and 1980s, through my PhD studies at the University of Bath in the latter half of the 1980s (under the invaluable supervision of Prof Peter Redfern), then back to the industry with Wyeth-Ayerst in 1989 before returning to the University of Bath in 1995 where I have remained ever since. Throughout that time in industry and academia, I have worked with a wide range of wonderful, highly skilled, individuals and made life-long friends too numerous to name individually here (but you should all know who you are on both sides of the Atlantic Ocean). I shall remain eternally grateful for all your help, guidance, encouragement, patience, comments, critique (usually constructive), and tutelage throughout my career in pharmacology.

## Statistical Packages

You will note that at the end of most of the chapters in this book, I have been able to provide screenshots from the software packages that I used to analyse the examples used in the book. This was for two purposes. First, this allowed me to check my own calculations for every single example and statistics test described herein (yes; every example has been analysed in the good old-fashioned way by hand and a good calculator – good God, what a geek I hear you cry – and you'd be right as my academic colleagues keep telling me!), and second, I hope that when you run your own data analysis you will now be forewarned about what to expect (and not be surprised) by the output from the software you have used. To that end, I am most grateful to the software companies concerned for permission to reproduce screenshots from their software. Consequently, screenshots from GraphPad – Prism®Statistics software version 8.2 and above are printed with permission of GraphPad Software, San Diego, California, USA; screenshots from MiniTab software version 18 and above are printed with permission of MiniTab, LLC; screenshots from InVivoStat are reprinted with permission of the InVivoStat team (specifically Simon Bate); and finally screenshots from IBM® SPSS® Statistics software (SPSS) version 26 and above are printed with permission from International Business Machines Corporation (IBM).

## Homo Sapiens – Part 2

I've been very lucky to have a number of very close friends who have remained loyal regardless of where my career has taken me, so a special mention to Dave Bragg ('Braggy'), John Clapham (JC), and Alan Rainbird for your unwavering friendship (which I value more than words can ever express) since we first met over 45 years ago, John Kelly (*see above*), and more recently to Kevin McDermott for dragging me out most Saturday mornings to the golf course to clear our heads for a few therapeutic hours away from the stress of our professional lives, see you on the first tee mate!

Finally (!), all my love to my wife Angela and my children Matthew and Samantha – how you all ever put up with such a cantankerous old git as myself (especially during the last four years or so while I worked on this manuscript) I shall never know. You are all my rock, and I will always be forever grateful.

# Foreword

For the last 25 years or so, I have become increasingly involved in teaching the fundamentals of statistical analysis of experimental data to, initially, pharmacy and pharmacology undergraduates but, more lately, undergraduates in other disciplines (e.g. natural sciences, biomedical sciences, biology, biochemistry, psychology, and toxicology) and postgraduate students and early researchers in these and more specific areas of pharmacological research (e.g. neuropharmacology). Throughout this time, I have become increasingly aware of the statistical rigour required by scientific journals for publication of scientific papers to be approved. However, this has been coupled with increased anxiety on the part of both new and experienced researchers as to whether their statistical approach is correct for the data generated by their studies. These observations suggest that in the past the teaching of experimental design and statistical analysis has been poor across the sector. Indeed, if I mention stats (sic) to most researchers, they hold their hands to their face and perform an imitation of Edvard Munch's *Der Schrei der Natur* ('The Scream of Nature', or more commonly known as just 'The Scream')! Statistical analysis is often viewed as burdensome and an inconvenient chore, generally borne out of ignorance and a lack of appreciation of how useful rigorous statistical analysis may be.

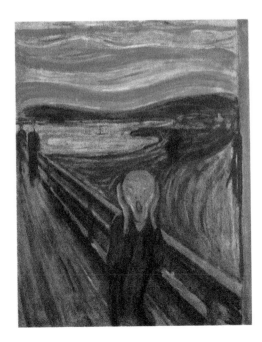

**Der Schrei der Natur (circa 1893), Edvard Munch (1863–1944)**

I'll give you three examples:

**Example 1:** On various occasions, I have had final year undergraduate students bang on my office door; I say bang – it was definitely more than just a polite knock, probably borne out of fear (of me? Never!), frustration, or sheer panic, holding a raft of printed data in one hand and a mug of coffee in the other (*so how did they bang on the door?*). After a period of trying to quell their anxiety, it seems that the student had been sent to me to gain advice on how to analyse the plethora of data generated by their final year project. My initial response has always been 'I'm sorry, I can't help you!'. At this point, the student invariably looks at me incredulously and dissolves in floods of tears, sobbing 'but you must help me, my project report is due in tomorrow (*why is it always tomorrow?*), and my supervisor said you are the stats guru and would be happy to help – I have nobody else to turn to and I really want a first' (*don't they always*)! I then explain to them that good scientific research is achieved by good experimental technique. This involves high-quality experimental design not only of the experimental protocol involved but also the identification of how the resulting data are to be analysed. I then tell them to return to their supervisor and explain that the data are worthless and should be binned forthwith, that they need to sit down and go over their experimental design and build into their protocols the exact method by which they will analyse the resulting data *before* they perform any of the planned experiments. Good experimental design requires knowledge about the expected experimental output; what type of data will my experiment generate? It is only with this knowledge that the appropriate statistical techniques may be identified. The statistical tests used are an important component of the *Methodology*, and as such must be identified before *getting your hands dirty* and performing the experiments. Once the student and supervisor have identified the appropriate statistical approach, then the student can perform the experiments and gather the resulting data. The student's response (in between further floods of tears and sobs) is something along the lines of 'so all this data is worthless (*yes*)? I need to identify the stats tests to use (*yes!*)? And then I do the experiments (*yes!!*)? BUT MY REPORT IS DUE IN TOMORROW (*Tough! Not my problem*)!!' Whereupon the student invariably storms out of my office, reams of paper in one hand, coffee mug in t'other, slamming the door behind them (*how do they do that if their hands are full?*). 300 ms later either my phone rings or there are further knocks on my office door - it's the supervisor concerned, and rather irate! (I exaggerate here - I've never known an academic move that fast.) After carefully explaining the requirements of good experimental design and statistical analysis (to somebody who, let's face it, should know this anyway!), I finally agree to look at the student's data and provide advice as to how the data may be analysed. Interestingly, in subsequent years, it is the same supervisor's students who bang on my door seeking advice (again, too late in my opinion), so perhaps you can't teach an old dog new tricks. Most importantly, however, it is a lesson learnt by the student, so at least the next generation of pharmacologists have a fair chance of getting it right!

The principle problem here is ignorance that rigorous statistical analysis is a component of good experimental design. Consequently, the statistical methodology to be employed in research must be decided before the experiments are performed. In my experience, this is due to historically very poor teaching of statistics in pharmacology across the sector, such that those now with the responsibility of teaching pharmacology to current undergraduates or newly qualified graduates (whether they be in academia or the pharmaceutical industry) are themselves at a disadvantage and too naive to understand the importance of rigorous statistical analysis. Consequently, they are unable to provide high-quality supervision to enable less experienced individuals to develop and hone their experimental technique.

**Example 2:** I was once stopped in the corridor by a fellow post-doc (and close friend) who described a series of experiments involving cell culture in different mediums which they were unsure how to analyse. Essentially, the post-doc had a single flask of a particular CHO cell line and was trying to determine which of three mediums promoted the best cell growth. Three further flasks were prepared each one containing a different medium, and a sample of the cell line was decanted into each of the three test flasks. Sometime later, three samples were taken from each flask (so nine samples in total) and the number of cells per unit volume determined. The question was; 'how do I analyse the data? Do I do a number of $t$-tests (are they paired)? Do I do ANOVA? And if so, which *post hoc* test (*don't worry I'll explain all these terms later in the book*)'. I looked at the data, checked I had the right information about the design of this simple experiment and said 'Sorry, you don't have enough data for statistical analysis – you only have an $n$ of one in each case'. The post-doc stared at me quizzically and said, 'Don't be daft, I have $n$ of 3 for each medium!'. 'Er…, no!', I replied, 'You estimated the cell numbers in triplicate, but that only gives you $n = 1$ in each case, all you've done is obtain an estimate of precision and hopefully accuracy of your estimates, but that doesn't change the fact that you've only got $n = 1$ for each flask'. 'No, no, no!' the post-doc strenuously exclaimed, 'I have $n = 3$ in each case, three samples from each flask for the different mediums!'. 'Er, no!', I replied (at the risk of repeating myself ), 'If you wanted to do this properly then you should have prepared three flasks for each medium (so nine flasks in total), and decanted the same volume of CHO cells into each flask. Sometime later, you should then have taken 3 samples from each flask (so 27 samples) and estimated the cell number in each case. You would then calculate the average for each flask so that you get an improved accurate measure of the cell concentration in each flask (thanks to the measures in triplicate). This will then give you three measures for each medium which you can analyse by one-way ANOVA followed by a Tukey All Means *post hoc* test (*don't worry about these terms; all will become clear later in the book. I just included them to impress you, whet your appetite for what is to come and to try and convince you I know what I'm talking about!*). The post-doc looked at me aghast! 'I don't have time for that!', came the reply, 'I have a group meeting with my Prof. this afternoon and I need to present this data so we can discuss which medium to use in our future studies – our latest grant proposal depends on demonstrating that one of

these mediums is significantly different from the others, so I need to subject these data to statistical analysis!'. I looked at the summary bar chart the post-doc had prepared from the data and it was clear from the eye-ball test (*this is probably one of the best tests to use to appreciate data and is very simple to perform – I'll reveal how later in the book!*) that one of the mediums showed clear advantages in terms of cell growth than the others. 'Just look at your data', I said, 'Medium $X$ is clearly better than $Y$ or $Z$, that's all you have to say!'. (This statement refers to one of the other very common statistical test; the IBO test. Er…, IBO is defined as 'It's Bloody Obvious'). 'That's no good', replied the post doc 'Prof likes to see stars (*so thump him, I thought but didn't say out loud*), and the more stars the better and happier he'll be'. (*So, thump him harder? At this point, I'm left with the thought, what is the difference between a five years old starting Primary School and a 50 years old Prof leading a prestigious research group? Answer = absolutely nothing, they both like stars, preferably gold!*] 'Not with these data', I said resignedly, 'you've only got $n = 1$ for each medium and you can't perform rigorous statistical analysis with such a paucity of data.' 'Never mind' said the post doc 'I'll do it my way. Thanks.' and disappeared down the corridor repeatedly muttering '1-way ANOVA and some bloody *post hoc* test'. My words were left hanging in the ether!

The problem here is ignorance about $n$ numbers leading to poor experimental design, a lack of understanding of the term 'triplicate' and the consequences that this has for statistical analysis. This is a very simple error that is commonly seen.

**Example 3:** Publication of research in scientific journals depend on the peer review system (where experienced researchers act as referees on papers submitted to journals for publication). A friend of mine excitedly showed me a paper he had just been requested to review from a very reputable journal. He was thrilled on two counts; first, the fact that he had been asked to act as referee by this journal was a form of tacit recognition of his own expertise. Second, the paper was written by a group he had long admired and indeed, I think he hoped he could join this group in the future to further his own career. The following day we met, and he looked very downcast. It transpired that he had spent a couple of hours looking through the manuscript the previous evening and it soon became apparent that the statistical analysis used by the authors was not appropriate according to the experimental design and the type of data generated by the studies described. It was clear that he was going to have to reject the paper in its current state and advise that publication would only be acceptable if the statistical analysis was completely revised. He duly submitted his report to the journal. I didn't hear anything more for a month or so, but eventually he showed me a letter he had subsequently received from the journal. The letter thanked him for his time and effort in reviewing the manuscript, the tactful way he had written his review and the conscientious and constructive way he had dealt with the statistical shortcomings of the paper. Included also were the comments made by other referees (they were all in agreement in rejecting the manuscript and for the same reasons) and the subsequent response from the authors. To cut a long story short, the authors rejected the comment made by the editor and referees and, in particular, were scathing about the comments regarding their statistical analysis. Their final comment was (and I paraphrase here), 'This is the way we've always analysed our data. We see no reason to change now and so we'll continue to do it our way!'. The paper was rightly rejected by the journal. However, six months later (or so) my friend barged into my office and threw a paper on my desk. 'Look at this!', he exclaimed (getting increasingly louder as he muttered words which I can't repeat here but which seriously questioned the marital status of the parents of those unfortunate individuals related in some way to the document now lying in front of me). The paper was the manuscript he (and others) had rejected earlier but published almost word for word in a different journal! So, while it may be difficult to teach a dog new tricks (see above), success probably depends on the dog willing to learn something afresh – it's just unfortunate that some dogs are too arrogant and set in their ways to consider and adopt new methods or to accept that perhaps what they did in the past was not the best approach.

The problem here is that we all get set in our ways and once we know that a particular technique works then we are loath to change it – even in the face of convincing arguments that our methodology could (should?) be improved or that our current methods are just plain wrong! The use of statistics in pharmacology has improved markedly over the last 15–20 years and bears little resemblance to the techniques used when I first started my career in pharmacology over 45 years ago. Even so, I still see example after example of manuscripts submitted to reputable scientific journals where the statistical analysis employed is wrong; indeed, the majority of manuscripts that I reject (I would estimate about 90%) are rejected on the basis of inappropriate (wrong) statistical analysis.

Experimental design and statistical analysis is not a burdensome and an inconvenient chore – stats is fun and very rewarding! In fact, statistics is only burdensome and an inconvenient chore to those who don't know what they're doing (or why) and are not prepared to learn or understand a few simple basic rules. I am an experimental pharmacologist with over 45 years' experience in designing a wide range of preclinical experiments in pharmacology (both *in vitro* and *in vivo*) and through those years I have learnt the basic rules of statistical analysis and how such analyses should be coupled with the process of experimental design. Statistics, to me, is not an academic exercise but simply, in general terms, a tool by which I better understand the data generated by my experiments that enables me to make clear, concise and accurate conclusions about the change in data (usually induced by drug treatment – I am a pharmacologist after all)

I observe. Statistics is a tool (not in the derogatory terminology), and just as a cabinet maker knows his tools to produce exquisite pieces of furniture (with each tool having a specific purpose), so the scientist needs to understand his statistical tools to analyse data and draw appropriate conclusions.

I have taught statistics for the better part of 25 years and during throughout this time I have always focused on three points.

**1** There are different types of data. Identification of the type of data you have is important since this directly determines the type of statistical analysis which may be used on that data.

**2** Once both the type of data and statistical test are identified, then it is just a simple matter of running the appropriate test on the data. These days with current computing power and the plethora of statistical analysis packages available, it is no longer necessary to perform statistical tests by hand and use lookup tables; it is simply a matter of ensuring the data is input into the stats package in the right format and then press the right button. This book will provide screen images of the output from some of the most common statistical packages commercially available (principally GraphPad Prism, Invivo Stat. MiniTab, and SPSS) so you'll know what to expect and look for when you use these packages to analyse your own experimental data.

**3** Each statistical test you perform will produce an output. But how do you interpret that output? This book will explain how and help you to draw the appropriate conclusions from the statistical analysis of your own data.

So, you have a set of data and you know what type of data it is and what type of test you need to use to analyse that data. That directly leads to the correct conclusions – easy, isn't it! Well, perhaps not quite that easy, but this book will show you how. It will demystify statistical analysis so that, hopefully, if at some time in the future I said to you 'Stats', you wouldn't run into the distance under a tumultuous orange sky with your hands held to your face and your mouth in the shape of a polo mint, but instead you will smile benignly and, with a glint in your eye, say 'Bring it on!'.

PJM 04/01/2021

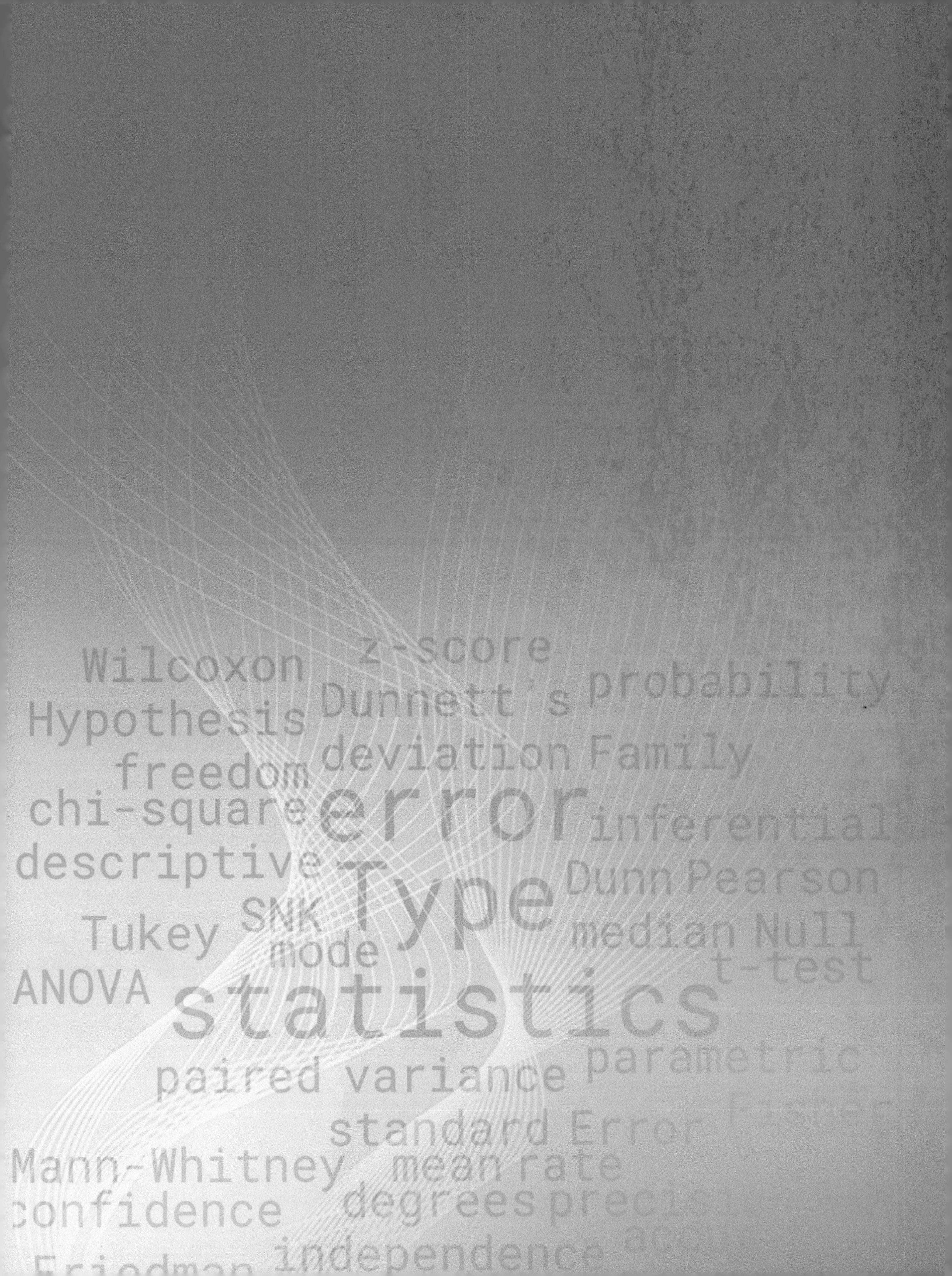

Wilcoxon

z-score

probability

Hypothesis

Dunnett's

deviation Family

freedom

error

chi-square

inferential

descriptive

Dunn Pearson

Tukey SNK Type

median Null

mode

t-test

ANOVA

statistics

paired variance parametric

standard Error

Mann-Whitney mean rate

confidence degrees precision

independence

# 1 Introduction

## Experimental design: the important decision about statistical analysis

Whenever you make plans for your annual holiday, you do not just pack your suitcase willy-nilly without first making plans about what you want to do, where you want to go, how you are going to get there, etc. For example, if your idea is to go trekking around the coast of Iceland, then you would look really stupid if, on arrival in Reykjavik, you opened your suitcase only to find beachwear and towels! Indeed, identifying what you want to do on holiday and where you intend to go determines what you need to take with you and what travel arrangements you need to make. In fact, what you do on holiday can be viewed as the final output of your holiday arrangements. The same can be said for the design of any well-planned, robust, scientific experiment. The final output of your experiment, i.e. the communication of your results, whether it be a figure (scatter graph, bar chart, etc) or table, largely determines every single step in the preceding experimental design, including the strategy of your statistical analysis.

Figure 1.1 shows the final output of an experiment which examined the effect of pre-treatment with mesulergine (an antagonist at 5-HT$_{2C}$ receptors) on the ability of $m$-chlorophenylpiperazine ($m$CPP; a 5-HT$_{2C}$ receptor agonist) to reduce the locomotor activity of rats.

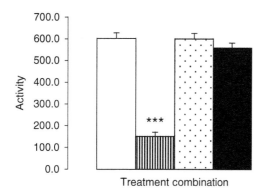

**Figure 1.1** **The effect of mesulergine on *m*CPP-induced hypolocomotion.** Vertical bars indicate mean locomotor activity counts ± Standard Error of the Mean. Saline-pre-treated animals were subcutaneously treated with either saline (open bar) or *m*CPP (vertical lines), while mesulergine-pre-treated subjects received either saline (stippled bar) or *m*CPP (solid bar). Two-way ANOVA revealed main effects of pre-treatment [$F(1,28) = 74.799$] and challenge treatment [$F(1,28) = 110.999$] and an interaction between pre- and challenge treatments [$F(1,28) = 76.095$], $p < 0.001$ in all cases. *Post hoc* analysis (Tukey) revealed that saline + *m*CPP combination-treated animals exhibited significantly lower levels of activity than the other three treatment combination groups (∗∗∗, $p < 0.001$ in all cases). For all other pairwise comparisons, $p > 0.05$. Data on file.

The bar chart contains four bars, each corresponding to the treatment combination administered to the subject animals, which are aligned along the x-axis and whose height equates to the calculated **arithmetic mean** value of the corresponding locomotor activity as indicated on the y-axis. Below the figure is the **legend** which describes the contents of the bar chart. The legend is divided into three sections. The first part is the **figure number** and the **title,** and usually these are in bold type. The second part is first half of the legend text in normal type and is a summary of the **axis parameters** arising from the **experimental protocol,** together with a summary of the **Descriptive Statistics** used to produce the bars and the **key** to differentiate each bar in the figure. The last part of the legend is a summary of the **Inferential Statistics** and includes, in this example, the data arising from both the **ANOVA model** and *post hoc* **tests** used to analyse the data (including an explanation of any indicators in the Figure, for example, the stars, used to identify significant differences between data sets); Screenshots of the statistical analysis are provided at the end of Chapter 17. This final output of your experiment is the last in a series of steps that comprise the complete experimental design process, and just as if you were planning your holiday to Iceland (the island, not the frozen food store!) or a sunny Mediterranean beach, it is easy to identify these steps in reverse order. Thus:

- The step immediately prior to producing such a summary of experimental data is the **Inferential Statistical** tests employed to analyse the data. In the example provided here, this would be the **two-way ANOVA test** followed by a suitable *post hoc* test (here the **Tukey** test was used); why these tests were deemed appropriate will be explained later (see Chapter 17). The statistical test employed, however, is determined by the type and number of data sets produced by the experiment, but may include tests of data distribution and skewness, pairwise comparisons, other models of ANOVA, etc.

- The step immediately prior to the Inferential Statistical analysis is the calculation of the **Descriptive Statistics**. These are the calculated summary values used to describe the data which are subsequently used to generate the data in the figure (e.g. bar height, etc.). Most experimental data are generally summarised by a measure of **central tendency**, such as the **Mean** (of which there are three types – but more about that later), together with the Standard Deviation or Standard Error of the Mean, **Median** (together with the range or semi-quartile ranges), or **Mode**. However, note here that the measure of central tendency you report must be appropriate to the data your experiment has generated (see Chapters 5, 8, and 9).

- The step prior to the statistical procedures is the **input** of your experimental data into your favourite statistical package. All statistical packages differ slightly from each other, but the most common method is to use a data spreadsheet similar to that seen with Microsoft Excel (see Figure 1.2).

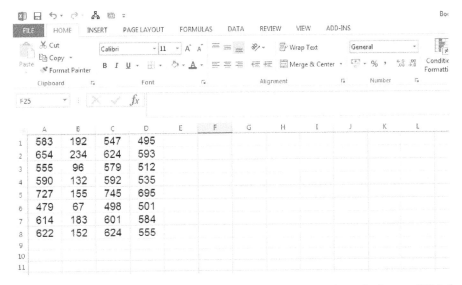

**Figure 1.2** **Excel spreadsheet showing original rodent locomotor activity data examining the effect of mesulergine on *m*CPP-induced hypolocomotion (see Figure 1.1).** The functionality of spreadsheets such as Microsoft Excel allows the calculation of simple Descriptive Statistics such as Mean, Standard Deviation, Standard Error of the Mean. Data on file.

- Of course, you must generate your data before you are able to input such data into the spreadsheet and to achieve this you must decide on your **experimental methodology** – the process which generates a series of values which eventually allows you to draw conclusions about your experiment.
- Before you decide on your methodology, however, you must have a **working hypothesis** which, in turn, is the result of your
- **experimental aims** that address the
- **problem** you have identified and is the raison d'etre of the whole experimental design process.

If we reverse these stages, then we have a list of events that summarise the experimental design process;

## Experimental design process

1 What is the problem?
2 What is the aim?
3 Hypothesis
4 Experimental methodology
5 Data collection
6 Data input
7 Descriptive Statistical data
8 Inferential Statistical data
9 Final output

Notice that the Descriptive and Inferential Statistical steps (steps 7 and 8) are integral to the overall experimental design process. It is absolutely vital, therefore, that you decide on your statistical approach, both how you are going to convey (i.e. your summary figure or table) and analyse your data (Descriptive Statistics and Inferential Statistics, respectively) *before* you perform your experiment! It is fundamentally unacceptable to complete your experiment, obtain your data, and then scratch your head wondering what statistical strategy you need to adopt to analyse your data; all this demonstrates is very poor experimental technique. (*At this point refer back to Example 1 in the Foreword.*)

## Statistical analysis: why are statistical tests required? The eye-ball test!

But why do we need statistics? Surely life would be so much easier, less complicated, and with reduced levels of anxiety if we just did not bother. However, as scientists we have a duty to communicate the results of our studies to the wider world, and so we need to have confidence in the data generated by our studies. Consequently, we must provide evidence that supports the conclusions derived from our studies, and that support is provided by the statistical analysis of our data – but we should not rely purely upon our statistical analysis. The statistical data generated by our analysis is there to **support** our observations and not to replace what we can see with our own eyes. So, the first stage in analysing your data is to just look at it – but look at it with a critical eye. In Figure 1.1, it is quite clear that saline-pre-treated animals subsequently treated with *m*CPP exhibit far lower levels of locomotor activity than any of the other three treatment combinations – this simple observation is an example of the **eye-ball** test (sometimes also known as the B.O. test – Bloody Obvious!). Importantly, the data also suggest that subjects pre-treated with mesulergine subsequently fail to respond as expected to acute treatment with *m*CPP (i.e. they fail to show *m*CPP-induced hypolocomotion); the main conclusion here, therefore, is that mesulergine blocks the behavioural effect of *m*CPP supporting the notion that because mesulergine is a 5-HT$_{2C}$ receptor antagonist, then the hypolocomotor activity induced by *m*CPP is most likely mediated via agonist activity at 5-HT$_{2C}$ receptors. The subsequent Inferential Statistical analysis simply supports this observation; this is important since the results of our statistical analysis should always be consistent with what we can see with our own eyes. If your statistical analysis contradicts what you can see, then there is something wrong in the presentation of your data, the statistical analysis used, or in the interpretation of the statistical results.

Another example of where the B.O. test alone provides confidence in our observations is the classical concentration–effect curve obtained with receptor agonists in isolated tissue experiments *in vitro*. Figure 1.3 summarises the effect of increasing concentrations of the $\alpha_1$ adrenoceptor agonist, phenylephrine, on the rat anococcygeus muscle.

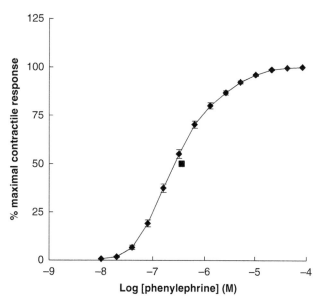

**Figure 1.3 Phenylephrine-induced contraction of the rat anococcygeus muscle.** Values show Mean $\pm$ S.E.M ($N = 70$) of the percentage maximal response (Y-axis) plotted according to $Log_{10}$ of the phenylephrine concentration (X-axis). The mean $EC_{50}$ value for phenylephrine (solid square) $= 3.6$ (2.8, 4.7) $\times$ $10^{-7}$ M. Mauchly's test indicated that the assumption of sphericity had been violated, $\chi^2$ (90) $= 1903.64$, $p < 0.001$. Subsequent Greenhouse–Geisser corrected ($\varepsilon = 0.156$) Repeated Measures ANOVA revealed significant variation between the responses according to dose [$F$(2.027, 139.862) $= 1618.36$, $p < 0.001$]. *Post hoc* analysis (repeated Paired $t$-test with Bonferroni correction) revealed significant difference between successive concentrations ($p < 0.01$) in all cases except between the highest two concentrations examined ($p > 0.05$). Data on file.

Clearly phenylephrine induces contractions of this smooth muscle, the magnitude of which is obviously related to drug concentration until a maximal response is achieved. Do we really need high-powered statistical analysis to tell us what our eyes can clearly see? Probably not, but for completeness, I have included a suitable analysis in the figure legend.

However, life, and the data we generate, is not always so clear-cut. The problem occurs when we are presented with data that are somewhat equivocal such that the eye-ball test starts to fail. In such cases we then rely heavily on the results of our statistical approach – that is perfectly acceptable, as long as we stick to a few basic rules that ensure we use the correct statistical approach to analyse and understand our data. If we fail to do so, then we severely run the risk of making erroneous, unsubstantiated conclusions. As scientists we need to have a robust, objective approach to data analysis, so we can arrive at our conclusions with confidence. It is important to acknowledge that nothing is ever proven with statistical analysis in the scientific world. Statistical analysis is all about **probability,** and the most we can hope for is to demonstrate the likelihood that two or more groups are either similar or different.

## The structure of this book: Descriptive and Inferential Statistics

The process of statistical analysis is broadly divided into two principle divisions. The first, and smaller, division is entitled **Descriptive Statistics** and provides a range of values which allows the appropriate summary of experimental data. Such values include, for example, the **Mean, Median, Mode, Variance, Standard Deviation, semi-quartile range values,** etc. and will be described in more detail in **Chapters 5, 8 and 9**. The second, and by far the larger division, concerns all the statistical tests that are employed to analyse data in order to draw appropriate conclusions about the relationship between different groups of values, and this division is entitled **Inferential Statistics** and will be the focus of the remainder of this book (from **Chapter 10** onwards).

Before we continue this journey of discovery into the mystical world of experimental design and statistical analysis, I would just like to make a few comments about the approach and design taken throughout the book. To an experimental pharmacologist, statistical analysis simply provides a tool by which data obtained through robust experimentation may be understood. The purpose of this book is therefore to show the experimental pharmacologist how to use this tool: how to decide which statistical approach is appropriate for their data, how to prepare for and perform statistical analysis, and how to interpret the resulting output from the analysis. Consequently, this is very much a **how-to, hands-on** book; what it is clearly not is an academic text focused on the vagaries of statistical theory – I really have little interest in why such tests work, I just need to know which test to use and when!

You will notice that the book is organised into (I hope, at least that is the plan) logical sections. Each section will contain a description of the test being described with some examples of experimental data and their statistical analysis. There are a range of software packages available to analyse scientific data, and I dare say, you, your lecturers, Department, or Institution will each have their favourite. Each of the analysis chapters, therefore, conclude with a number of **Screenshots** showing the appropriate output from a limited number of statistical packages (notably GraphPad Prism, InVivo Stat, MiniTab, and IBM SPSS) of the example data. My aim (or, at least, hope!) is that you will be able to perform you own analysis of the data examples and recognise the similarity between what you see herein and from your own efforts.

Throughout this Introduction, there is one word that pops up repeatedly, and that is the term **data**. So, what are data? Considering that the aim of this book is to show you how to subject data to appropriate statistical analysis, it is probably most important before we go any further that you understand exactly what data are and appreciate that there are different types of data.

So, sit back and tighten your safety belt as we start our journey into the realm of data.

**Write Your Own Notes**

6 |

Experimental Design and Statistical Analysis for Pharmacology and the Biomedical Sci...

# 2 So, what are data?

As far as the experimental pharmacologist is concerned, data are simply numbers generated by our experimental observations. In some cases, the answer may be 'Yes' or 'No', 'Present' or 'Absent', where the observation has no discernible magnitude, but subsequently we assign value to these observations to allow statistical analysis. In other experiments, the data may simply be recorded as the number of times a particular event has occurred within a certain time period, for example, when a specific behaviour (e.g. head-shake) is exhibited by rodents in behavioural experiments; such data are known as **quantal** data. In other cases, data may be described as a continuous variable, such as height or blood pressure. So, data may have different characteristics, and it is important to ascertain the type of data obtained from our observations since this determines the subsequent approach for the Descriptive and Inferential Statistical analysis and the presentation of such data. For the time being, let us just consider how you are going to present your data.

## Data handling and presentation

Whatever the type of data our experiment has generated, we need to present our results in some form or other such as text, tables, or figures. The form that is chosen depends on the type of data you have and the message you wish to convey.

### Text

Typically, data presented as **text** in the body of a manuscript (e.g. your laboratory report or that paper you wish to submit to the British Journal of Pharmacology). The following is a description of the phenylephrine data provided in the previous chapter (see Figure 1.3).

Figure 1.3 summarizes the ability of increasing concentrations of the $\alpha_1$-adrenoceptor agonists, phenylephrine, to induce contractions of the isolated anococcygeus muscle of male Wistar rats *in vitro* ($N = 70$). Data were analysed by Repeated Measures ANOVA. However, initial Mauchly's test indicated that the assumption of sphericity had been violated, $\chi^2 (90) = 1903.64$, $p < 0.001$; therefore the degrees of freedom in the subsequent Repeated Measures ANOVA test were corrected using Greenhouse–Geisser estimates of sphericity ($\varepsilon = 0.156$). The Repeated Measures ANOVA revealed significant variation between the contractile responses according to the final organ bath concentration of phenylephrine [$F(2.027, 139.862) = 1618.36$, $p < 0.001$]. *Post hoc* analysis (repeated Paired *t*-test with Bonferroni correction) revealed significant differences between successive concentrations in all pairwise comparisons ($p < 0.01$) except between the highest two concentrations examined ($p > 0.05$). These data clearly show that the response of the anococcygeus muscle is dependent on the concentration of phenylephrine to which it is exposed. The threshold concentration to significantly induce a response was $2 \times 10^{-8}$ M with a maximum response achieved at $4.1 \times 10^{-5}$ M. The mean $EC_{50}$ for phenylephrine was 3.6 (2.8, 4.7) $\times 10^{-7}$ M, $pEC_{50} = 6.44$.

Note that the manuscript description of the data contains the same factual information as the legend for the figure (see Figure 1.3) but allows the opportunity to provide some extra detail, and the language used does not have to be so concise.

### Tables

Generally, tables are used by experimental pharmacologists for two principal purposes in reporting experimental data; either as a means of summarizing their own data from a series of experiments or to summarize a substantial collection of data or information from a series of previously published studies already in the public domain.

Table 2.1 summarises the potency of atropine, a muscarinic cholinergic antagonist, and mepyramine, a histamine $H_1$ receptor antagonist, to block the contractile responses to acetylcholine and histamine in the isolated guinea pig ileum *in vitro*.

**Table 2.1** The relative potency of atropine and mepyramine on muscarinic and histaminic responses in the isolated guinea pig ileum.

|  | **Atropine** | **Mepyramine** |
| --- | --- | --- |
| Acetylcholine | 9.0 | >5.0 |
| Histamine | 5.8 | 9.3 |

Summary of $pA_2$ values for atropine and mepyramine for acetylcholine- and histamine-induced contractile responses in isolated guinea pig ileum *in vitro*. Data on file.

The table summarizes the $pA_2$ values ($-Log_{10}$ of the antagonist concentration, expressed in M values, estimated to double the $EC_{50}$ concentration of the respective agonist); the magnitude of the $pA_2$ value reflects antagonist potency on the receptor system stimulated by each agonist. The data indicate that atropine is about $1000 \times$ more potent on muscarinic M3 receptor than on histaminic $H_1$ receptors, while mepyramine may be up to $10\,000 \times$ times more selective for $H_1$ receptors. This table demonstrates the phenomenon of **differential antagonism** expressed by atropine and mepyramine for these two receptor systems, and the relationships between these values are far easier to see in the table compared with when the values are buried in a paragraph of text.

In contrast, Table 2.2 summarizes the association of neuropathic pain with various disease states in terms of its classification and aetiology according to NICE clinical guidelines. This table simply shows how a wealth of information may be summarized efficiently; to describe all the relevant clinical studies within the body of a manuscript would be laborious and time-consuming to prepare and, most likely, extremely boring to read.

**Table 2.2** Disease associated with neuropathic pain.

| Disease | Classification | Aetiology |
| --- | --- | --- |
| Painful diabetic neuropathy | Peripheral | Metabolic |
| Cancer pain due to surgery or chemotherapy | Peripheral | Paraneoplastic |
| HIV-related neuropathy | Peripheral | Infection |
| Post-herpetic neuralgia | Peripheral | Infection |
| Radiculopathy (nerve compression) | Peripheral | Trauma |
| Spinal cord injury | Central | Trauma |
| Multiple sclerosis | Central | Neurodegeneration |
| Post-stroke pain | Central | Neurotoxic |
| Phantom limb | Peripheral/central | Trauma |
| Cancer | Peripheral/central | Paraneoplastic |

Classification is based on originating lesion. NICE clinical guideline 173 (2013).

## Figures

In most cases, experimental data may be most efficiently communicated by the use of figures.

- **Line charts** are useful to show trends in categories. Care must be taken to ensure that the use of line charts is not confused with scatter plots. While the magnitude of the data (shown on the Y-axis) may be a continuous variable, the values on the X-axis in line charts are not, and the data are plotted at set intervals or individual categories along the X-axis; line charts are therefore **wholly inappropriate for plotting information where the X-axis reflects the magnitude of a continuous variable**.

- **X-Y Scatter plots** should be used when you wish to show the relationship between the magnitude of two sets of continuous variables. Figure 1.3 is an example of an X-Y scatter plot, where $Log_{10}$ of the molar drug concentration is plotted along the X-axis and the magnitude of the ensuing response (expressed as % maximal response) is plotted up the Y-axis. In both cases the sets of values may take any value within the range set along each axis.

- **Bar charts** are typically used to compare values across a few categories. Figure 1.1 is an example of a bar chart where the height of each bar represents the magnitude of the parameter measured (i.e. locomotor activity) according to the category of drug treatment combination administered to the animals used in the study. Consequently, bar charts are very similar to line charts and just convey a different visual impression of the data.

- **Histograms** are similar to bar charts where the frequency of continuous data (Y-axis) is plotted against the pre-defined ranges of the values (X-axis).

- **Box–whisker plots** provide a representation of the key features of a univariate sample of data. The whiskers indicate the range while the box indicates the median and upper and lower quartiles.

- **Pie charts** may be used when you wish to express and compare categories of observations as proportions of a whole. So, if you can set your total to 100%, then each category should reflect a proportion of the total and be expressed as a percentage. I have used pie charts in my explanation of the theory behind Analysis of Variance, where the total size of the chart reflects the total sample variance in the data while the size of the segments reflects the relative sizes of the Between and Within sample variances (see Chapter 15).

# 3 Numbers; counting and measuring, precision, and accuracy

When we obtain data in our experiments, we either count the occurrence of an event or we make measurements of a specific parameter.

A **count** can only be a whole number (i.e. an **integer**), while a **measurement** may have any number of decimal places depending on either the accuracy of the instrumentation of the equipment used to make the measurement or any subsequent calculation that uses such measurements. So, if we use a typical home room thermometer to measure temperature, then we should be able to observe whole degree Celsius differences in temperature. If we use a laboratory thermometer then, hopefully, we should achieve an accuracy of half a degree Celsius, and accuracy may be further improved to 0.1 of a degree Celsius by using a reasonably priced digital thermometer. However, if we have access to a high-quality industrial thermometer for use with thermocouples or resistance thermometer probes to measure temperature, then the accuracy may be improved even further. However, no number of decimal places will yield the true temperature as we will always be unsure of what number lies beyond the last digit. Perhaps the best we can hope for, no matter what we are measuring, is to achieve data with the highest level of precision and accuracy available to us.

## Precision and accuracy

The term **precision** reflects the consistency of a series of measurements and is therefore the ability to obtain the same value on multiple occasions. So, the measure of precision is related to the spread of the data; the higher the precision of the data, then the less the spread of the values. The measurement of precision is provided by the **coefficient of variation** while **accuracy** reflects the nearness of the measurement to the true value.

- **Coefficient of variation** is calculated as follows; (see Chapter 5 for information regarding calculation of the mean and standard deviation).

$$(\text{Standard Deviation/Mean}) \times 100 \qquad (3.1)$$

- **% Accuracy is** calculated by dividing the **measured value** by the **true value** and is expressed as a percentage.

$$(\text{Measured value/True value}) \times 100 \qquad (3.2)$$

Consider the following example.

## Example 3.1

Two groups of students were asked to make 10 measurements of the pH of a solution (with a known pH of 8.0). The resulting data is shown in the table below.

**Table 3.1** Estimation of pH.

| Observation | Group 1 | Group 2 |
|---|---|---|
| 1 | 6.0 | 8.4 |
| 2 | 8.7 | 8.6 |
| 3 | 9.2 | 8.7 |
| 4 | 10.0 | 8.9 |
| 5 | 6.5 | 8.8 |
| 6 | 7.5 | 8.5 |
| 7 | 9.7 | 8.3 |
| 8 | 8.8 | 8.4 |
| 9 | 6.5 | 8.4 |
| 10 | 7.1 | 8.9 |
| Mean | 8.0 | 8.59 |
| St dev | 1.453 | 0.223 |
| Coefficient of variation (%) | 18.2 | 2.6 |
| % Accuracy | 100.0 | 107.4 |

The respective coefficients of variation show that Group 2 was more precise in their pH measurements compared with the data obtained by Group 1; however, their estimation of the solution's pH was quite poor with a % accuracy of 107.4%. In contrast, Group 1 was 100% accurate in their estimation of the pH, but their measurements were highly variable. Consequently, while Group 2 was very precise, in contrast Group 1 was highly accurate *but did not know it* due to the inherent variation in their data (see Figure 3.1)!

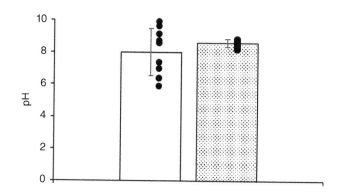

**Figure 3.1** **Estimation of pH: precision and accuracy.** Summary of data from Table 3.1. Group A (open bar) pH = 8.0 ± 1.453 (mean ± St. dev). Group B (shaded bar) pH = 8.59 ± 0.223. Closed circles indicate raw data values for each group.

*Experimental Design and Statistical Analysis for Pharmacology and the Biomedical Sciences*, First Edition. Paul J. Mitchell.

So, you can have precision without accuracy, but you will never know how accurate you are without precision.

## Errors in measurement

In all our experimental measurements, there will be various levels of accuracy and precision – as experimental pharmacologists, it is our responsibility to reduce as far as possible these potential sources of error in our observations. The problem is, however, no matter how hard we try, there will always be the possibility for error in our observations such that all measurements will have some degree of error.

The different sources of measurement error are as follows:

- A **blunder** is where there is a gross mistake in recording data by, for example, recording the wrong value, misreading a scale. All blunders should be eliminated by recording data carefully. Blunders should not be included in the analysis of data.
- An **observer error** may simply be an incorrect reading of a measurement or device. This is similar to a blunder but may be due to inexperience of the observer (e.g. recording the incorrect units of measurement; mg instead of g) or the incorrect recording of someone else's measurements. Such observational errors should be eliminated from any subsequent analysis unless the level of error can be accurately corrected.
- A **systematic error** may occur if a machine is incorrectly calibrated. However, this may be compensated for if the degree of error is known. Systematic errors may be eliminated or corrected by the careful calibration of your equipment.
- **Random errors** are positive and negative fluctuations in the data that are generally beyond the control of the experimenter. These may be unpredictable changes in ambient temperature, humidity, or lighting conditions or variations in human reaction time during manual measurement of time variables. The level of error may be reduced or even eliminated by taking repeated measurements (e.g. taking measurements in duplicate, triplicate, or more depending on the size of the error) to increase the accuracy of the reported, *single*, observation.
- An **instrumental error** may occur if a piece of equipment is faulty and provides an incorrect reading. Generally, such issues are not apparent until after completion of the experiment. Such error data should be discarded.

So, the data we obtain from our experiments will always be a balance between our striving for accuracy and precision on one side against the possibility of an error in our measurements on the other side.

One method we may adopt to reduce error in our measurements and increase the precision of the data is to take repeated readings *from the same sample*. Unfortunately, however, such a process is often interpreted as producing independent observations, thereby increasing the number of samples in our data group(s). So, let us look at this more carefully and try to clear up any misunderstandings about this important issue.

## Independent observations or duplicate/triplicate/quadruplicate? That is the question!

### Example 3.2

Consider a simple experiment where you are trying to assess the effect of a drug or serum on the population growth of cells in culture. You carefully prepare two flasks containing equal volumes of identical growth medium, except that one flask also contains the drug or serum you are interested in. From your stock flask of cells in culture, you carefully remove an exact volume and add the aliquot to one of the flasks. As carefully as possible you repeat the process and add another aliquot to the second flask. The assumption here is that you have added the same number of cells to each flask so that the cell concentration in each flask is the same. You then leave the flasks to incubate. After a suitable incubation period (e.g. three days) you take four samples from each flask and estimate the cell concentration using a haemocytometer. This process is summarised in Figure 3.2.

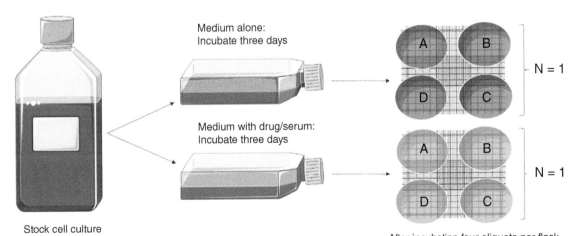

Figure 3.2 **Measurement of cell population in quadruplicate.**

In this example, the cell population in each flask is measured **in quadruplicate**. This is a process whereby the precision of the final population value is improved by taking more than just one reading. It is important to note, however, that these are not independent readings as in each case the four samples are taken at the **same** time from the **same** flask. Consequently, the four values are averaged to provide a **single** value which is the best estimate of the population of cells in each flask, i.e. $n = 1$ for each flask. Such a process has often been erroneously misinterpreted as providing an $n = 4$, but this is incorrect simply because the four values for each flask are not independent. *[See also Chapter 20, Example 20.3.]*

## Example 3.3

In contrast, consider a second, albeit similar, experiment. Here the initial set-up is different in that six aliquots from the stock solution are placed in a multi-well plate. Drug or serum is then added to three of the wells, the other three wells are the controls. All wells are then left to incubate for three days. At the end of the incubation period, four samples from each of these wells are placed on a haemocytometer and the cells were counted. This process is summarised in Figure 3.3, but note the important step of adding drug or serum to three samples independently **prior** to incubation.

In this latter example, the cell population from each initial aliquot is subsequently measured **in quadruplicate** to improve the precision of the final population value by taking more than just one reading. However, the fact that samples were taken from flask and drug or serum added **prior** to incubation now means that there are three independent wells containing medium alone or with drug or serum during the incubation period. Consequently, we now have **three** independent estimates of the cell population each of which has been estimated in **quadruplicate**, i.e. we now have $n = 3$ estimations of cell growth over the three days of incubation.

Note that the measurements in quadruplicate still only provide an $n$ of 1 for each original aliquot, but the fact that we now prepared three aliquots means that we now have $n = 3$ for each flask. This is useful because we can now perform some meaningful analysis of the cell populations exposed to drug or serum compared with our control group.

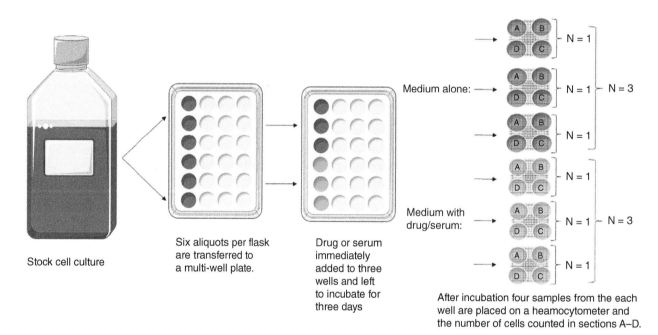

Stock cell culture

Six aliquots per flask are transferred to a multi-well plate.

Drug or serum immediately added to three wells and left to incubate for three days

Medium alone:

Medium with drug/serum:

After incubation four samples from the each well are placed on a heamocytometer and the number of cells counted in sections A–D.

**Figure 3.3  Multiple estimates of cell population in quadruplicate.**

# Example 3.4

There is a further situation using a similar experimental scenario which we need to consider. Here your laboratory has just purchased two new *p*H metres, and you wish to compare their accuracy and precision. You prepare two solutions of 0.1 mM HCl and 0.1 mM NaOH, *p*H values of 4.0 and 10.0, respectively, from which you carefully decant a small volume of each solution into two small beakers. You then use each *p*H metre, in turn, to obtain three measurements of the *p*H of each solution. You very carefully ensure that the *p*H electrode is cleaned between each measurement so as not to contaminate subsequent readings. This process and resulting *p*H readings are summarised in Figure 3.4.

There is an argument here that these two sets of samples simply reflect a single measurement in triplicate, similar to that described in the first example above (see Figure 3.2). However, this situation is slightly different since here we are interested in the performance of the two *p*H metres. Consequently, it is

perfectly reasonable to treat these measurements as independent and so $n = 3$ in for both *p*H metre for each solution, whereupon the average *p*H (with the spread of data described by the standard deviation) for each set of data may be calculated. This may appear inconsistent with the earlier example, but to understand why this is permissible, then you need to understand the questions being asked in both situations. In the first, we were interested in the effect of the drug or serum on the population growth of the cells and not our consistency in measuring the number of cells. In this latter situation, however, it is the relative performance of the equipment being used, in terms of accuracy, consistency, precision, and variability, that is being investigated.

The take-home message here is that as with everything in data analysis, the question being asked is of paramount importance and is a direct consequence of the aim of the experiment.

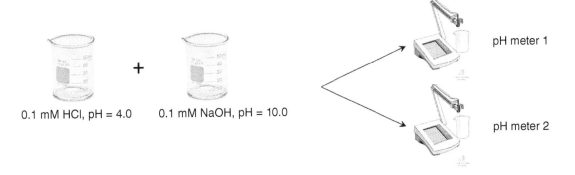

| | Solution | Measurement | | | Mean | Standard Deviation | Coefficient of Variation (%) | Accuracy (%) |
| --- | --- | --- | --- | --- | --- | --- | --- | --- |
| | | 1 | 2 | 3 | | | | |
| pH meter 1 | 0.1mM HCl | 4.01 | 4.01 | 4.00 | 4.007 | 0.00577 | 0.144 | 100.167 |
| | 0.1 mM NaOH | 10.0 | 9.99 | 9.99 | 9.993 | 0.00577 | 0.058 | 99.933 |
| pH meter 2 | 0.1 mM HCl | 3.92 | 3.91 | 3.94 | 3.923 | 0.01528 | 0.389 | 98.083 |
| | 0.1 mM NaOH | 9.91 | 9.93 | 9.95 | 9.930 | 0.02000 | 0.201 | 99.300 |

Figure 3.4  **Comparison of the accuracy and precision of two *p*H metres.**

## Independent and paired data sets

I have used the term 'independent' on a few occasions so far, and it is a term that is often used in statistics (independent observations, independent groups, independent data), and so it is important that we understand the true meaning of this term.

Consider the situation where you are interested in the heights of female students compared with those of age-matched male students (see Chapter 5, Tables 5.1 and 5.2 for example data). There is a clear distinction between these groups based on their gender, and so the groups of female and male students are clearly **independent** from each other as they contain different participants or subjects and consequently produce independent data sets. Similarly, if we compared the heights of male students when they started secondary school to a different group of students at university, then these groups would also be independent since they clearly contain different participants.

In contrast, a different situation arises where a group of male students had their heights measured both on starting secondary school and again when they started university. In this situation the heights of the *same* participants are examined but at different time points; in such circumstances the resulting data is said to be **paired**.

This distinction between independent and paired groups is important since, as we shall see later, it informs our decision on the inferential statistical tests subsequently used to analysis data.

Of course, some data measurements include both independent and paired data sets. Consider the situation where the heights of female and male students are measured when they start secondary school and again when they are at university. Such data will include independent groups (based on their gender) and paired data (based on the time at which the heights were measured).

In addition to these terms, statisticians also use the terms '**Between**' and '**Within**' to describe different variables and factors in an experiment. The term 'Between group variable' refers to clear differences between independent groups used in an experiment; in the examples above then gender is a Between-Group Variable. In contrast, the term 'Within group variable' refers to experimental changes experienced by the same group of participants or subjects during the course of an experiment and always occurs as a function of time; in the examples above, then the time at which the height measurements were obtained is a Within-Group Variable.

**Write Your Own Notes**

# 4 Data collection: sampling and populations, different types of data, data distributions

## Sampling and populations

Whenever we perform an experiment, we obtain measurements according to our observations, and as described in earlier chapters our aim is to collect data in a precise and accurate manner. Statistics may be defined as the science of **collecting**, **summarising**, **presenting**, and **interpreting** such data. A collection of data on their own is not information, but a valid summary and description of that data set derive information by putting the data into context. Statistics therefore involves summarising a collection of data in a clear and understandable way such that our reader or audience may see clearly the similarity or differences between the groups in our experiment.

One very important issue we need to accept in statistics is that in almost all cases, we only work with **samples** taken from whole **populations** of subjects. Consequently, we are almost always faced with the situation in which we estimate population parameters from the samples we have obtained.

For example, suppose we wanted to determine the height of students at your university or institution. We would not be able to determine the height of every single student, so we would choose a '**representative sample**' of students, measure their height, and then *estimate* the average height from these values.

- A statistical **population**, therefore, is the set of all possible values (our observations/measurements) that could possibly be measured.
- A **sample** is the subset of the population for which we have a limited number of observations drawn at random from the population that will be used to describe the parent population (see Figure 4.1).

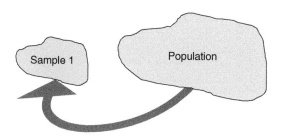

**Figure 4.1** A data sample is a random set of values drawn from the parent population.

By necessity this process involves the tacit assumption that the sample group is truly representative of the parent population. Furthermore, if we take a large number of samples from the population and divide those randomly into subgroups of equal size, then each subgroup should truly represent the parent population. Furthermore, if the last statement is true, then each subgroup should be equal to each other. In reality, of course, there will be some differences not only between the subgroups but also to the parent population, and it is determining the importance of those differences where we rely on statistical analysis.

## The Central Limit Theorem

Luckily, however, the small differences that arise as a result of taking samples from a population are not a huge issue thanks to what is known as the **Central Limit Theorem**, which states that, *given a large enough sample size, then the sampling distribution of the sample mean will approximate to a normal distribution regardless of the variable's distribution in the given population.* I know I have not described or explained the nature of the normal distribution as yet (sorry!), but have a quick look at Figure 4.7 later in this chapter and compare the shape to the distributions of data sets shown in Figures 5.3 and 5.4 in Chapter 5; can you see the differences in shape?

**So, what does this theorem mean? Well, for any set of observations we can easily produce a scatterplot of the *magnitude* of the observation on the x-axis against the *frequency* of occurrence for each value on the y-axis. The resulting scatterplot is called the frequency distribution for that variable. Interestingly, the values of a variable in any given population may follow different distributions including a normal distribution (Figure 4.7) or distributions that show a right or left skew (Figures 5.3 and 5.4, respectively) in the frequency distribution scatterplot.**

**However, if we take a sufficiently large number of random samples from a population and record the mean of those samples (i.e. this is what is known as the sample mean) and then repeat this process a number of times (making sure we replace the random values each time to maintain the population size and distribution), then the distribution of the sample means (if plotted as a histogram) will approximate to a normal distribution, irrespective of the inherent distribution of all the samples in the original population. The shape of the resulting histogram is known as the sampling distribution of the mean.**

**Unfortunately, the shape of the sampling distribution depends on the number of samples taken each time from the population. In most cases a sample size of 30 is sufficient for the sampling distribution of the mean to approximate to a normal distribution. However, with smaller sample sizes, the resulting sampling distribution is generally different from the normal distribution and instead approximates to a *t*-distribution where the shape of the sampling distribution depends on the sample size (see Figure 4.9; notice that as the sample size increases, so the shape of the curve approximates to a normal distribution!). The Central Limit Theorem is important in statistics since it links the distribution of the variable in the population to the sampling distribution of the mean. Furthermore, it is vital**

to understand the theorem when we start to consider the confidence intervals of different statistical parameters (see later in Chapter 22).

## Types of data

In the majority of our experiments, the data we obtain will be numerical in nature. However, it is important to carefully distinguish the nature of the data being analysed since not all data may be treated similarly. Consequently, the type of statistical analysis we employ depends on the type of data obtained; i.e. statistical tests are generally specific for the kind of data we wish to analyse.

In general terms, there are three kinds of data, although as can be seen below, there may be further differences within measurement data depending on form and scale.

### 1 Nominal (categorical) data

Such data are where either numerals are applied to attributes or categories that are not strictly measures but allow accurate identification, or where the number of observations in a category may be recorded. For example, hair colour may be a category and the frequency of individuals with black, brown, red, blonde, or brunette hair is recorded. The results of survey data are typically categorical.

### 2 Ordinal data

Such data are where a scale with ranks is employed to order the observations. The rationale behind the ranks is that the values may be ranked in order (which makes it an ordinal scale) of magnitude. Data obtained from well-being scales are examples of ordinal (ranked) data.

### 3 Measurement data

Numerical data may exist in two forms and in three types of scale.

### Form of measurement data

**i Discrete** data (aka **meristic**) are generally counts and may only be discrete values normally represented by integers.
**ii** In contrast, **continuous** data are those observations or measurements where the precision is only limited by the experimenter and the equipment used.

### Types of scale

**i** An **interval scale** is where the values are measured on a scale where the differences are uniform but ratios not so. For example, on the Celsius temperature scale, the difference between 5° and 10° is the same as between 10° and 15°, but the ratio between 5° and 15° does not imply that the latter is three times as warm as the former.
**ii** A **ratio scale** is where the values have a meaningful zero point. Examples here include length, weight, and volume. Thus, 15 cm is three times longer than 5 cm, 2 kg is twice as heavy as 1 kg, and 200 ml is four times the volume of 50 ml.
**iii** A **circular scale** may be used when one measures annual dates, clock times, etc. Generally, neither differences nor ratios of data obtained from circular scales are sensible or useful derivatives, and consequently special methods are employed for such data; such methods are outside the scope of this book.

A further issue we need to consider before deciding which statistical methods are appropriate to apply to our experimental data concerns the distribution of our data sets.

## Classification of data distributions

If we collect a large number of observations in an experiment and from these data produce a histogram plot (where the frequency of the observations is plotted against magnitude), then the resulting figure represents a summary of the distribution of the data. With sufficient number of observations, then the frequency of occurrence of each observation is closely related to the *probability* that future observations will have a particular value. Furthermore, the distributions created by our data often map to distributions that are mathematically generated. Each distribution is defined by an equation, and this allows the probability of a given score to be calculated. Probability distributions depend on the form of the data obtained (see **form of measurement data**, above) and consequently are either discrete or continuous; in both cases **discrete probability distributions** and **continuous probability distributions** are statistical functions that provide a way of mapping out the likelihood that an observation will have a given value.

The different types of theoretical mathematical distributions are summarised in Table 4.1. Some of these probability distributions are outside the remit of this book and are only included here for completeness.

Table 4.1 Classification of probability distributions.

| Probability distributions | |
| --- | --- |
| **Discrete distributions** | **Continuous distributions** |
| Uniform distribution | Uniform distribution |
| Bernoulli distribution | Exponential distribution |
| Binomial distribution | Gamma distribution |
| Poisson distribution | Normal distribution |
| Geometric distribution | Chi-square distribution |
| Negative binomial distribution | Student-$t$ distribution |
| Hypergeometric distribution | $F$ distribution |
| | Beta distribution |
| | Weibull distribution |
| | Gumbel distribution |

In contrast, the discrete and continuous probability distributions described briefly below are either of theoretical interest or are distributions which may inform our decisions regarding which statistical methods we use to describe and analyse data from our experiments. Care must be taken, however, to ensure that we interpose our experimental data on the correct mathematical distribution, since if we make an incorrect decision, then we risk arriving at erroneous conclusions.

### i Discrete uniform distribution (Figure 4.2)

This is a very simple distribution where the probability of each equally spaced possible integer values is equal. An example would be rolling fair six-sided dice; here the probability of each side occurring would be equal, i.e. there would be six equally like probabilities. In standard statistical nomenclature, $p$ is the variable used to denote probability. So here $p = 1/6 = 0.167$.

### ii Bernoulli distribution (Figure 4.3)

Whenever you toss a coin, then the only outcomes are either the coin lands heads or tails uppermost; the question being asked here is '*will this single trial succeed*'. This is an example of the most basic of random events where a single event may only have one or two possible outcomes with a fixed probability of each occurring. The Bernoulli distribution has only one controlling parameter which is the probability of success according to whether you call heads or

16

Experimental Design and Statistical Analysis for Pharmacology and the Biomedical S...

tails; in both cases the probabilities of success or failure *in a single trial* are equal and will have a probability of 0.5 (i.e. $p = 0.5$).

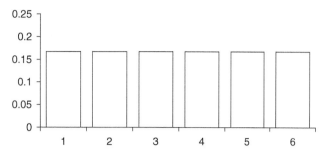

**Figure 4.2 The discrete uniform distribution.** X-axis values indicate the resulting number shown on the throw of a six-sided dice. Y-axis values indicate the relative probability density.

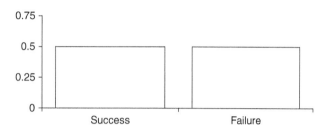

**Figure 4.3 The Bernoulli distribution.** X-axis values indicate the resulting outcome from only two possibilities, e.g. success or failure to throw a heads on the toss of a coin. Y-axis values indicate the relative probability density.

### iii Binomial distribution (Figure 4.4)

The binomial distribution is an extension of the Bernoulli distribution to include multiple success or failure trials with a fixed probability. Consequently, the binomial distribution addresses the question 'out of a given number of trials, how many will be successful'? So, if you tossed a coin 10 times, in how many of these trials would the coin land heads? With a fair coin you would expect five heads and five tails as the outcomes of the 10 trials. But what is the probability of only two heads, or nine heads, or no heads at all? For those who are interested (!), the probability of obtaining exactly $k$ success in $n$ trials is given by the **binomial probability mass function** and is discussed in detail in Appendix A.1.

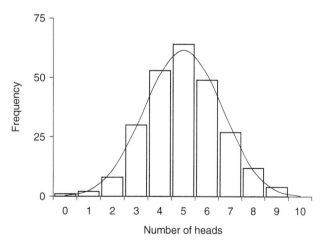

**Figure 4.4 The binomial distribution.** 250 undergraduate students were asked to toss a coin 10 times and count the number of times the coin landed heads uppermost. The X-axis indicates the number of times the coin was successfully tossed to land heads from 10 trials. The Y-axis indicates a) the predicted number of students for each level of success according to probability mass function for the binomial distribution (thin solid line) and b) the observed number of students for each level of outcome (open bars). For further discussion and calculation of the binomial probability mass function, see Appendix A.1.

### iv Poisson distribution

The Poisson distribution (which is very similar to the binomial distribution) examines how many times a discrete event will occur within a given period of time.

### v Continuous uniform distribution

This is very simple distribution where (as with the discrete uniform distribution, see Figure 4.2) the probability densities for each value are equal. In this situation, however, the measured values are not limited to integers.

### vi Exponential distribution (Figure 4.5)

The exponential distribution is used to map the time between independent events that happen at a constant rate. Examples of this include the rate at which radioactive particles decay and the rate at which drugs are eliminated from the body according to first-order pharmacokinetic principles (Figure 4.6). For calculation of the **exponential probability mass function,** see Appendix A.2.

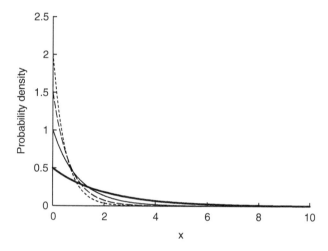

**Figure 4.5 The exponential distribution.** The probability density function of the exponential distribution for events that happen at a constant rate, $\lambda$. Curves shown are for rate values of $\lambda = 0.5$ (bold line), 1.0 (thin line), 1.5 (dashed line), and 2.0 (dotted line). X-axis values indicate the stochastic variable, x. Y-axis values indicate probability (see also Appendix A.2).

### vii Normal Distribution (Figure 4.7)

The Normal Distribution (also known as the **Gaussian distribution**) is the most widely used distribution, particularly in the biological sciences where most (but not all) biologically derived data follow a Normal Distribution. A Normal Distribution assumes that all measurement/observations are tightly clustered around the **population** mean, $\mu$, and that the frequency of the observations decays rapidly and equally the further the observations are above and below the mean, thereby producing a characteristic bell shape (see Figure 4.7; for calculation of the probability density of the Normal Distribution, see Appendix A.3.). The spread of the data either side of the population mean is quantified by the variance, $\sigma^2$; where the square root of the variance is the Standard Deviation, $\sigma$ (see Chapter 5). The normal distribution with these parameters is usually denoted as $N$ with the values of the population mean and standard deviation immediately following in parenthesis, thus; $N(\mu, \sigma)$. Every normal distribution is a version of the simplest case where the mean is set to zero and the standard deviation equals 1; this is denoted as $N(0, 1)$ and is known as the **Standard Normal Distribution** (see Chapter 7). Furthermore, the area under the curve of the Standard Normal Distribution is equal to 1, the consequence of which means that sections defined by multiples of the standard deviation either side of the mean equate to specific proportions of the total area under the curve. Because Normal

Distribution curves are *parameterised* by their corresponding Mean and Standard Deviation values, then such data are known as **parametric**. Consequently, **parametric statistics** (both Descriptive and Inferential Statistics) assume that sample data sets come

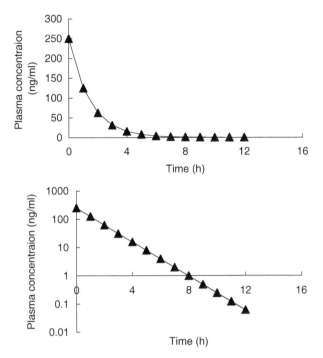

Figure 4.6 **Plasma concentration of drug X following intravenous administration.** Upper panel: X-axis values indicate time post-administration. Y-axis values indicate plasma concentration (ng/ml) plotted on a linear scale. Lower panel: X-axis values indicate time post-administration. Y-axis values indicate plasma concentration (ng/ml) plotted on a $Log_{10}$ scale. Half-life ($t_{1/2}$) of drug X equals 1 hour.

from data populations that follow a fixed set of parameters. In contrast, **non-parametric** data sets, and their corresponding Descriptive and Inferential Statistics, are also called **distribution-free** because there are no assumptions that the data sets follow a specific distribution. Appreciation of the qualities of the Normal Distribution (and the Standard form) and differences to non-parametric data are fundamental in informing our strategy to analyse

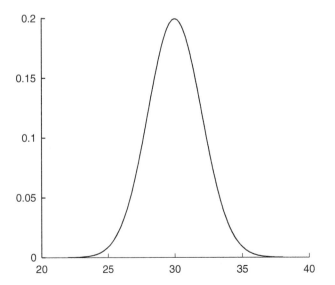

Figure 4.7 **The Normal Distribution curve, N(30,2).** The Normal Distribution curve has a Mean of 30 and a Standard Deviation of 2. X-axis values indicate magnitude of the observations, while the Y-axis indicates the probability density function (see also Appendix A.3).

experimental pharmacological data. As we shall see later, there are numerous statistical tests available to analyse data that is Normally Distributed, and these provide very powerful, robust, procedures the results of which in turn allow us to derive conclusions from our experimental data.

### viii Chi-square distribution (Figure 4.8)

The Chi-squared distribution is used primarily in hypothesis testing (see appropriate sections in **Inferential Analysis**) due to its close relationship to the normal distribution and is also a component of the definition of the *t*-distribution and the *F*-distribution (see below). In the simplest terms, the Chi-squared distribution is the square of the standard normal distribution. The Chi-squared distribution is used in Chi-squared tests of independence in contingency tables used for categorical data (see Pearson's Chi-squared test, Chapter 21), to determine how well an observed distribution of data fits with the expected theoretical distribution of the data if the variables are independent and in Chi-squared tests for variance in a population that follows a normal distribution.

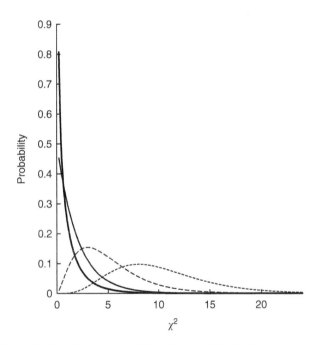

Figure 4.8 **The Chi-square distribution.** The probability density function for the Chi-squared distribution with 1 (bold solid line), 2 (thin solid line), 5 (dashed line), and 10 (dotted line) degrees of freedom. X-axis values indicate Chi-squared ($\chi^2$) and Y-axis indicates probability (see also Appendix A.4).

### ix Student-t distribution (Figure 4.9)

The Student *t*-distribution is derived from the Chi-square and normal distributions. The distribution is symmetrical and bell-shaped, very much like the Normal Distribution (see Figure 4.7) but with greater area under the curve in the tails of the distribution. The *t*-distribution arises when the mean of a set of data that follows a normal distribution is estimated where the sample size is small and the population standard deviation ($\sigma$) is unknown. As the sample size increases so the *t*-distribution approximates more closely to the standard normal distribution. The *t*-distribution plays an important role in assessing the probability that two sample means arise from the same population, in determining the confidence intervals for the difference between two population means (see Chapters 11 and 12) and in linear regression analysis (see Chapter 20).

## x F distribution (Figure 4.10)

The F distribution (named after Sir Ronald Fisher, who developed the F distribution for use in determining the critical values for the **Analysis of Variance** (ANOVA) models; see Chapters 15, 16 and 17) is a function of the ratio of two independent random variables (each of which has a Chi-square distribution) divided by its respective number of **Degrees of Freedom**. It is used in several applications including assessing the equality of two or more population variances and the validity of equations following multiple regression analysis. The F-distribution has two very important properties; first, it is defined for positive values only (this makes sense since all variance values are positive!), and second, unlike the t-distribution, it is not symmetrical about its mean but instead is positively skewed.

## So why do we need to understand data distribution?

Of the data distributions briefly described above, the majority are only of value to understand the theoretical basis of statistical analysis (the Chi square, t- and F-distributions are important once we get into inferential statistics, but only if we wish to understand the process of how such tests work). In contrast, the most important distribution for the experimental pharmacologist is the Normal Distribution which shall be discussed in detail later (see Chapters 6 and 7).

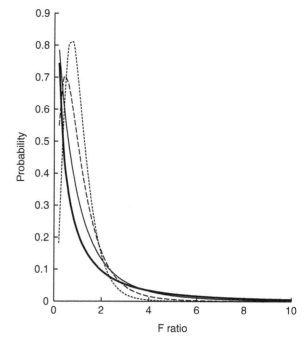

**Figure 4.10 The F distribution.** The probability density function of the F distribution with 1, 4 (bold solid line), 2, 8 (thin solid line), 4, 20 (dashed line), and 8, 32 (dotted line) degrees of freedom. X-axis values indicate the F ratio, while Y-axis values indicate probability density function (see also Appendix A.6)

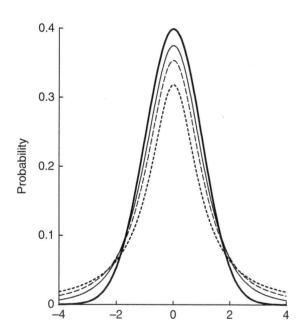

**Figure 4.9 The t-distribution.** The probability density function of the t-distribution with 1 (dotted line), 2 (dashed line), and 4 (thin solid line) degrees of freedom compared with the Standard Normal Distribution (bold solid line; N (0,1)). For the t-distribution data the X-axis values indicate the value of t. For the Standard Normal Distribution, the X values indicate the mean of zero with standard deviations either side of the mean. Y-axis indicates probability in all cases. Note as the degrees of freedom increase so the probability density function of the t-distribution approximates towards the Standard Normal Distribution (see also Appendix A.5).

# Write Your Own Notes

# 5 Descriptive statistics; measures to describe and summarise data sets

I argued in Chapter 1 that statistical analysis may be divided into Descriptive and Inferential Statistics. So, let's take a set of values and examine how such data may be described by **Descriptive Statistics**.

The following discussion refers to **height data** obtained from a group of young adults to demonstrate how Descriptive Statistics may be used to describe and summarise experimental data. Table 5.1 below lists the various heights of 40 female undergraduate students obtained in 2016 and 2017; I've only included female students since, as we shall see later, sex is important even in statistics!

**Table 5.1** Height (m) of 40 female undergraduate students.

| | Ht (m) | | Ht (m) | | Ht (m) | | Ht (m) |
|---|---|---|---|---|---|---|---|
| 1 | 1.641 | 11 | 1.581 | 21 | 1.624 | 31 | 1.677 |
| 2 | 1.578 | 12 | 1.602 | 22 | 1.794 | 32 | 1.524 |
| 3 | 1.753 | 13 | 1.702 | 23 | 1.742 | 33 | 1.681 |
| 4 | 1.588 | 14 | 1.568 | 24 | 1.731 | 34 | 1.731 |
| 5 | 1.644 | 15 | 1.698 | 25 | 1.659 | 35 | 1.631 |
| 6 | 1.602 | 16 | 1.613 | 26 | 1.580 | 36 | 1.645 |
| 7 | 1.556 | 17 | 1.683 | 27 | 1.663 | 37 | 1.705 |
| 8 | 1.666 | 18 | 1.556 | 28 | 1.614 | 38 | 1.744 |
| 9 | 1.482 | 19 | 1.692 | 29 | 1.652 | 39 | 1.647 |
| 10 | 1.743 | 20 | 1.698 | 30 | 1.613 | 40 | 1.743 |

There are some descriptive values which we can obtain easily from such a set of data;

• **Minimum:** the lowest value in the set. Here the minimum value is 1.482 m.
• **Maximum:** the highest value in the set. Here the maximum value is 1.794 m.
• **Range:** the range is the difference between the minimum and maximum values. Here the range is 1.794 − 1.482 = 0.312 m.

However, these values provide little useful information about the data set, especially if we wish to compare this set to the heights of another set of students. For example, Table 5.2 lists the

**Table 5.2** Height (m) of 33 male undergraduate students.

| | Ht (m) | | Ht (m) | | Ht (m) |
|---|---|---|---|---|---|
| 1 | 1.796 | 12 | 1.765 | 23 | 1.720 |
| 2 | 1.852 | 13 | 1.795 | 24 | 1.770 |
| 3 | 1.792 | 14 | 1.889 | 25 | 1.795 |
| 4 | 1.865 | 15 | 1.785 | 26 | 1.816 |
| 5 | 1.853 | 16 | 1.863 | 27 | 1.805 |
| 6 | 1.920 | 17 | 1.745 | 28 | 1.732 |
| 7 | 1.835 | 18 | 1.762 | 29 | 1.670 |
| 8 | 1.811 | 19 | 1.833 | 30 | 1.761 |
| 9 | 1.812 | 20 | 1.795 | 31 | 1.705 |
| 10 | 1.881 | 21 | 1.870 | 32 | 1.840 |
| 11 | 1.909 | 22 | 1.780 | 33 | 1.830 |

corresponding heights of the male students taken from the same student cohort.

The minimum, maximum, and range vales of these data are, 1.670 m, 1.920 m, and 0.250 m, respectively. Comparison of these two sets of data suggests that the shortest and tallest of the male students are both taller than their equivalent counterparts in the female cohort, while the range of the male heights is slightly less than that of the female heights. Does this infer that the males are generally taller than the females? If so, then how can we be sure?

One descriptive statistic we could easily obtain is where the centre of the frequency distribution lies (this is known as a measure of **central tendency** of the data sets). In general terms, there are three measures of central tendency;

## 1 The Mode

The mode is easy to identify in a frequency distribution since it is the score associated with the tallest bar in the histogram. However, one problem with the mode is that it can often take more than one value; frequency distributions with one mode are known as unimodal, while those with two modes (where there are two values with an equal and highest score) are known as bimodal, and those with more than two modes are known as multimodal.

## 2 The Median

The median is the middle score when the observations are ranked in order of magnitude, such that there are an equal number of observations below the median as there are above it.

For example, Table 5.3 lists the number of head shake behaviours exhibited by 15 male Wistar rats during a 10-minute observation period ranked according to the magnitude of the behaviour shown by each rat. The median score is 15 (see lighter cells). In comparison, the arithmetic mean is 18.2. Furthermore, the distribution of this data set is multimodal, with modes at 9, 11, and 15 head shakes.

**Table 5.3** Head shake behaviour exhibited by male Wistar rats.

| No | Head shakes | No | Head shakes | No | Head shakes |
|---|---|---|---|---|---|
| 1 | 7 | 6 | 11 | 11 | 23 |
| 2 | 9 | 7 | 12 | 12 | 28 |
| 3 | 9 | 8 | 15 | 13 | 31 |
| 4 | 10 | 9 | 15 | 14 | 34 |
| 5 | 11 | 10 | 20 | 15 | 38 |

## 3 The Mean

The mean of a set of data is the measure of central tendency that most people are aware of and is simply the average score calculated as the sum of all the observations divided by the number of subjects in the data set. One important point to note is that the symbol used to denote the mean differs according to whether you are dealing with population data (where the mean is denoted by $\mu$) or sample

*Experimental Design and Statistical Analysis for Pharmacology and the Biomedical Sciences*, First Edition. Paul J. Mitchell.
© 2022 John Wiley & Sons Ltd. Published 2022 by John Wiley & Sons Ltd

data (where the mean is denoted by $\bar{x}$). However, unless you are a mathematician, most people do not realise that there are three different means that may be calculated depending on the nature of the scores used in the calculation.

### I Arithmetic mean

As stated above, the arithmetic mean is simply the **sum** of the observed scores divided by the **number** of observations. The arithmetic mean is calculated for data where the measurements are derived from a linear scale (e.g. height, weight). So, for the female height data presented above (see Table 5.1), the arithmetic mean is equal to 1.651 m, while the arithmetic mean of the corresponding male height is (Table 5.2) 1.808 m.

### II Geometric mean

In contrast to the arithmetic mean, the geometric mean is calculated by using the **product** of the observations and is used to calculate the mean value for observations or calculated data sets that follow a **geometric** progression. Technically, the geometric mean is defined as the **'n'th root of the product of 'n' numbers**. In practice, the geometric mean is most easily determined by calculating the arithmetic mean using the $\log_{10}$ of the scores in the data set rather than the raw scores. In experimental pharmacology, the geometric mean is typically used when calculating the mean of data derived from a logarithm scale, e.g. $EC_{50}$ values calculated from concentration–effect curves in isolated tissue experiments.

### III Harmonic mean

The harmonic mean is calculated by using the **reciprocal** values of the observations and is used in economics, when the data sample contains values related to speed or fractions, or when the sample contains outliers. It is not used very often in experimental pharmacology.

## Parametric Descriptive Statistics and the Normal Distribution

It is important to note that for data that follow a perfectly Normal Distribution, then the Mode, Median, and arithmetic mean all have the same value. In reality of course, and because we generally obtain *samples* from a population rather than complete population data, then our data sets generally only approximate to a Normal Distribution so there are usually some minor differences between these measures of central tendency. A further point to note is that, by design, none of these measures provide an indication of the spread of our data sets.

Consider the Normal Distribution curves in shown in Figure 5.1.

These three sets of data all have the same arithmetic mean, but the shapes of the distribution curves are different due to the spread of the data contained within each set. Clearly, therefore, relying just on the arithmetic mean is not a suitable parameter by which different groups may be differentiated; we also need to consider the *spread* of the data within each set.

One possible method to achieve this may be to calculate the sum of all the differences of each observation from the group mean; these values for the female height data are listed in Table 5.4. If we now sum all these difference values, then we get the following:

$$\sum (\bar{x} - x) = 0.000 \tag{5.1}$$

Clearly, this indicates that the sum of all the difference values where the height measurements are less than the mean is equal to the sum of all the difference values where the height measurements are greater than the mean, which is exactly what we would predict from a set of data that follows a Normal Distribution.

One technique that is used throughout statistics to rid ourselves of negative values is to calculate the square of the differences; these squared values for the female height data are also listed in Table 5.4. If we now sum all these squared values, then we get the following:

$$\sum (\bar{x} - x)^2 = 0.191 \text{ m}^2 \tag{5.2}$$

This value is known as the **Sum of Squares (SSQ)** and is extremely useful as it is directly related to the spread of the data around the arithmetic mean. However, the magnitude of the SSQ also reflects the number of terms used in the calculation. For example, the SSQ for the male cohort of height data = 0.109 m² (calculated from the values in Table 5.2). This appears to be less than the equivalent value for the female cohort, but there are fewer male students than female students in these data sets, so it is impossible to tell whether the differences between the two SSQ values reflect differences in the spread of the original height data or simply differences in the number of measurements in each cohort.

To correct for the differences in group size, it should be a simple matter of dividing each SSQ value by the corresponding number of observations in each data set. Indeed, if we were dealing with total populations, then that is exactly what we would do. However, since we are dealing with sample sets of data, we take a more conservative view and divide each cohort's SSQ value by $n - 1$, where $n$ equals the number of observations in each cohort. This $n - 1$ value is known as the **Degrees of Freedom**. The definition of the Degrees of Freedom is *the number of values or entities in a final statistical calculation that are free to vary*, and no, I don't understand that terminology either so, bear with me and let me try a simple explanation!

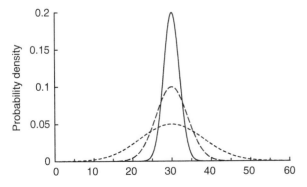

**Figure 5.1 Normal Distribution curves**. The probability density function of three Normal Distribution curves each with Mean = 30 and Standard Deviation values of 2 (solid line), 4 (dashed line), and 8 (dotted line), respectively. Relative area under each curve = 1. See also Appendix A.3.

**Table 5.4** Female height data.

| | Ht | $\bar{x}-x$ | $(\bar{x}-x)^2$ | | Ht | $\bar{x}-x$ | $(\bar{x}-x)^2$ |
|---|---|---|---|---|---|---|---|
| 1 | 1.641 | 0.010 | 0.000103 | 21 | 1.624 | 0.027 | 0.000737 |
| 2 | 1.578 | 0.073 | 0.005351 | 22 | 1.794 | −0.143 | 0.020406 |
| 3 | 1.753 | −0.102 | 0.010373 | 23 | 1.742 | −0.091 | 0.008254 |
| 4 | 1.588 | 0.063 | 0.003988 | 24 | 1.731 | −0.080 | 0.006376 |
| 5 | 1.644 | 0.007 | 0.000051 | 25 | 1.659 | −0.008 | 0.000062 |
| 6 | 1.602 | 0.049 | 0.002416 | 26 | 1.580 | 0.071 | 0.005062 |
| 7 | 1.556 | 0.095 | 0.009054 | 27 | 1.663 | −0.012 | 0.000140 |
| 8 | 1.666 | −0.015 | 0.000221 | 28 | 1.614 | 0.037 | 0.001380 |
| 9 | 1.482 | 0.169 | 0.028612 | 29 | 1.652 | −0.001 | 0.000001 |
| 10 | 1.743 | −0.092 | 0.008436 | 30 | 1.613 | 0.038 | 0.001455 |
| 11 | 1.581 | 0.070 | 0.004921 | 31 | 1.677 | −0.026 | 0.000668 |
| 12 | 1.602 | 0.049 | 0.002416 | 32 | 1.524 | 0.127 | 0.016167 |
| 13 | 1.702 | −0.051 | 0.002586 | 33 | 1.681 | −0.030 | 0.000891 |
| 14 | 1.568 | 0.083 | 0.006914 | 34 | 1.731 | −0.080 | 0.006376 |
| 15 | 1.698 | −0.047 | 0.002195 | 35 | 1.631 | 0.020 | 0.000406 |
| 16 | 1.613 | 0.038 | 0.001455 | 36 | 1.645 | 0.006 | 0.000038 |
| 17 | 1.683 | −0.032 | 0.001014 | 37 | 1.705 | −0.054 | 0.002900 |
| 18 | 1.556 | 0.095 | 0.009054 | 38 | 1.744 | −0.093 | 0.008621 |
| 19 | 1.692 | −0.041 | 0.001669 | 39 | 1.647 | 0.004 | 0.000017 |
| 20 | 1.698 | −0.047 | 0.002195 | 40 | 1.743 | −0.092 | 0.008436 |

Summary of raw height data (m) of 40 female undergraduate students together with absolute differences and the squared differences from the group arithmetic mean. The sum of the absolute differences is 0.000 m, while the sum of the squared differences is 0.191 m².

## Degrees of Freedom – a simple analogy

My wife, Angela, and I have two children, Matthew and Samantha. When they were young (a long time ago now) they used to get their pocket money from their Nana (my mother-in-law) and their Grandma (my mother) by cheque every week or so – I couldn't afford to give them pocket money as you'll never be rich if you're a young academic! One Saturday morning when Samantha was about 9 she turned to me and said, 'Dad, you know I get my pocket money from Nana?'. 'Yes....', I replied (immediately wondering where this conversation was going to lead). 'Well', Sam continued, 'my cheque hasn't arrived yet and I've no money to go and buy some sweets from the village shop so I was wondering if you'd lend me a pound until Nana's cheque arrives; I'll pay you back.......... honest!'. It's at this point, experienced by all Fathers, where you feel as though you have M.U.G. tattooed on your forehead! Anyway, I gave (!) Sam a pound coin on the proviso that she gave me the change on her return from the shop. So off she went skipping down the lane to the village and returned about 45 minutes later happily grasping a bag of sweets in her hand. She even gave me the change from her purchase; 15p. So, my question to you is; 'How much did the sweets cost?' To which you confidently (!) reply, '85p', and you'd be correct (phew!).

The following weekend Sam came up to me again and said, 'Dad, unfortunately Nana's cheque still hasn't arrived!' Like any good Father my immediate response was, 'So? Live with it, life can be tough sometimes!' Actually, I just thought this and instead just looked at her with raised eyebrows! Sam quickly continued before I could draw breath, 'So I was wondering if you'd lend me another pound, so I could go and buy some sweets, like last week.' All I could think about at this stage was the future dental bills that would no doubt ensue – however, I rapidly capitulated (which Dad doesn't?) and gave her the required coin. So off she went skipping down the lane. On her return sometime later, she presented me with 20p change. So how much were the sweets this week? To which you reply 80p. OK, but this week she bought two bags of sweets, so how much was each bag? Well, if the bags were identical then each would cost 40p. But if they were different, then you'd need to know the cost of one bag to work out the cost of the other.

These examples may be summarised mathematically as follows:

1  a = b1 + c; where a = £1, b1 = cost of sweets, c = change
2  a = b1 + b2 + c where b1 and b2 = cost of each bag of sweets

In both cases, you need to know $n - 1$ pieces of information (i.e. 2 and 3 pieces of information, respectively) to allow you to complete the whole data set, and it doesn't matter which $n - 1$ pieces of information you know since which observations you use are free to vary! Degrees of freedom values are very important in statistics and we will come across them repeatedly, so it is important you know what they mean and how they are derived; and you won't forget as you'll always have the image of a little girl skipping off to buy her bag(s) of sweets!

Let's return to the height data to continue our descriptive analysis.

## Variance

If we take the Sum of Squares for a set of data and correct for the number of observations by dividing through by either $n$ (for population data) or the Degrees of Freedom (for sample data sets, $n - 1$), then the resulting value is known as the **Variance**, denoted by the symbol $\sigma^2$ (population variance) or $s^2$ (sample variance), respectively.

While the mathematical equation for the population variance calculation is

$$\sigma^2 = \frac{\sum (\mu - x)^2}{n} \quad (5.3)$$

note that the equivalent equation for the sample variance calculation is slightly different, thus,

$$s^2 = \frac{\sum (\bar{x} - x)^2}{n - 1} \quad (5.4)$$

So, the corresponding sample variance values for the two sets of height data for the undergraduate male and female students are

$$\text{Female}: \quad s^2 = 0.191/39 = 0.004897 \text{ m}^2$$
$$\text{Male}: \quad s^2 = 0.109/32 = 0.003406 \text{ m}^2 \quad (5.5)$$

Proportionately, these values are somewhat closer to each other than when we compared the respective Sum of Squares values, but they still suggest that the female height data have a slightly greater spread than the corresponding data from the male students.

## Standard Deviation

When we first started looking at the spread of the height data, we squared the differences of each observation from the arithmetic mean to produce the Sum of Squares. Consequently, the Variance is based on data derived from squared values. We need to correct for this to arrive at the standard value that reflects the spread of the data in any Normal Distribution, the **Standard Deviation**.

Mathematically, the Standard Deviation is simply the square root of the Variance, thus,

$$\text{Population Standard Deviation} \quad \sigma = \sqrt{\sigma^2} = \sqrt{\frac{\sum (\mu - x)^2}{n}} \quad (5.6)$$

$$\text{Sample Standard Deviation} \quad s = \sqrt{s^2} = \sqrt{\frac{\sum (\bar{x} - x)^2}{n - 1}} \quad (5.7)$$

It is important to note here that the Standard Deviation values of data sets are in the same units of measurement as the original data. The corresponding sample Standard Deviation values for our two groups of height data are

$$\text{Female}: \quad s = \sqrt{0.004897} = 0.06999 \text{ m}$$
$$\text{Male}: \quad s = \sqrt{0.003406} = 0.05836 \text{ m} \quad (5.8)$$

Knowing the mean and standard deviation values of these data sets allows comparison of the stylised distribution of the male and female data sets of height data assuming they both follow a Normal Distribution (see Figure 5.2). Thus; whether inferential statistical tests may suggest if there is a real, meaningful, difference between the female and male heights.

There is one further measure of descriptive statistics that we need to consider that is routinely used to describe experimental data, and that is the **Standard Error of the Mean**.

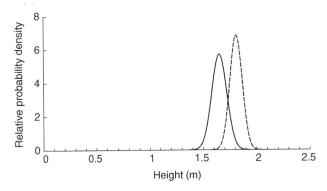

**Figure 5.2 Predicted Normal Distribution curves for undergraduate female ($n = 40$) and male ($n = 33$) height data.** X-axis indicates height (m) and Y-axis indicates relative probability density. Arithmetic mean ± standard deviation for female cohort = 1.651 ± 0.06999 m (solid line), for male cohort = 1.808 ± 0.05836 m (dashed line). This figure suggests that the male cohort are generally taller than their female counterparts. Later, we shall examine these data sets more closely to see if female heights differ significantly from the male heights.

## Standard Error of the Mean

Because the Standard Error of the Mean (S.E.M.) for a set of data is derived from the Standard Deviation (which in turn is derived from the Variance and, consequently, the Sum of Squares values, as described above), it is often erroneously assumed that the Standard Error of the Mean reflects the spread of the values in the data set. This assumption is understandable when you consider how the Standard Error of the Mean is calculated, thus,

$$\text{Standard Error of the Mean} = \frac{\text{Standard Deviation}}{\sqrt{n}} \quad (5.9)$$

Interestingly, it is more common for error bars in scientific figures to represent the Standard Error of the Mean rather than the Standard Deviation. It seems to me that the main reason for this is that the S.E.M. bars are smaller than the Standard Deviation bars and therefore convey the impression that the data is tighter, i.e. less spread of the values, thereby increasing our confidence in the accuracy of the data. However, the Standard Error of the Mean, as the term implies, is more to do with our confidence in the value or position of the Mean value rather than the spread of the data *around* the mean.

So, for sets of data where the values follow a Normal Distribution, then the accepted Descriptive Statistics to describe such data in terms of central tendency and spread of the values are

1 the **Mean**,
2 the **Variance**,
3 the **Standard Deviation**,
4 the **Standard Error of the Mean**.

The following table summarises these Descriptive Statistics for our female and male height data sets:

Table 5.5 Descriptive statistics summary table (Parametric data).

| | Mean (m) | Variance (m²) | St dev (m) | S.E.M. (m) |
|---|---|---|---|---|
| Female | 1.651 | 0.004897 | 0.06999 | 0.01105 |
| Male | 1.808 | 0.003406 | 0.05836 | 0.01016 |

Summary descriptive statistics for female and male height data calculated from Tables 5.1 and 5.2, respectively.

The generally accepted format for reporting these values is

- Mean ± Standard Deviation, or
- Mean ± Standard Error of the Mean

Note that for normally distributed data sets then **the Mode = Median = Mean**, and for such data the mean is the preferred measure of central tendency.

Unfortunately, life is not so simple that all sets of data follow a Normal Distribution (oh that it was so, life would be so much easier). Indeed, it is not unusual in pharmacology (or any biological science for that matter) to be presented with data sets whose frequency distributions deviate from a symmetrical normal distribution. There are two main ways in which a frequency distribution may deviate from normal;

**1 Lack of symmetry**. This is termed **skew** (or **skewness**) and indicates that the most frequent observations occur at one end of the distribution resulting in a long tail of less frequent observations towards the opposite end of the distribution. A skewed distribution may be either **positively skewed** (where the less observed values are at the higher or more positive end of the distribution; Figure 5.3) or **negatively skewed** (where the less observed values are at the lower or more negative tail of the distribution; Figure 5.4). The degree of skewness in the distribution of a data set is given by the adjusted **Fisher–Pearson (F-P) skewness coefficient** according to the formula:

$$G_1 = \frac{\sqrt{N(N-1)}}{N-2} \frac{\sum (x-\bar{x})^3/N}{s^3} \qquad (5.10)$$

where $\bar{x}$ is sample mean, $s$ is the sample standard deviation (although it is generally computed with $N$ in the denominator rather than $N-1$), and $N$ is the number of data points. The first part of the equation is an adjustment for sample size and approaches 1 as $N$ gets large. The skewness for a normal distribution is 0 and that for any symmetrical distribution should approach 0. In contrast, positively and negatively skewed distributions will have positive and negative Fisher–Pearson skewness coefficients, respectively, and the greater the degree of skewness will result in greater coefficient values.

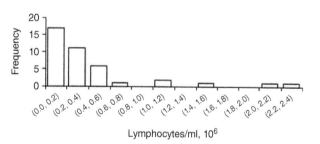

**Figure 5.3** **Positively skewed distribution of blood lymphocytes (10⁶ cells per ml) obtained from 40 HIV patients.** Adjusted Fisher–Pearson coefficient = 2.357 (calculated z-score = 6.302, p < 0.001).

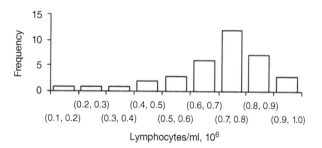

**Figure 5.4** **Negatively skewed distribution of blood lymphocytes (10⁶ cells per ml) obtained from 36 leukaemic patients**. Adjusted Fisher–Pearson coefficient = −1.245 (calculated z-score = −3.168, p < 0.01).

One important aspect of the Normal Distribution is that the three measures of central tendency are equal. Thus, the Mode = Median = Mean. However, when the distribution of a data set is highly positively or highly negatively skewed, as shown in Figures 5.3 and 5.4, respectively, then the equality of these measures no longer holds true. Thus, in a positively skewed set of data, the Mode < Median < Mean. In contrast, for a negatively skewed set of data, the opposite is true; thus, the Mode > Median > Mean. In both cases, the greater the skewness of the data, the greater the differences between these three important measures of central tendency; clearly, the extreme outliers in both positively and negatively skewed distributions have profound effects on these Descriptive Statistics (see Table 5.6). Because skewed distributions of data sets show such deviation from the normal distribution, it is not appropriate to use parametric measures such as the Mean, Variance, Standard Deviation, and Standard Error of the Mean to describe such data nor it is appropriate to apply parametric inferential statistics to analyse such data. At this point, we must make an important decision as to how to proceed in the analysis of the data. Essentially, we need to decide whether to transform our data set so that the distribution of the transformed data approximates to that of a normal distribution (see Chapter 6) or accept that the distribution of our data is too far removed from a normal distribution and proceed to analyse the data by applying non-parametric Descriptive and Inferential Statistics.

**Table 5.6** Summary of Mean, Median and Mode values for positively and negatively skewed distributions.

|  | Mode | Median | Mean |
| --- | --- | --- | --- |
| Positively skewed | 0.18 | 0.27 | 0.43 |
| Negatively skewed | 0.77 | 0.73 | 0.69 |

Note how the outlier values pull the Mean value away from the Median and Mode for each data set. Values calculated for data in Figures 5.3 and 5.4.

**2 Pointedness**. This is termed **kurtosis** and indicates how much the observed scores cluster in the tails of the distribution which is reflected in how pointy the distribution looks. A distribution with positive kurtosis has relatively more observations in the tails of the distribution and consequently looks sharper and more pointed; this is known as a **leptokurtic distribution**. In contrast, a distribution with negative kurtosis has proportionately less observations in the tails and, as a consequence, looks flatter and more rounded near the centre; this is known as a **platykurtic distribution**. The formula for kurtosis is

$$\text{kurtosis} = \frac{\sum (x-\bar{x})^4/N}{s^4} \qquad (5.11)$$

where $\bar{x}$ is sample mean, $s$ is the sample standard deviation (as with the Fisher–Pearson skewness coefficient $s$ is generally computed with $N$ in the denominator rather than $N-1$), and $N$ is the number of data points. The kurtosis value for a Normal Distribution is 3, but most software packages reset the calculated kurtosis score to 0 for a standard normal distribution. Consequently, most reported kurtosis values are lower (by 3) than the calculated value (known as excess kurtosis). By convention, therefore, a positive kurtosis value indicates a leptokurtic distribution, while a negative value indicates a platykurtic distribution.

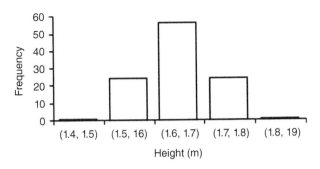

Figure 5.5 **A leptokurtic distribution shown by 106 undergraduate female students.** Excessive kurtosis = 0.768 (calculated $z$-score = 2.053, $p < 0.05$).

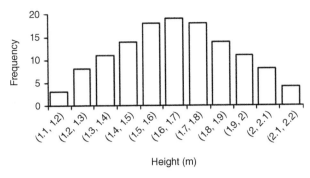

Figure 5.6 **A platykurtic distribution shown by 128 male and female 6th form students.** Excessive kurtosis = −0.656 (calculated $z$-score = −2.102, $p < 0.05$).

# Example output from statistical software

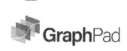 

## A

|   |  | A<br>Female | B<br>Male |
|---|---|---|---|
| 1 | Number of values | 40 | 33 |
| 2 |  |  |  |
| 3 | Minimum | 1.482 | 1.670 |
| 4 | 25% Percentile | 1.602 | 1.768 |
| 5 | Median | 1.650 | 1.805 |
| 6 | 75% Percentile | 1.701 | 1.853 |
| 7 | Maximum | 1.794 | 1.920 |
| 8 | Range | 0.3120 | 0.2500 |
| 9 |  |  |  |
| 10 | Mean | 1.651 | 1.808 |
| 11 | Std. Deviation | 0.07006 | 0.05827 |
| 12 | Std. Error of Mean | 0.01108 | 0.01014 |

## B

|   |  | A<br>Head shake | B |
|---|---|---|---|
| 1 | Number of values | 15 |  |
| 2 |  |  |  |
| 3 | Minimum | 7.000 |  |
| 4 | 25% Percentile | 10.00 |  |
| 5 | Median | 15.00 |  |
| 6 | 75% Percentile | 28.00 |  |
| 7 | Maximum | 38.00 |  |
| 8 | Range | 31.00 |  |
| 9 |  |  |  |
| 10 | Mean | 18.20 |  |
| 11 | Std. Deviation | 10.19 |  |
| 12 | Std. Error of Mean | 2.630 |  |

## C

|   |  | A<br>positive | B<br>negative | C<br>leptokurtic | D<br>platykurtic |
|---|---|---|---|---|---|
| 1 | Number of values | 40 | 36 | 106 | 128 |
| 2 |  |  |  |  |  |
| 3 | 25% Percentile | 0.1230 | 0.6225 | 1.600 | 1.450 |
| 4 | Median | 0.2723 | 0.7339 | 1.660 | 1.654 |
| 5 | 75% Percentile | 0.5150 | 0.8275 | 1.692 | 1.850 |
| 6 |  |  |  |  |  |
| 7 | Mean | 0.4336 | 0.6980 | 1.648 | 1.656 |
| 8 | Std. Deviation | 0.5263 | 0.1900 | 0.07086 | 0.2472 |
| 9 | Std. Error of Mean | 0.08322 | 0.03167 | 0.006883 | 0.02185 |
| 10 |  |  |  |  |  |
| 11 | Skewness | 2.357 | -1.245 | -0.3054 | 0.01617 |
| 12 | Kurtosis | 5.560 | 1.994 | 0.7684 | -0.6565 |

Summary descriptive statistics from GraphPad Prism, v8. Panel A shows the summary descriptive statistics for the female and male height data provided in Tables 5.1 and 5.2, respectively. Panel B shows the summary descriptive statistics for the rodent head shake data provided in Table 5.3.

Panel C shows the summary descriptive statistics for the positively and negatively skewed data shown graphically in Figures 5.3 and 5.4, respectively, together with the summary descriptive statistics for the leptokurtic and platykurtic data distributions shown graphically in Figures 5.5 and 5.6, respectively.

*Source*: GraphPad Software.

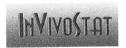

**A**

InVivoStat v4.0.2   My Data   Statistics ▾   My Analyses

View Analysis Log   Export to Html   Export Images

## InVivoStat Summary Statistics

### Variable selection

Responses Female,Male,Head shake are analysed in this module.

### Summary statistics

#### Summary statistics for Female

| Response | Mean | N | Variance | Std dev | Std error | Min | Max | Median | Lower quartile | Upper quartile |
|---|---|---|---|---|---|---|---|---|---|---|
| Female | 1.6512 | 40 | 0.0049 | 0.0701 | 0.0111 | 1.4820 | 1.7940 | 1.6495 | 1.6020 | 1.7000 |

#### Summary statistics for Male

| Response | Mean | N | Variance | Std dev | Std error | Min | Max | Median | Lower quartile | Upper quartile |
|---|---|---|---|---|---|---|---|---|---|---|
| Male | 1.8076 | 33 | 0.0034 | 0.0583 | 0.0101 | 1.6700 | 1.9200 | 1.8050 | 1.7700 | 1.8520 |

#### Summary statistics for Head shake

| Response | Mean | N | Variance | Std dev | Std error | Min | Max | Median | Lower quartile | Upper quartile |
|---|---|---|---|---|---|---|---|---|---|---|
| Head shake | 18.2000 | 15 | 103.7429 | 10.1854 | 2.6299 | 7.0000 | 38.0000 | 15.0000 | 10.0000 | 28.0000 |

**B**

## InVivoStat Summary Statistics

### Variable selection

Responses positive,negative,leptokurtic,platykurtic are analysed in this module.

### Summary statistics

#### Summary statistics for positive

| Response | Mean | N | Std dev | Lower 95% CI | Upper 95% CI |
|---|---|---|---|---|---|
| positive | 0.4336 | 40 | 0.5263 | 0.2653 | 0.6019 |

#### Summary statistics for negative

| Response | Mean | N | Std dev | Lower 95% CI | Upper 95% CI |
|---|---|---|---|---|---|
| negative | 0.6980 | 36 | 0.1900 | 0.6337 | 0.7623 |

#### Summary statistics for leptokurtic

| Response | Mean | N | Std dev | Lower 95% CI | Upper 95% CI |
|---|---|---|---|---|---|
| leptokurtic | 1.6482 | 106 | 0.0709 | 1.6346 | 1.6619 |

#### Summary statistics for platykurtic

| Response | Mean | N | Std dev | Lower 95% CI | Upper 95% CI |
|---|---|---|---|---|---|
| platykurtic | 1.6557 | 128 | 0.2472 | 1.6125 | 1.6989 |

Summary descriptive statistics from InVivoStat, v4.0.2. Panel A shows the summary descriptive statistics for the female and male height data provided in Tables 5.1 and 5.2, respectively, together with the summary descriptive statistics for the rodent head shake data provided in Table 5.3.

Panel B shows the summary descriptive statistics for the positively and negatively skewed data shown graphically in Figures 5.3 and 5.4, respectively, together with the summary descriptive statistics for the leptokurtic and platykurtic data distributions shown graphically in Figures 5.5 and 5.6, respectively.

*Source*: InVivoStat.

 Minitab

**A**

| Variable | Mean | SE Mean | St Dev | Median | Mode | N for mode |
|---|---|---|---|---|---|---|
| Female | 1.6511 | 0.0111 | 0.0701 | 1.6495 | 1.556, 1.602, 1.613, 1.698 | 2 |
| Male | 1.8076 | 0.0101 | 0.0583 | 1.8050 | 1.795 | 3 |
| Head shake | 18.20 | 2.63 | 10.19 | 15.00 | 11.15 | 2 |

**B**

| Variable | N | N* | Mean | Median | Mode | N for mode | Skewness |
|---|---|---|---|---|---|---|---|
| Positive | 40 | 0 | 0.4336 | 0.2723 | * | 0 | 2.36 |
| Negative | 36 | 0 | 0.6980 | 0.7339 | 0.77 | 3 | −1.24 |
| Leptokurtic | 106 | 0 | 1.6482 | 1.6600 | 1.67 | 9 | −0.31 |
| Platykurtic | 128 | 0 | 1.6557 | 1.6540 | 1.45 | 13 | 0.02 |

Summary descriptive statistics from MiniTab, v19. Panel A shows the summary descriptive statistics for the female and male height data provided in Tables 5.1 and 5.2, respectively, together with the summary descriptive statistics for the rodent head shake data provided in Table 5.3.

Panel B shows the summary descriptive statistics for the positively and negatively skewed data shown graphically in Figures 5.3 and 5.4, respectively, together with the summary descriptive statistics for the leptokurtic and platykurtic data distributions shown graphically in Figures 5.5 and 5.6, respectively.

*Source*: Minitab, LLC.

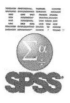

**A**

**Statistics**

|  |  | Female | Male |
|---|---|---|---|
| N | Valid | 40 | 33 |
|  | Missing | 88 | 95 |
| Mean |  | 1.6511 | 1.8076 |
| Std. Error of Mean |  | .01108 | .01014 |
| Median |  | 1.6495 | 1.8050 |
| Mode |  | 1.56[a] | 1.80 |
| Std. Deviation |  | .07006 | .05827 |
| Variance |  | .005 | .003 |
| Skewness |  | -.176 | -.194 |
| Std. Error of Skewness |  | .374 | .409 |
| Kurtosis |  | -.359 | -.112 |
| Std. Error of Kurtosis |  | .733 | .798 |
| Percentiles | 25 | 1.6020 | 1.7675 |
|  | 50 | 1.6495 | 1.8050 |
|  | 75 | 1.7010 | 1.8525 |

a. Multiple modes exist. The smallest value is shown

**B**

**Statistics**

Head_shake

| N | Valid |  | 15 |
|---|---|---|---|
|  | Missing |  | 113 |
| Mean |  |  | 18.2000 |
| Std. Error of Mean |  |  | 2.62987 |
| Median |  |  | 15.0000 |
| Mode |  |  | 9.00[a] |
| Std. Deviation |  |  | 10.18542 |
| Variance |  |  | 103.743 |
| Skewness |  |  | .803 |
| Std. Error of Skewness |  |  | .580 |
| Kurtosis |  |  | -.765 |
| Std. Error of Kurtosis |  |  | 1.121 |
| Minimum |  |  | 7.00 |
| Maximum |  |  | 38.00 |
| Percentiles | 25 |  | 10.0000 |
|  | 50 |  | 15.0000 |
|  | 75 |  | 28.0000 |

a. Multiple modes exist. The smallest value is shown

**C**

**Statistics**

|  |  | Positive | Negative | Leptokurtic | Platykurtic |
|---|---|---|---|---|---|
| N | Valid | 40 | 36 | 106 | 128 |
|  | Missing | 88 | 92 | 22 | 0 |
| Mean |  | .4336 | .6980 | 1.6482 | 1.6557 |
| Std. Error of Mean |  | .08322 | .03167 | .00688 | .02185 |
| Median |  | .2723 | .7339 | 1.6600 | 1.6540 |
| Mode |  | .02[a] | .77 | 1.67 | 1.45 |
| Std. Deviation |  | .52632 | .19002 | .07086 | .24724 |
| Variance |  | .277 | .036 | .005 | .061 |
| Skewness |  | 2.357 | -1.245 | -.305 | .016 |
| Std. Error of Skewness |  | .374 | .393 | .235 | .214 |
| Kurtosis |  | 5.560 | 1.994 | .768 | -.656 |
| Std. Error of Kurtosis |  | .733 | .768 | .465 | .425 |
| Minimum |  | .02 | .10 | 1.40 | 1.10 |
| Maximum |  | 2.33 | .98 | 1.85 | 2.19 |
| Percentiles | 25 | .1230 | .6225 | 1.6000 | 1.4500 |
|  | 50 | .2723 | .7339 | 1.6600 | 1.6540 |
|  | 75 | .5150 | .8275 | 1.6920 | 1.8500 |

a. Multiple modes exist. The smallest value is shown

Summary descriptive statistics from SPSS, v27. Panel A shows the summary descriptive statistics for the female and male height data provided in Tables 5.1 and 5.2, respectively. Panel B shows the summary descriptive statistics for the rodent head shake data provided in Table 5.3.

Panel C shows the summary descriptive statistics for the positively and negatively skewed data shown graphically in Figures 5.3 and 5.4, respectively, together with the summary descriptive statistics for the leptokurtic and platykurtic data distributions shown graphically in Figures 5.5 and 5.6, respectively.

*Source*: IBM Corporation.

# Write Your Own Notes

# 6 Testing for normality and transforming skewed data sets

Parametric statistical methods assume that the data to be analysed are drawn from a population that has a normal distribution which is characterised by the Mean and Variance. Furthermore, the symmetry of the normal distribution is such that the Mode, Median, and Mean values are equal (see sections 4.vii and Chapter 5). However, when the distribution of data sets is highly skewed, then the equality of these measures of central tendency is lost (see Table 5.6) and the assumption of normality no longer holds.

There are two principle assumptions that justify the use of parametric analysis of data sets that can be formally examined. These are tests for normality (the **Kolmogorov–Smirnov** and **Shapiro–Wilk** tests) and for homogeneity of variance (**Levene's** test).

## 1 Kolmogorov–Smirnov (K–S) and Shapiro–Wilk (S–W) tests

These tests both compare the values of the data set to a normally distributed set of scores with the same mean and standard deviation. The output of both tests comprises of a test statistic (denoted by D for the K–S test and W for the S–W test) with corresponding degrees of freedom and a significance level, $p$. Remember, these tests (and hence the $p$-value) reflect the relationship of the test data to a normal distribution, so if $p > 0.05$ then the distribution of the data is not different from a normal distribution. Conversely, if $p < 0.05$, then the test data are not normally distributed. These tests essentially provide the same information regarding the normality of a data set except that the S–W test has more power and may indicate a significant deviation from normality when the K–S test does not (see negative skew, original data in Table 6.2)!

## 2 Levene's test

This test examines the assumption that the variances of different groups of experimental data are equal, known as **homogeneity of variance** (see Figure 6.1). In contrast, different groups of data that exhibit **heterogeneity of variance** (where the variances differ markedly between the groups, see Figure 6.2) violate a basic assumption of parametric data and consequently it is inappropriate to analyse such data sets using parametric analysis. Heterogeneity of variance is often observed in data generated by behavioural pharmacological studies where low scores of behavioural observations are tightly clustered (low variance), but the spread of the data increases as the magnitude of the observations increases (see Figure 6.2). Levene's test is only appropriate where there are multiple groups of data.

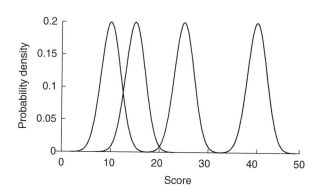

**Figure 6.1 Homogeneity of variance.** Normal distribution curves for data sets with mean values of 10, 15, 25, and 40 each with a standard deviation of 2. Note that the spread of the data sets does not change as the magnitude of the mean value increases.

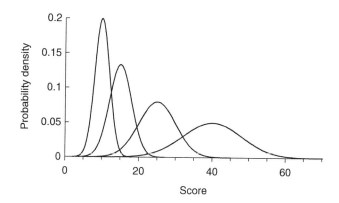

**Figure 6.2 Heterogeneity of variance.** Normal distribution curves for data sets with mean values of 10, 15, 25, and 40 with standard deviation values of 2, 3, 5, and 8, respectively. Note that the spread of the data sets increases as the magnitude of the mean value increases.

## Care!

Sometimes, the results of the K–S, S–W, and Levene's tests may be misleading. When the data sets contain a large number of samples, then each of these tests may indicate significant differences (i.e. $p < 0.05$), indicating either deviations from normality or heterogeneity of variance, as discussed above. Consequently, these tests should be interpreted in conjunction with histogram plots and the values for skewness and kurtosis.

*Experimental Design and Statistical Analysis for Pharmacology and the Biomedical Sciences*, First Edition. Paul J. Mitchell.
© 2022 John Wiley & Sons Ltd. Published 2022 by John Wiley & Sons Ltd.

The output of the Levene's test comprises of the test statistic (denoted by the letter F) with two different degrees of freedom and a significance level, $p$. Here, the basic assumption is that the data groups exhibit homogeneity of variance and so if $p > 0.05$ then the variances across the groups may be assumed to not differ significantly. In contrast, if $p < 0.05$, then this would indicate that the variances are significantly different between the different groups and consequently the assumption of homogeneity of variance is violated. Alternatively, the **Brown–Forsythe** or **Bartlett's** tests for equal variances provided by some statistical software may be used.

## Transforming skewed data sets to approximate a normal distribution

The distributions of the positively and negatively skewed data sets described in Chapter 5 (see Figures 5.3 and 5.4, respectively) clearly do not suggest that these sets of data may be described by a normal distribution, and thus it would be inappropriate to describe and analyse such data sets using parametric descriptive and inferential statistics. The use of parametric analysis is always attractive, however, as there is a greater variety of tests available to analyse data sets and such tests are generally stronger than the equivalent tests used in non-parametric analysis. Whenever you are presented with skewed data sets, however, all is not lost since it is perfectly acceptable in statistics to transform the data sets to overcome problems with normality, outliers, or unequal variances. Data transformation is acceptable since the process is applied to all the values in the data sets thereby changing the **form** of the relationship between the values while maintaining the relative differences between the values. Table 6.1 summarises a variety of data transformations (known as the **Tukey Ladder of Transformations**) that *may* (no guarantees here!) result in an approximation to a normal distribution.

Table 6.1 Tukey ladder of transformations.

| Transformation | Effect | Applied to: |
|---|---|---|
| $1/x^3$ | Stronger | |
| $1/x^2$ | Strong | |
| $1/x$ | Strong | |
| $1/\sqrt{x}$ | Strong | Positive skew |
| $\log_{10} x$ | Mild | |
| $\sqrt{x}$ | Mild | |
| X | No change | |
| $x^2$ | Mild | Negative skew |
| $x^3$ | Strong | |
| $\text{Antilog}_{10} x$ | Stronger | |

Summary of the mathematical functions used to transform data together with the effect on the data distribution and their application.

## Transforming positive skew

In the previous chapter, Figure 5.3 summarised the positively skewed distribution of blood lymphocyte number (expressed as $10^6$ lymphocytes per ml of blood) obtained from 40 HIV patients. In order to transform the skewed distribution of the raw values to a distribution that approximates a normal distribution the successful process must essentially tease apart the values at the lower end of the data range, while at the same time it must condense those values at the upper end of the data range. The two most common methods used to transform such positively skewed distributions are to calculate either the square root or the $\log_{10}$

values of the original values in the data set. Figure 6.3 shows the resulting distribution of the lymphocyte data following a $\log_{10}$ transformation.

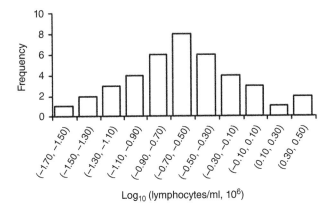

Figure 6.3 **Histogram plot of lymphocyte number per ml of blood following $\log_{10}$ transformation of the data from 40 HIV patients** (see Figure 5.3 for original data). Adjusted Fisher–Pearson coefficient = −0.089 (calculated $z$-score = −0.238, $p > 0.05$).

Visual inspection of the resulting distribution suggests that the transformed data are now more equally spread around the centre values. Indeed, calculation of the adjusted Fisher–Pearson coefficient indicates no significant skew in the data distribution, while the K–S test indicates no significant difference from a normal distribution (see Table 6.2). Clearly, subjecting the original values to a $\log_{10}$ transformation has resulted in a distribution that successfully approximates very closely to a normal distribution.

## Transforming negative skew

Figure 5.4 in Chapter 5 summarised the negatively skewed distribution of blood lymphocyte number (expressed as $10^6$ lymphocytes per ml of blood) obtained from another group of 36 leukaemic patients. In this situation, a successful transformation must essentially condense the values at the lower end of the data range, while at the same time it must tease apart those values at the upper end of the data range (i.e. the exact opposite from the process required to transform a positive skew). The two most common methods used to transform such negatively skewed distributions are to calculate either the square or the $\text{antilog}_{10}$ values of the original values in the data set. Figures 6.4 and 6.5 show the resulting distribution of the lymphocyte data following a square and an $\text{antilog}_{10}$ transformation, respectively.

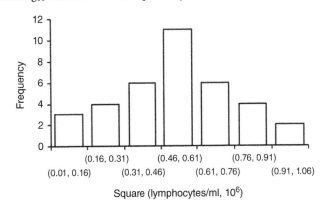

Figure 6.4 **Histogram plot of lymphocyte number per ml of blood following square transformation of the data from 36 leukaemic patients** (see Figure 5.4 for original data). Adjusted Fisher–Pearson coefficient = −0.293 (calculated $z$-score = −0.736, $p > 0.05$).

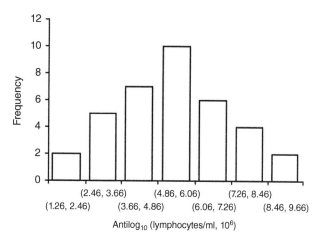

**Figure 6.5** **Histogram plot of lymphocyte number per ml of blood following antilog10 transformation of the data from 36 leukaemic patients** (see Figure 5.4 for original data). Adjusted Fisher–Pearson coefficient = −0.006 (calculated $z$-score = −0.015, $p > 0.05$).

In both cases, visual inspection of the resulting distributions shows that the transformed data sets are now more equally spread around the respective centre values. Indeed, calculation of the adjusted Fisher–Pearson coefficients indicates no significant skew in the data distributions in both cases, while the K–S test indicates that neither distribution now shows a significant difference from a normal distribution (see Table 6.2). Clearly, subjecting the original values to either a square or antilog$_{10}$ transformation of the original data values resulted in a distribution that successfully approximates very closely to a normal distribution.

Table 6.2 summarises the measures of central tendency (mode, median, and mean) and various statistics related to skewness, kurtosis, and normality determined prior to and following various methods of data transformation appropriate to normalise either

positive and negative skew in the distribution of the raw data. For both the positively and negatively skewed data, notice the relatively large differences between the measures of central tendency coupled with the significant skewness, kurtosis, and significant differences from a normal distribution. In all cases, the data transformation used here corrected the issues of skewness, kurtosis, or deviation from normality seen in the frequency distributions of the original data sets.

There is no guarantee that a particular data transformation will solve issues with skewness or kurtosis; just use whatever transformation is successful. However, note that all subsequent analysis must be performed on the transformed data sets!

## Removing outliers: Grubbs's test

Of course, in some cases, the distribution of a data set may appear to be slightly skewed simply by the presence of outlier data values. **Grubbs's test** is used to detect outliers in sets of data assumed to be sampled from a normally distributed population; consequently, the data distribution should be examined to ensure it approximates to normality before applying the test. Grubbs's test identifies one outlier at a time which is then removed from the data set. The test is run repeatedly until no outliers are detected. The problem with the test is that with small sample sizes ($n \leq 6$), most of the observations may be identified as outliers and consequently removed from the data set (which may leave you with no useable values in your data set if used excessively – so take care if you use this test)!

## QQ plots

A quantile–quantile plot (**QQ plot**) is a scatterplot of quantile probability values which allow the quantile values of two distributions to be plotted against each other, thereby providing a visual technique to examine if two data sets have a common underlying distribution. If the two data sets have a similar distribution, then

**Table 6.2** Comparison of measures of central tendency and distribution analysis prior to and following data transformation.

|  | Positive skew | | Negative skew | | |
|---|---|---|---|---|---|
|  | **Original** | **Log$_{10}$** | **Original** | **Square** | **Antilog$_{10}$** |
|  | (Figure 5.3) | (Figure 6.3) | (Figure 5.4) | (Figure 6.4) | (Figure 6.5) |
| **Mode** | 0.18 | −0.53 | 0.77 | 0.59 | 5.89 |
| **Median** | 0.272 | −0.565 | 0.734 | 0.539 | 5.4190 |
| **Mean** | 0.434 | −0.612 | 0.698 | 0.5223 | 5.401 |
| **F–P skew** | 2.357 | −0.089 | −1.245 | −0.293 | −0.006 |
| Std Error | 0.374 | 0.374 | 0.393 | 0.393 | 0.393 |
| $Z$-score | 6.302 | −0.238 | 3.168 | −0.746 | −0.015 |
| $p$-Value | $p < 0.001$ | $p > 0.05$ | $p < 0.01$ | $p > 0.05$ | $p > 0.05$ |
| **Kurtosis** | 5.560 | −0.201 | 1.994 | −0.201 | −0.161 |
| Std error | 0.733 | 0.733 | 0.768 | 0.768 | 0.768 |
| $Z$-score | 7.585 | −0.274 | 2.596 | −0.262 | −0.210 |
| $p$-Value | $p < 0.001$ | $p > 0.05$ | $p < 0.01$ | $p > 0.05$ | $p > 0.05$ |
| **K–S test; D** | 0.241 | 0.076 | 0.136 | 0.079 | 0.068 |
| df | 40 | 40 | 36 | 36 | 36 |
| $p$-Value | $p < 0.001$ | $p = 0.200$ | $p = 0.089$ | $p = 0.200$ | $p = 0.200$ |
| **S–W test; W** | 0.696 | 0.987 | 0.917 | 0.985 | 0.992 |
| df | 40 | 40 | 36 | 36 | 36 |
| $p$-Value | $p < 0.001$ | $p = 0.919$ | $p = 0.010$ | $p = 0.899$ | $p = 0.995$ |

Summary values were calculated using SPSS v24 software. Z-scores for both Fisher–Pearson skewness and kurtosis were calculated by dividing the coefficient values by respective standard error values. Threshold values for $z$ (irrespective of sign); if $z > 1.96$ then $p < 0.05$, if $z > 2.58$ then $p < 0.01$, and if $z > 3.29$ then $p < 0.001$ (for further explanation of $z$-scores, see Chapter 7). K–S and S–W indicate Kolmogorov–Smirnov (D) and Shapiro–Wilk (W) test statistics, respectively for normality.

the quantile values of the first data set will be very similar to those of the second; that is each quantile value for data set x will approximately equal that of data set y and if the two distributions are identical then x = y for all quantile values. QQ plots are commonly used to compare observed data sets (y-axis) to a theoretical standard normal distribution (x-axis) (see Chapter 7); linearity indicates the observed data are normally distributed, while deviation from linearity in the tails may indicate a skewed distribution of the data. Examples of QQ plots are provided in the following screen shots from various statistical software packages.

# Example output from statistical software

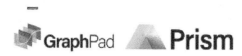

A

| | | A | B | C | D | E |
|---|---|---|---|---|---|---|
| | | positive | negative | Log10 positive | Square negative | Antilog negative |
| 1 | Number of values | 40 | 36 | 40 | 36 | 36 |
| 2 | | | | | | |
| 3 | Minimum | 0.02000 | 0.1000 | -1.699 | 0.01000 | 1.259 |
| 4 | Maximum | 2.330 | 0.9800 | 0.3674 | 0.9604 | 9.560 |
| 5 | Range | 2.310 | 0.8800 | 2.066 | 0.9504 | 8.291 |
| 6 | | | | | | |
| 7 | Mean | 0.4336 | 0.6980 | -0.6116 | 0.5223 | 5.401 |
| 8 | Std. Deviation | 0.5263 | 0.1900 | 0.4854 | 0.2288 | 1.947 |
| 9 | Std. Error of Mean | 0.08322 | 0.03167 | 0.07674 | 0.03814 | 0.3245 |
| 10 | | | | | | |
| 11 | Skewness | 2.357 | -1.245 | -0.08940 | -0.2932 | -0.006416 |
| 12 | Kurtosis | 5.560 | 1.994 | -0.2013 | -0.2006 | -0.1613 |

B

| Normality and Lognormality Tests Tabular results | A | B | C | D | E |
|---|---|---|---|---|---|
| | positive | negative | Log10 positive | Square negative | Antilog negative |
| **Test for normal distribution** | | | | | |
| Shapiro-Wilk test | | | | | |
| W | 0.6966 | 0.9166 | 0.9870 | 0.9851 | 0.9921 |
| P value | <0.0001 | 0.0100 | 0.9186 | 0.8991 | 0.9954 |
| Passed normality test (alpha=0.05)? | No | No | Yes | Yes | Yes |
| P value summary | **** | * | ns | ns | ns |
| | | | | | |
| Kolmogorov-Smirnov test | | | | | |
| KS distance | 0.2406 | 0.1363 | 0.07598 | 0.07943 | 0.06774 |
| P value | <0.0001 | 0.0887 | >0.1000 | >0.1000 | >0.1000 |
| Passed normality test (alpha=0.05)? | No | Yes | Yes | Yes | Yes |
| P value summary | **** | ns | ns | ns | ns |
| | | | | | |
| **Number of values** | 40 | 36 | 40 | 36 | 36 |

C

Normal QQ plot

D

Normal QQ plot

E

Normal QQ plot

F

Normal QQ plot

G

Normal QQ plot

Summary descriptive statistics from GraphPad Prism, v8. Panel A shows the summary descriptive statistics for the positively and negatively skewed data shown graphically in Figures 5.3 and 5.4, respectively, together with the summary descriptive statistics following $Log_{10}$ transformation of the positively skewed data (see Figure 6.3) and both square and antilog transformation of the negatively skewed data (see Figures 6.4 and 6.5, respectively). Panel B summarises the results of the Shapiro–Wilk and Kolmogorov–Smirnov tests of normality for both skewed and transformed data sets.

Panel C shows the normal QQ plot of the positively skewed data from Figure 5.3; note how the normal QQ plot deviates from unity at the tails of the data. Panel D shows the normal QQ plot following $Log_{10}$ transformation of the positively skewed data. Panel E shows the normal QQ plot of the negatively skewed data from Figure 5.4; note how the normal QQ plot deviates from unity at the tails of the data. Panel F shows the normal QQ plot following square transformation of the negatively skewed data. Panel G shows the normal QQ plot following antilog transformation of the negatively skewed data. Note how the normal QQ plots of the transformed data sets lie on or near the line of unity in all cases.

*Source*: GraphPad Software.

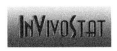

**A**

View Analysis Log | Export to Html | Export Images

## InVivoStat Summary Statistics

### Variable selection

Responses positive,negative,$Log_{10}$ positive,Square negative,Antilog negative are analysed in this module.

### Summary statistics
### Summary statistics for positive

| Response | Mean | N | Std Dev | Median | Lower quartile | Upper quartile |
|---|---|---|---|---|---|---|
| Positive | 0.4336 | 40 | 0.5263 | 0.2723 | 0.1259 | 0.5100 |

### Summary statistics for negative

| Response | Mean | N | Std Dev | Median | Lower quartile | Upper quartile |
|---|---|---|---|---|---|---|
| Negative | 0.6980 | 36 | 0.1900 | 0.7339 | 0.6250 | 0.8250 |

**B**

### Summary statistics for $Log_{10}$ positive

| Response | Mean | N | Std Dev | Median | Lower quartile | Upper quartile |
|---|---|---|---|---|---|---|
| $Log_{10}$ positive | −0.6116 | 40 | 0.4854 | −0.5650 | −0.9004 | −0.2925 |

### Summary statistics for Square negative

| Response | Mean | N | Std Dev | Median | Lower quartile | Upper quartile |
|---|---|---|---|---|---|---|
| Square negative | 0.5223 | 36 | 0.2288 | 0.5386 | 0.3907 | 0.6806 |

### Summary statistics for Antilog negative

| Response | Mean | N | Std Dev | Median | Lower quartile | Upper quartile |
|---|---|---|---|---|---|---|
| Antilog negative | 5.4006 | 36 | 1.9469 | 5.4190 | 4.2172 | 6.6839 |

**C** **D** **E** **F** **G**

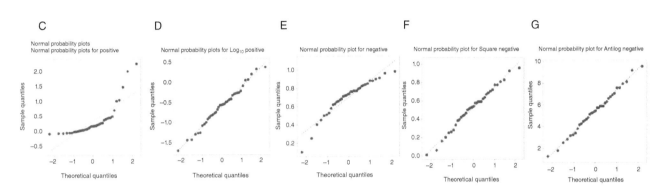

Summary descriptive statistics from InVivoStat, v4.0.2. Panel A shows the summary descriptive statistics for the positively and negatively skewed data shown graphically in Figures 5.3 and 5.4, respectively. Panel B shows the summary descriptive statistics following $Log_{10}$ transformation of the positively skewed data (see Figure 6.3) and both square and antilog transformation of the negatively skewed data (see Figures 6.4 and 6.5, respectively).

Panel C shows the normal probability plot of the positively skewed data from Figure 5.3; note how the normal probability plot deviates from unity at the tails of the data. Panel D shows the normal probability plot following $Log_{10}$ transformation of the positively skewed data. Panel E shows the normal probability plot of the negatively skewed data from Figure 5.4; note how the normal probability plot deviates from unity at the tails of the data. Panel F shows the normal probability plot following square transformation of the negatively skewed data. Panel G shows the normal probability plot following antilog transformation of the negatively skewed data. Note how the normal probability plots of the transformed data sets lie on or near the line of unity in all cases. Finally, note that the axes are reversed compared to the normal QQ plots provided by GraphPad Prism.

*Source*: InVivoStat.

**Minitab**

**A**

Statistics

| Variable | Mean | SE Mean | St Dev | Median | Mode | N for Mode | Skewness | Kurtosis |
|---|---|---|---|---|---|---|---|---|
| +ve | 0.4336 | 0.0832 | 0.5263 | 0.2723 | * | 0 | 2.36 | 5.56 |
| $Log_{10}$ +ve | −0.6116 | 0.0767 | 0.4854 | −0.5650 | * | 0 | −0.09 | −0.20 |
| −ve | 0.6980 | 0.0317 | 0.1900 | 0.7339 | 0.77 | 3 | −1.24 | 1.99 |
| Sq −ve | 0.5223 | 0.0381 | 0.2288 | 0.5386 | 0.5929 | 3 | −0.29 | −0.20 |
| Antilog -ve | 5.401 | 0.324 | 1.947 | 5.419 | 5.88844 | 3 | −0.01 | −0.16 |

**B**

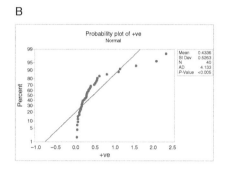

**C**

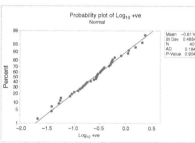

**D**

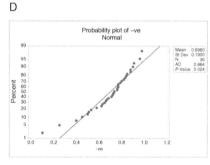

**E**

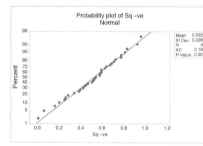

**F**

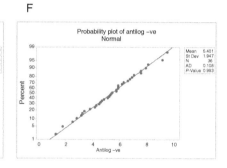

Summary descriptive statistics from MiniTab, v19. Panel A shows the summary descriptive statistics for the positively and negatively skewed data shown graphically in Figures 5.3 and 5.4, respectively, together with the summary descriptive statistics following $Log_{10}$ transformation of the positively skewed data (see Figure 6.3) and both square and antilog transformation of the negatively skewed data (see Figures 6.4 and 6.5, respectively).

Panel B shows the normal probability plot of the positively skewed data from Figure 5.3; note how the normal probability plot deviates from unity at the tails of the data. Panel C shows the normal probability plot following $Log_{10}$ transformation of the positively skewed data. Panel D shows the normal probability plot of the negatively skewed data from Figure 5.4; note how the normal probability plot deviates from unity at the tails of the data. Panel E shows the normal probability plot following square transformation of the negatively skewed data. Panel F shows the normal probability plot following antilog transformation of the negatively skewed data. Note how the normal probability plots of the transformed data sets lie on or near the line of unity in all cases.

*Source*: Minitab Inc.

A

**Descriptive Statistics**

| | N | Mean | | Std. Deviation | Skewness | | Kurtosis | |
| --- | --- | --- | --- | --- | --- | --- | --- | --- |
| | Statistic | Statistic | Std. Error | Statistic | Statistic | Std. Error | Statistic | Std. Error |
| Positive | 40 | .4336 | .08322 | .52632 | 2.357 | .374 | 5.560 | .733 |
| Negative | 36 | .6980 | .03167 | .19002 | -1.245 | .393 | 1.994 | .768 |
| Log10_positive | 40 | -.6116 | .07674 | .48536 | -.089 | .374 | -.201 | .733 |
| Square_negative | 36 | .5223 | .03814 | .22884 | -.293 | .393 | -.201 | .768 |
| Antilog_negative | 36 | 5.4006 | .32449 | 1.94692 | -.006 | .393 | -.161 | .768 |
| Valid N (listwise) | 36 | | | | | | | |

B

**Tests of Normality**

| | Kolmogorov-Smirnov[a] | | | Shapiro-Wilk | | |
| --- | --- | --- | --- | --- | --- | --- |
| | Statistic | df | Sig. | Statistic | df | Sig. |
| Positive | .285 | 36 | .000 | .664 | 36 | .000 |
| Negative | .136 | 36 | .089 | .917 | 36 | .010 |
| Log10_positive | .085 | 36 | .200* | .982 | 36 | .819 |
| Square_negative | .079 | 36 | .200* | .985 | 36 | .899 |
| Antilog_negative | .068 | 36 | .200* | .992 | 36 | .995 |

*. This is a lower bound of the true significance.

a. Lilliefors Significance Correction

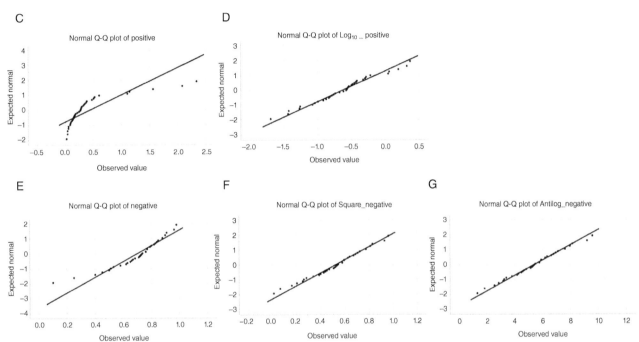

C — Normal Q-Q plot of positive

D — Normal Q-Q plot of Log₁₀_positive

E — Normal Q-Q plot of negative

F — Normal Q-Q plot of Square_negative

G — Normal Q-Q plot of Antilog_negative

Summary descriptive statistics from SPSS, v27. Panel A shows the summary descriptive statistics for the positively and negatively skewed data shown graphically in Figures 5.3 and 5.4, respectively. Panel B shows the summary descriptive statistics following Log₁₀ transformation of the positively skewed data (see Figure 6.3) and both square and antilog transformation of the negatively skewed data (see Figures 6.4 and 6.5, respectively).

Panel C shows the normal probability plot of the positively skewed data from Figure 5.3; note how the normal probability plot deviates from unity at the tails of the data. Panel D shows the normal probability plot following Log₁₀ transformation of the positively skewed data. Panel E shows the normal probability plot of the negatively skewed data from Figure 5.4; note how the normal probability plot deviates from unity at the tails of the data. Panel F shows the normal probability plot following square transformation of the negatively skewed data. Panel G shows the normal probability plot following antilog transformation of the negatively skewed data. Note how the normal probability plots of the transformed data sets lie on or near the line of unity in all cases.

*Source*: IBM Corporation.

# 7 The Standard Normal Distribution

At this point, it is important to further our understanding of the Normal Distribution curve. I've stated already that most biologically derived data sets follow a Normal Distribution (see Chapter 4 vii). Every normal distribution is a variation of the simplest case where the mean is set to 0 and the standard deviation equals 1, denoted as N(0, 1), which is known as the **Standard Normal Distribution**. We may think of this in another way where the normal distribution of our data set is simply where the domain of the standard normal distribution has been stretched by the standard deviation ($\sigma$) and then translated by the mean value ($\mu$). Thus, any set of sampled data that follows a normal distribution may be converted to a data set that has a mean of 0 and a standard deviation of 1 as follows:

**1** The data may be centred around 0 by taking each score ($x$) and subtracting from it the sample mean value of all the scores ($\bar{x}$); this essentially translates all the scores so that the mean is 0.

**2** The resulting scores are then divided by the standard deviation ($s$) of the original data set to ensure the translated data now have a standard deviation of 1.

The resulting scores are known a $z$-scores, denoted by the letter $z$, and the whole process is summarised as follows:

$$z = \frac{x - \bar{x}}{s} \tag{7.1}$$

Graphically, the normal distribution curve of the sampled data is identical to that following translation to the standard normal distribution (see Figure 7.1).

As described in Chapter 4, there are many different data distributions that have been characterised and each has a specific probability density function. The Standard Normal Distribution is very important because the shape of the distribution curve is precisely described by a mathematical power density function (see Appendix A.3) and, consequently, the area under the curve (AUC) (which, remember, is equal to 1) provides information regarding the probability of the occurrence of a particular value. Furthermore, this also enables the AUC of different sections to be calculated. The probability values for the standard normal distribution have been calculated and are provided in Appendix B. Table 7.1 provides a selected number of values appropriate for the following discussion.

The bottom panel of Figure 7.1 includes vertical gridlines appropriate to integer values of the $z$-scores. If we consider a $z$-score of 1 (so this is equal to 1 standard deviation above the mean), then Table 7.1 indicates that 0.84131 (i.e. 84.131%) of the AUC lies to the left of +1, while 0.15866 (i.e. 15.866%) lies to the right of +1. Of course, the standard normal distribution is perfectly symmetrical so that if $z = -1$ then 15.866% lies to the left of $-1$ while 84.131% lies to the right. Consequently, this means that 68.27% (i.e. $1-(2 \times$

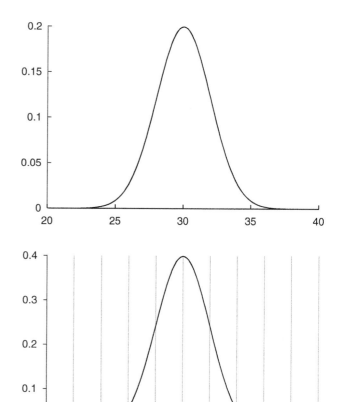

**Figure 7.1** Comparison of the normal distribution curve, N(30, 2), (top panel) with the equivalent Standard Normal Distribution, N(0, 1), (bottom panel).

**Table 7.1** Relationship between selected $z$-scores and AUC for the Standard Normal Distribution.

| $z$-score | Area | | |
|---|---|---|---|
| | Larger | Smaller | $-z$ to $+z$ (= % of total AUC) |
| 0 | 0.5000 | 0.5000 | |
| +1.00 | 0.84134 | 0.15866 | 0.68268 (=68.3%) |
| +1.64 | 0.94950 | 0.05050 | 0.89900 (=89.9%) |
| +1.96 | 0.97500 | 0.02500 | 0.95000 (=95.0%) |
| +2.00 | 0.97725 | 0.02275 | 0.95450 (=95.5%) |
| +2.33 | 0.99010 | 0.00990 | 0.98020 (=98.0%) |
| +2.58 | 0.99506 | 0.00494 | 0.99012 (=99.0%) |
| +3.00 | 0.99865 | 0.00135 | 0.99730 (=99.7%) |
| +3.29 | 0.99950 | 0.00050 | 0.99900 (=99.9%) |

*Experimental Design and Statistical Analysis for Pharmacology and the Biomedical Sciences*, First Edition. Paul J. Mitchell.
© 2022 John Wiley & Sons Ltd. Published 2022 by John Wiley & Sons Ltd.

0.15866) = 0.68268) of the values lie between one standard deviation either side of the mean (i.e. from $z$-scores of $-1$ to $+1$; see Figure 7.2).

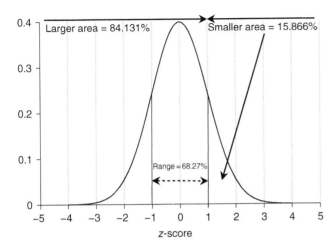

**Figure 7.2** Areas under the curve of the standard normal distribution corresponding to one standard deviation above and/or below mean zero.

Correspondingly, if $z = +2$ then 0.97725 (97.725%) lies below $z$ and 0.02275 (2.275%) lies above (so 95.45% lies between two standard deviations either side of the mean) (see Figure 7.3), while if $z = +3$ then 0.99865 (99.865%) lies below $z$ and 0.00135 (0.135%) lies above (with 99.73% lying between three standard deviations either side of the mean) (see Figure 7.4).

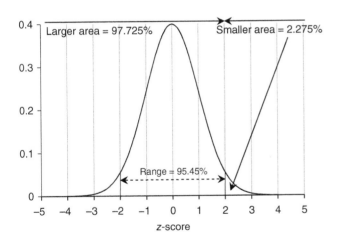

**Figure 7.3** Areas under the curve of the standard normal distribution corresponding to two standard deviations above and/or below mean zero.

The relationship between $z$-scores and probability is very important as it allows us to determine the $z$-scores for specific proportions of the data set. Thus, 5% of the population lies above a $z$-score of $+1.64$, 2.5% lies above $z = +1.96$, and 1% lies above $z = +2.33$. Furthermore, 95% of the values lie between $z$-scores of $-1.96$ and $+1.96$ (see Figure 7.5).

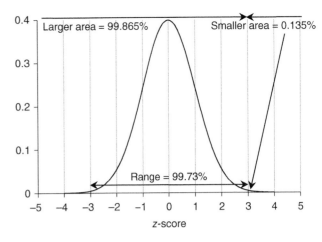

**Figure 7.4** Areas under the curve of the standard normal distribution corresponding to three standard deviations above and/or below mean zero.

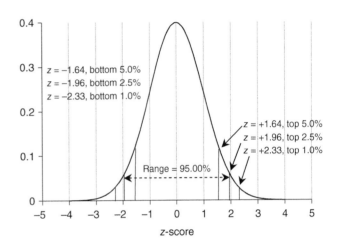

**Figure 7.5** Areas under the curve of the standard normal distribution corresponding to the top and bottom 5% (dashed line), 2.5% (solid line), and 1% (dotted line) of the sample population.

The important point to remember here is that the relationship between the $z$-scores (and hence any standard deviation value) and the AUC (and hence the probability scores) applies to all normal distribution curves. Thus, consider the data of student heights summarised in Figure 5.2. From the summary descriptive statistics for the male and female data sets (i.e. sample mean and sample standard deviations for each data set), we can calculate the corresponding height values that contain 95% of the observations for both sets of data. This calculation may be summarised as follows:

$$95\% \text{ range} = \bar{x} - (1.96s) \text{ to } \bar{x} + (1.96s) \qquad (7.2)$$

where $\bar{x}$ is the sample mean and $s$ is the standard deviation. Thus,

Female group : $1.651 \pm 0.06999$ m.

$$1.651 - (1.96 \times 0.06999) \text{ to } 1.651 + (1.96 \times 0.06999) \qquad (7.3)$$

$$95\% \text{range} = 1.514 - 1.788 \text{ m}$$

Male group : $1.808 \pm 0.05836$ m

$$1.808 - (1.96 \times 0.05836) \text{ to } 1.808 + (1.96 \times 0.05836) \quad (7.4)$$

95%range = 1.694 – 1.942 m

Furthermore, the probability of the $z$-scores allows us to answer questions such as:

*What is the probability of students being at least 1.70 m?*

We need to calculate this separately for the female and male cohorts. In both cases, we need to calculate the AUC corresponding to that greater than the calculated $z$-score appropriate for 1.7 m for the two student cohorts.

**1** Female students:

Calculate difference from the sample mean;

$$1.70 - 1.651 = 0.049 \text{ m} \quad (7.5)$$

Now express this as a $z$-score by dividing by the sample standard deviation; $\quad 0.049/0.06999 = 0.701 \quad (7.6)$

The table of the standard normal distribution (see Appendix A.2) indicates that the probability of $z = 0.701$ or greater is 24.2%; note that this is the smaller section above the dotted line in Figure 7.6, below.

**2** Male students:

Calculate difference from the sample mean;

$$1.70 - 1.808 = -0.108 \text{ m} \quad (7.7)$$

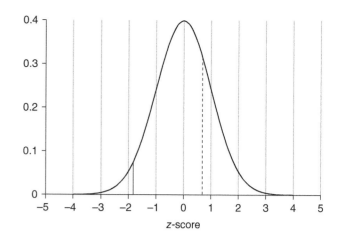

**Figure 7.6 Probability of male and female students being at least 1.7 m in height**. Female students are $1.651 \pm 0.06999$ m ($\bar{x} \pm$ St Dev). Female $z$-score for 1.7 m = +0.701 (dotted line). Area above $z$ = +0.701 is 24.2%. Male students are $1.808 \pm 0.05836$ m (($\bar{x} \pm$ St Dev). Male $z$-score for 1.7 m = −1.85058 (solid line). Area above $z$ = −1.85058 is 96.8%.

Now express this as a $z$-score by dividing by the sample standard deviation; $\quad -0.108/0.05836 = -1.85058$

$$(7.8)$$

The table of the standard normal distribution (see Appendix B) indicates that the probability of $z = -1.851$ or greater is 96.8%; note that this is the larger section above the solid line in Figure 7.6, below.

# Write Your Own Notes

# 8 Non-parametric descriptive statistics

In Chapter 5, I introduced various measures of central tendency (Mode, Median, and Mean), measures related to the spread of data whose distribution approximates that of a normal distribution (Range, Sum of Squares, Variance, and Standard Deviation), and a measure related to our confidence in the value of the mean (Standard Error of the Mean), i.e. parametric descriptive statistics. However, not all data sets follow a normal distribution (see Figures 5.3 and 5.4). It may be possible to transform a data set such that the distribution approximates to a normal distribution (see Chapter 6), whereupon reporting parametric descriptive statistical values using the transformed data is perfectly acceptable (note here that any subsequent inferential statistical test(s) should also be performed on the transformed data, only). In some cases, however, applying parametric analysis to either raw or transformed data may not be appropriate – so what Descriptive Statistics are available to us to provide a measure of central tendency and measures related to the spread of the data in such circumstances?

## Non-parametric descriptive statistics

Measures of central tendency are useful descriptive statistics because they provide a value where half of the observations are greater than the measure, while half are less than the measure. For data sets that are normally distributed, the Mean is an acceptable measure of central tendency because it approximates to the Median value, which is defined as the middle score when the observations are ranked in order of magnitude.

However, consider the positively skewed data set shown in Figure 5.3. Calculation of the Mode, Median, and Mean (see Table 6.2) of the original raw data indicated that the Mean ($0.434 \times 10^6$ lymphocytes per ml) is larger than the Median ($0.272 \times 10^6$ lymphocytes per ml) which is larger than the Mode ($0.18 \times 10^6$ lymphocytes per ml). In such cases, the Mean is inappropriate to use as a measure of central tendency because, in terms of the number of scores, it fails to divide the data set into two equal subsets of values. Indeed, in such circumstances, only the **Median** should be used as a measure of central tendency.

However, like other measures of central tendency, the Median fails to provide any measure related to the spread of the data. We could, of course, use the **Range** (see Chapter 5), but because this uses the highest and lowest values it is dramatically affected by extreme values (outliers). One way around this is to exclude a certain proportion of the highest and lowest scores. By convention, it is acceptable to exclude the top and bottom 25% of the observations such that we are left with the middle 50% of the observations. Calculation of the difference between the remaining scores after exclusion provides a range value known as the **interquartile range**.

To calculate the interquartile range, we first need to calculate what are known as quartiles which are three values that divided the number of observations into four equal parts. We already know the middle quartile (also known as the second quartile) which we call the median divides our data set into two equal parts. The lower quartile (or first quartile) is the median of the lower half of the data

set, while the upper quartile (or third quartile) is the median of the upper half of the data set. Note that the median of the complete data set is not included in the calculation of the upper and lower quartiles once the data is split into two equal halves.

The table below (Table 8.1) lists the number of head shake behaviours that I previously used in Chapter 5 (see Table 5.3).

**Table 8.1** Head shake behaviour exhibited by male Wistar rats.

| No | Head shakes | No | Head shakes | No | Head shakes |
|----|-------------|----|-------------|----|-------------|
| 1 | 7 | 6 | 11 | 11 | 23 |
| 2 | 9 | 7 | 12 | 12 | 28 |
| 3 | 9 | 8 | 15 | 13 | 31 |
| 4 | 10 | 9 | 15 | 14 | 34 |
| 5 | 11 | 10 | 20 | 15 | 38 |

Number of head shake behaviours exhibited by 15 male Wistar rats during a 10-minutes observation period ranked according to the magnitude of the behaviour shown by each rat. The lighter area indicates the median.

There are 15 observations in the data set, so the median value is the number of head shakes shown by the 8th animal once the data is ranked in order of magnitude. Consequently, the median equals 15 head shakes (you may call this the middle or second quartile, if you wish).

The lower quartile is the median of the lowest half of the data. Here, there are seven observations (excluding the 8th, see above) so that the middle value is the 4th observation. Consequently, the lower quartile equals 10 head shakes (which you may also call the first quartile).

The upper quartile is the median of the highest half of the data. Here, there are also seven observations (what a surprise!), so that the middle value is the 12th observation. Consequently, the upper quartile = 28 head shakes (yes, I know – you can call this the third quartile if you really want to). Collectively, the upper and lower quartile values are referred to as the **semi-quartile values**, and the difference between these is called the **interquartile range** (although some authors refer to this as the semi-interquartile range).

So, to summarise

1 **Median** = 15 head shakes
2 **Lower quartile** = 10 head shakes
3 **Upper quartile** = 28 head shakes
4 **Interquartile range** = 18 head shakes

The generally accepted **format** for reporting these values is
**Median (lower quartile, upper quartile)** = 15 (10, 28) head shakes.

There is one very important aspect to note here in that the values of the lower and upper quartiles are not equally spread around the median value, i.e. the lower quartile is only five head shakes less than the median, while the upper quartile is 13 head shakes greater than the median. In contrast, standard deviation values are always equally spread around the mean because of the symmetry of the normal distribution (i.e. $\bar{x} \pm$ St Dev).

It is acceptable to graphically represent non-parametric data as a bar chart (see Figure 8.1 below); however, note the asymmetry of the upper and lower bars which represent the values of the upper and lower quartiles (the asymmetry is produced by the skewed data distribution).

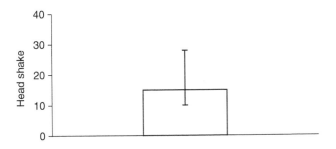

**Figure 8.1  Head shake behaviour exhibited by 15 male Wistar rats during a 10-minutes observation period.** Bar indicates the median of the number of head shakes, while the upper and lower error bars indicate the upper and lower semi-quartile values, respectively. Note the asymmetry of the interquartile range bars.

Perhaps a more accurate graphical representation of descriptive statistics related to non-parametric data sets is the **Box and Whisker plot** (see Figure 8.2).

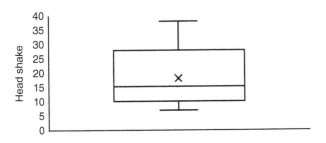

**Figure 8.2  Box and Whisker plot of head shake behaviour exhibited by 15 male Wistar rats during a 10-minutes observation period.** The box represents the upper and lower quartile values of the data, while the line across the box indicates the median value. The upper and lower error bars indicate the maximum and minimum values in the data set, respectively. The x represents the position of the mean value of the data (but should always be omitted in formal reporting of non-parametric data).

Here all the descriptive statistical values just described are included. The height of the Box summarises the interquartile range of the data set, where the upper extent of the box equals the upper quartile, the lower extent represents the lower quartile, and the line across the middle of the box represents the median of the data. In addition, the height of the upper error bar represents the maximum value of the data, while the bottom of the lower error bar represents the minimum value of the data. Some graphical packages also include an indicator of the mean value (denoted by x in Figure 8.2). This is useful for data inspection purposes **only** as it gives a good idea on the skewness of the data set. If the mean lies above the median, then the data most likely show a positive skew in distribution, whereas if the mean lies below the median then the data probably show a negative skew in distribution; furthermore, the greater the difference between the median and the mean, the

greater the degree of skew in the data set. However, in any final report (e.g. laboratory report, publication in the scientific literature), the position of the mean in Box–Whisker plots should be omitted as the use of parametric descriptive statistical values is inappropriate in reporting non-parametric data!

As we have seen, calculating the median value of an odd number of observations is straightforward. But how do you deal with an even number of observations. Consider the following set of data taken from an experiment using the Morris Water maze where rodents are trained to locate a submerged platform using their spatial memory.

**Table 8.2  Time (s) to locate submerged platform in Morris Water maze achieved by 20 Wistar rats.**

| No | Time (s) | No | Time (s) | No | Time (s) | No | Time (s) |
|----|----------|----|----------|----|----------|----|----------|
| 1 | 56 | 6 | 63 | 11 | 70 | 16 | 99 |
| 2 | 57 | 7 | 64 | 12 | 74 | 17 | 102 |
| 3 | 58 | 8 | 67 | 13 | 79 | 18 | 108 |
| 4 | 58 | 9 | 67 | 14 | 84 | 19 | 111 |
| 5 | 59 | 10 | 69 | 15 | 94 | 20 | 113 |

Data are the times taken for male Wister rats ($n = 20$, 240–260 g) to locate a submerged platform during a 120-s swim test ranked according to the magnitude of the time taken.

If we divide the 20 observations into two equal parts, then we end up with 10 observations in each half. Consequently, the median is the value equidistant between the 10th and 11th observation (see lighter area in Table 8.2). Thus, the median score for this set of data is

$$\text{Median} = (69 + 70)/2 = 69.5 \qquad (8.1)$$

Calculation of the lower and upper quartiles proceeds in the same way in that each half set of observations must be further divided into two equal halves. Consequently, the lower quartile lies equidistant between the observations 5 and 6, while the upper quartile lies equidistant between the observations 15 and 16. As in the previous example, the interquartile range is the difference between the lower and upper quartiles. Thus,

$$\text{Lower quartile} = (59 + 63)/2 = 61 \qquad (8.2)$$

$$\text{Upper quartile} = (94 + 99)/2 = 96.5 \qquad (8.3)$$

$$\text{Interquartile range} = 96.5 - 61 = 35.5 \qquad (8.4)$$

These values are summarised in Table 8.3. However, there are alternative methods to calculate the lower and upper quartiles depending on whether there are an even or odd number of data points, which may include or exclude the median value. For example, in one such method, the lower quartile lies at a position equal to the 5th observation **plus** one quarter of the difference between the 5th and 6th observations, while the upper quartile lies at a position equal to the 16th observation **minus** one-quarter of the difference between the 15th and 16th observations (*in the screen shots at the end of this chapter compare the InVivoStat results to those from the other statistical programmes*).

**Table 8.3** Summary of descriptive statistics (non-parametric data).

| | Interquartile values | | | |
|---|---|---|---|---|
| | **Median** | **Lower** | **Upper** | **Range** |
| **Time (s)** | 69.5 | 61 | 96.5 | 35.5 |

Summary descriptive statistics for times taken to locate submerged platform in the Morris water maze. Data calculated from Table 8.2.

In both data sets summarised in Tables 8.1 and 8.2, note that the actual values took second place to their position in the data set once all the values are ranked in order of magnitude. For example, the 17th observation in Table 8.2 could have any value between 100 and 107; inclusively, it would still be the 17th observation in order of magnitude. Furthermore, such a change in magnitude would have no effect on the median, lower quartile, upper quartile, or interquartile range. In addition, the lowest value (in this case 56 s) is free to vary between 0 and 56 s (inclusive), while the highest observation could have any value from 112 to infinity! The only effect these latter changes in time value would have would be to change the minimum value, maximum value, and consequently the range of the scores which, as previously argued, we don't use

to provide information regarding the spread of non-parametric data sets (remember, in preference we use the interquartile range value). The same cannot be said for normally distributed data subjected to parametric analysis; here any change in the value of an observation would have an effect (however, small that may be) on the descriptive statistics we use to summarise the data set.

Throughout Chapters 5, 6, and 8, I have introduced a number of terms and values that fall under the general term descriptive statistics. However, it is important to remember that in most cases these values are appropriate for **either** normally distributed or non-parametric data sets, and **not** both. Unfortunately, most statistical programmes simply calculate all these values regardless of the distribution of the data being summarised. Consequently, it is up to **you**, the experimenter, to identify which values are appropriate for your data set.

Table 8.4 lists the variety of terms and values used to describe data together with two empty columns under headings parametric and non-parametric. As a simple exercise, I would like **you** to complete the table by indicating in the appropriate column which test or descriptive statistic is appropriate for which type of data.

In the following Chapter, I shall reveal which of the above tests and values are appropriate for either parametric data, non-parametric data, or even both!

**Table 8.4** Summary of descriptive statistics.

| | Parametric (Normal Distribution) | Non-parametric (Non-Normal Distribution) |
|---|---|---|
| **Data distribution** | | |
| Normality: Kolmogorov–Smirnov (D) | | |
| Normality: Shapiro–Wilk (W) | | |
| Skew: Fisher–Pearson coefficient | | |
| Kurtosis | | |
| **Measures of central tendency** | | |
| Mode | | |
| Median | | |
| Mean ($\bar{x}$) | | |
| Standard Error of the Mean (S.E.M) | | |
| **Spread of data** | | |
| Minimum | | |
| Maximum | | |
| Range | | |
| Lower quartile | | |
| Upper quartile | | |
| Interquartile range | | |
| Sum of Squares | | |
| Variance ($s^2$) | | |
| Levene's test | | |
| Standard Deviation ($s$) | | |

# Example output from statistical software

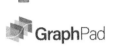 

A

| | A | B |
| | Head shake | Water maze |
|---|---|---|
| Number of values | 15 | 20 |
| Minimum | 7.000 | 56.00 |
| 25% Percentile | 10.00 | 60.00 |
| Median | 15.00 | 69.50 |
| 75% Percentile | 28.00 | 97.75 |
| Maximum | 38.00 | 113.0 |
| Range | 31.00 | 57.00 |

Summary descriptive statistics from GraphPad Prism, v8. Panel A shows the summary descriptive statistics for the head shake and water maze data from Tables 8.1 and 8.2, respectively. The correct format for reporting the descriptive statistics of non-parametric data sets is median (lower quartile and upper quartile). Thus, for the head shake data, 15 (10, 28), and for the water maze data, 69.50 (60.00, 97.75), note the asymmetry of the absolute difference between the median and the lower quartile compared to the median and the upper quartile. The mean, standard deviation, and standard error of the mean should not be used to summarise the descriptive statistics of non-parametric data sets.

*Source*: GraphPad Software.

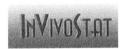

A

 Minitab

A

## Statistics

| Variable | Q1 | Median | Q3 | IQR |
|---|---|---|---|---|
| Head shake | 10.00 | 15.00 | 28.00 | 18.00 |
| Water maze | 60.00 | 69.50 | 97.75 | 37.75 |

Summary descriptive statistics from MiniTab, v19. Panel A shows the summary descriptive statistics for the head shake and water maze data from Tables 8.1 and 8.2, respectively. The correct format for reporting the descriptive statistics of non-parametric data sets is median (lower quartile and upper quartile). Thus, for the head shake data, 15 (10, 28), and for the water maze data, 69.50 (60.00, 97.75), note the asymmetry of the absolute difference between the median and the lower quartile compared to the median and the upper quartile. The mean, standard deviation, and standard error of the mean should not be used to summarise the descriptive statistics of non-parametric data sets.

*Source*: Minitab,LLC

A

## InVivoStat Summary Statistics

View Analysis Log | Export to Html | Export Images

### Variable selection

Responses Head shake,Water maze are analysed in this module.

### Summary statistics
#### Summary statistics for Head shake

| Response | N | Min | Max | Median | Lower quartile | Upper quartile |
|---|---|---|---|---|---|---|
| Head shake | 15 | 7.0000 | 38.0000 | 15.0000 | 10.0000 | 28.0000 |

#### Summary statistics for Water maze

| Response | N | Min | Max | Median | Lower quartile | Upper quartile |
|---|---|---|---|---|---|---|
| Water maze | 20 | 56.0000 | 113.0000 | 69.5000 | 61.0000 | 96.5000 |

Summary descriptive statistics from InVivoStat, v4.0.2. Panel A shows the summary descriptive statistics for the head shake and water maze data from Tables 8.1 and 8.2, respectively. The correct format for reporting the descriptive statistics of non-parametric data sets is median (lower quartile and upper quartile). Thus, for the head shake data, 15 (10, 28), and for the water maze data, 69.50 (61.00, 96.50), note the asymmetry of the absolute difference between the median and the lower quartile compared to the median and the upper quartile. Note also that InVivoStat reports for different lower and upper quartile values compared to

GraphPad Prism, MiniTab, and SPSS (see additional note below). The mean, standard deviation, and standard error of the mean should not be used to summarise the descriptive statistics of non-parametric data sets.

*Source*: InVivoStat.

## Statistics

| | | Head_shake | Water_maze |
|---|---|---|---|
| N | Valid | 15 | 20 |
| | Missing | 113 | 108 |
| Median | | 15.0000 | 69.5000 |
| Minimum | | 7.00 | 56.00 |
| Maximum | | 38.00 | 113.00 |
| Percentiles | 25 | 10.0000 | 60.0000 |
| | 50 | 15.0000 | 69.5000 |
| | 75 | 28.0000 | 97.7500 |

Summary descriptive statistics from SPSS, v27. Panel A shows the summary descriptive statistics for the head shake and water maze data from Tables 8.1 and 8.2, respectively. The correct format for reporting the descriptive statistics of non-parametric data sets is median (lower quartile and upper quartile). Thus, for the head shake data, 15 (10, 28), and for the water maze data, 69.50 (60.00, 97.75), note the asymmetry of the absolute difference between the median and the lower quartile compared to the median and the upper quartile. The mean, standard deviation, and standard error of the mean should not be used to summarise the descriptive statistics of non-parametric data sets.

*Source*: IBM Corporation.

# 9 Summary of descriptive statistics: so, what values may I use to describe my data?

## Introduction: the most important question to answer in statistical analysis!

Whenever I ask any group of students (not just those studying pharmacology), 'What is the most important question to ask in statistical analysis?', I get a variety of answers including 'What test should I use?', 'What is the value of $p$?', 'What is the Null Hypothesis?' and so on. In fact, none of these is the correct answer! I would argue most strongly that the most important question to ask is…….'What type of data set do I have?' since the answer to this question informs every step you take in, first, identifying which Descriptive Statistical values to report in the presentation of your data (see Chapters 5–8, and also Chapter 2) and, second, which Inferential Statistical tests you use to analyse your data. Decisions on whether the data approximate to a normal distribution, have an unknown distribution, or are categorical are absolutely critical for everything else you do with your data. If you get the correct answer to this question, then your life as an experimental pharmacologist will be so easy – get it wrong and everything will be downhill thereafter!

That one simple answer is the difference between euphoria and abject misery!

## What type of data do I have?

The answer to this question is in three parts.

**1** Are your data sets in categories? If the answer is 'Yes!', then you move to **chi-squared analysis** of contingency tables (see Chapter 21). If your answer is 'No!', then you move to the next question.
**2** Are your data normally distributed (see Chapter 6)? If the answer is 'Yes!', then you apply **Parametric Analysis** to your data. If the answer is 'No!', then you move to the next question.
**3** Are you able to transform your data so that your new values approximate to a normal distribution (see Chapters 5 and 6)? If the answer is 'Yes!', then transform your data as appropriate and apply Parametric Analysis to your *transformed* data. If the answer is 'No!', then you may assume that the distribution of your data is either unknown or is said to be distribution-free; consequently, you subject your data to **Non-Parametric Analysis** (see Chapter 8).

These sequential decisions may be summarized as shown in Figure 9.1, below.

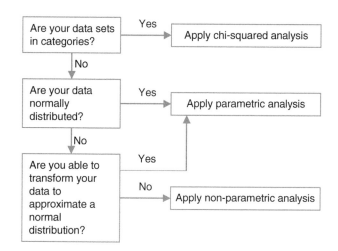

**Figure 9.1** Sequential decisions to identify data distribution.

Once you have allocated your non-categorical data to either Parametric analysis or Non-Parametric analysis, then similar decisions need to be made to identify the most appropriate strategy to analyse your data. However, although the identification of categorical data sets is generally obvious, most people struggle with differentiating between data sets that are normally distributed and those whose distribution is either unknown or distribution-free. The main problem here is that, as stated earlier (see Chapter 4), whenever we obtain experimental data, we only deal with samples of a population rather than the whole population. Furthermore, while the whole population may demonstrate a normal distribution, the distribution of our sample from that population may not be so readily apparent.

Figure 9.2 shows the histogram plot of the heights of 40 female undergraduate students. Just by looking at the histogram, we can see that the distribution of the height values takes up a bell-shaped curve which is consistent with what we would expect from data that is normally distributed.

*Experimental Design and Statistical Analysis for Pharmacology and the Biomedical Sciences*, First Edition. Paul J. Mitchell.
© 2022 John Wiley & Sons Ltd. Published 2022 by John Wiley & Sons Ltd

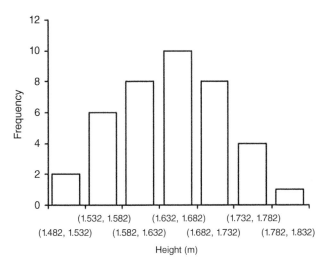

Figure 9.2 **Histogram of height data obtained from 40 undergraduate female students (2016–2017)**. X-axis values indicate bin width (m) for each bar. Data from Table 5.1

However, Figure 9.3 shows the resulting histogram for a random sample of 12 students. Clearly, the distribution of these data, which were taken for the earlier sample of 40 students, has lost that apparent relationship to a normal distribution.

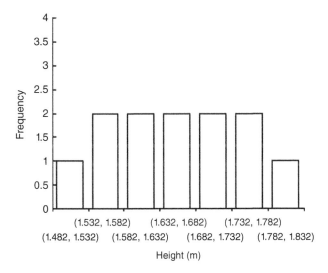

Figure 9.3 **Histogram of height data for 12 undergraduate female students (2016–2017)**. Data sampled at random from those values used for Figure 9.2 from Table 5.1.

The important point here is that as the sample size is reduced, it becomes more difficult to discern the distribution of the data. Of course, the reverse is also true; as the sample size increases, it becomes easier to determine the distribution of the data set and whether the parent population follows a normal distribution.

# Taking the first steps to data description and analysis

The most important question to ask about your data is, 'What type of data do I have?' The following table summarises the assumed properties of parametric and non-parametric data that may go some way to determining the type of data you have (Table 9.1). The table also includes the use of statistical tests to examine whether your data approximate to a normal distribution, have

significant skew or kurtosis, or have homogeneity of variance. These are very important steps in informing your decision. This is why the first section of Table 9.2 and the use of Levene's test (or alternatively the Brown–Forsythe or Bartlett's tests) for homogeneity of variance are common to both parametric and non-parametric data sets. Of course, the descriptive statistics you use in terms of central tendency and spread of data are dependent on the results of these analyses, and these values are summarised in Table 9.1.

Table 9.1 Assumptions of parametric and non-parametric data.

|  | **Parametric** | **Non-parametric** |
|---|---|---|
| Data type | Measurement | Ordinal (Ranks) Nominal (Categories) |
| Form | Continuous | Discrete |
| Scale | Interval and Ratio (theoretically without limit) | Limited |
| Spread | Homogeneity of variance | Heterogeneity of variance |
| Distribution | Approximately normally distributed | Non-normal distribution or distribution-free |
| Skewness (Fisher–Pearson) | F-P < ±2 $z$-score < 1.96, $p > 0.05$ | F-P > ±2 $z$-score > 1.96, $p < 0.05$ |
| Kurtosis | Kurtosis <5 $z$-score < 1.96, $p > 0.05$ | Kurtosis >5 $z$-score > 1.96, $p < 0.05$ |
| Shapiro–Wilk (W) | $p > 0.05$ | $p < 0.05$ |
| Kolmogorov–Smirnov (D) | $p > 0.05$ | $p < 0.05$ |
| Levene's test | $p > 0.05$ | $p < 0.05$ |

Table 9.2 Summary of descriptive statistics.

|  | **Parametric** | **Non-parametric** |
|---|---|---|
| **Data distribution** |  |  |
| Normality: Kolmogorov–Smirnov (D) | √ | √ |
| Normality: Shapiro–Wilk (W) | √ | √ |
| Skew: Fisher–Pearson coefficient | √ | √ |
| Kurtosis | √ | √ |
| **Measures of central tendency** |  |  |
| Mode | x | x |
| Median | (√) | √ |
| Mean ($\bar{x}$) | √ | x |
| **Spread of data** |  |  |
| Minimum | (√) | √ |
| Maximum | (√) | √ |
| Range | (√) | √ |
| Lower quartile | (√) | √ |
| Upper quartile | (√) | √ |
| Interquartile range | (√) | √ |
| Sum of Squares | √ | x |
| Variance ($s^2$) | √ | x |
| Levene's test | √ | √ |
| Standard Deviation (s) | √ | x |
| Standard Error of the Mean (S.E.M) | √ | x |

Summary of tests of data distribution and values related to Descriptive Statistics. Appropriate values are indicated by √, whereas inappropriate values are indicated by x. Note that √ in parenthesis, i.e. (√), indicates that the values generally used to describe non-parametric data may also be appropriate for parametric data.

Also remember that a distribution with significant positive or negative skew may be transformed so that the distribution of the transformed data approximates to a normal distribution; subsequent description and analysis would, of course, be performed on the transformed data.

There is one very important aspect to remember, however. As a general rule, it is inappropriate to apply parametric descriptive statistics or analysis to a set of data where the distribution clearly fails to follow a normal distribution or where the distribution is unknown. In contrast, however, it is perfectly legitimate to apply non-parametric descriptive statistics and analysis to data that follows a normal distribution (or at least approximates to a normal distribution such that any differences are of little consequence). This is why I have indicated, albeit in parentheses, that some non-parametric descriptive statistics may be applied to parametric data sets (see Table 9.2).

As previously stated, one big issue that you will come across time and time again is that statistical packages will routinely churn out a plethora of descriptive statistics when requested irrespective of the data distribution. Consequently, it is up to **you** to identify which values are appropriate. You should not, ever, just regurgitate these values without due consideration. In contrast, you must identify which values are appropriate for your data and only report those values.

## Strategy for descriptive statistics

Chapters 4–9 discussed the complexity of determining the type of data you have and the correct descriptive statistics to use to summarise that data. As stated earlier, however, everything we do with our data depends entirely on the type of data we have and, consequently, this is the foundation of every decision we subsequently make regarding our use of Descriptive and Inferential statistics. Table 9.3 summarises the legitimate use of Descriptive Statistics for different types of data sets you are likely to encounter; if you stick to these then you should never go far wrong!

Table 9.3 Legitimate use of descriptive statistics.

| Data type and/or distribution | Central tendency | Spread of data |
|---|---|---|
| Categorical | • Mode | |
| Parametric (raw or transformed data) | • Mean | • Sum of Squares<br>• Variance<br>• Standard Deviation<br>• Standard Error of the Mean |
| Non-parametric (or distribution unknown) | • Median | • Lower quartile<br>• Upper quartile<br>• Interquartile range |

Just to help clarify matters, I would like to provide a few examples of different types of data.

## Example data

### 1 Categorical data

One hundred forty-seven second-year Pharmacy and Pharmacology students at the University of Bath were shown a recording of an interview between a Psychiatrist and a patient suffering from depressive illness, following which the students were asked to score the level of depression using the Montgomery–Asberg Depression Rating Scale (MADRS). The MADRS consists of 10 categories, each of which is scored on a scale of 0 (absent) to 6 (maximum). Table 9.4 summarises the resulting data.

The most appropriate measure of central tendency to use here is the **Mode**, as this indicates the severity of each category chosen by most students. Summation of the Mode scores indicates severity of depressive illness suffered by the patient. The score of 35 shown in this example suggests that the patient was on the boarder of severe depressive illness.

Table 9.4 Summary of depression intensity scored by MADRS.

| | Intensity of each category | | | | | | | |
|---|---|---|---|---|---|---|---|---|
| | 0 | 1 | 2 | 3 | 4 | 5 | 6 | Mode |
| Apparent Sadness | 0 | 0 | 0 | 1 | 34 | **74** | 38 | 5 |
| Reported Sadness | 0 | 0 | 0 | 0 | 46 | **69** | 32 | 5 |
| Inner Tension | 2 | 3 | 2 | 7 | **61** | 53 | 19 | 4 |
| Reduced Sleep | 0 | 2 | 1 | 20 | **68** | 56 | 0 | 4 |
| Reduced Appetite | 57 | 48 | 25 | 10 | 4 | 2 | 1 | 0 |
| Concentration Difficulties | 1 | 5 | 16 | 41 | **59** | 20 | 5 | 4 |
| Lassitude | 7 | 0 | 1 | 13 | 31 | **69** | 26 | 5 |
| Inability to Feel | 7 | 10 | 43 | **66** | 10 | 8 | 3 | 3 |
| Pessimistic Thoughts | 6 | 0 | 5 | 12 | **65** | 50 | 9 | 4 |
| Suicidal Thoughts | 5 | **57** | 49 | 25 | 9 | 1 | 1 | 1 |
| | | | | | | | Total Score | 35 |

Values indicate the number of students choosing the intensity of each category within the MADRS. Values in bold indicate the mode value for clarity. Data on file.

### 2 Parametric data (use of arithmetic and geometric mean values)

Table 9.5 summarises the concentration-effect curves obtained by three students to determine the potency of a muscarinic receptor agonist to induce contractions of small lengths of isolated Guinea Pig Ileum mounted in an organ bath. The purpose of these experiments was to produce an average concentration-effect curve from the original data and also estimate the average potency of the muscarinic receptor agonist; drug potency in these studies is usually calculated by determining the concentration of receptor agonist which induces a half-maximal response, commonly referred to as the Effective Concentration 50% ($EC_{50}$).

**Table 9.5** Effect of a muscarinic receptor agonist to induce contractile responses in three preparations of isolated Guinea-Pig Ileum.

| [Drug] M | Log$_{10}$ [Drug] | Student No. 1 | 2 | 3 |
|---|---|---|---|---|
| $1 \times 10^{-10}$ | −10.0 | 0 | 0 | 0 |
| $3 \times 10^{-10}$ | −9.523 | 7 | 0 | 0 |
| $9 \times 10^{-10}$ | −9.046 | 20 | 5 | 0 |
| $2.7 \times 10^{-9}$ | −8.569 | 45 | 16 | 3 |
| $8.1 \times 10^{-9}$ | −8.092 | 70 | 40 | 7 |
| $2.43 \times 10^{-8}$ | −7.614 | 87 | 63 | 20 |
| $7.29 \times 10^{-8}$ | −7.137 | 95 | 83 | 42 |
| $2.19 \times 10^{-7}$ | −6.660 | 100 | 94 | 65 |
| $6.56 \times 10^{-7}$ | −6.183 | 100 | 97 | 83 |
| $1.97 \times 10^{-6}$ | −5.706 | 100 | 100 | 96 |
| $5.90 \times 10^{-6}$ | −5.229 | 100 | 100 | 100 |

Table values indicate calculated percentage of maximal response for each final bath concentration of the muscarinic receptor agonist for each tissue preparation.

There are three stages to the analysis of these data;

*a Calculation of individual drug potency by determining the EC$_{50}$ values from the raw data for each tissue*

Experimental EC$_{50}$ values are generally estimated by plotting the percentage maximal responses for each tissue (on the Y-axis) against the Log$_{10}$ of the agonist final bath concentration (on the X-axis) and then extrapolating the 50% response to the X-axis. There are 3 very important points to note here. First, the percentage maximal response values are plotted on a **linear** axis (Y-axis). Second, the final bath concentrations of the drug are plotted on a **logarithmic** axis (X-axis). However, this may be achieved in a couple of ways; either the Log$_{10}$ values of the final bath drug concentrations are calculated and plotted on a linear scale (see Figure 9.4), or the actual final bath drug concentrations are plotted on a Log$_{10}$ scale (see Figure 9.5). Whichever method of data plotting is chosen, the result is that the position of each data point is plotted in a logarithmic progression along the x-axis (notice the identical relative position of each vertical arrow in Figures 9.4 and 9.5). These figures are termed **Concentration-Effect Curves** and may be used to estimate either the Log$_{10}$ of the EC$_{50}$ values (from Figure 9.4) or the molar concentrations of the actual EC$_{50}$ values

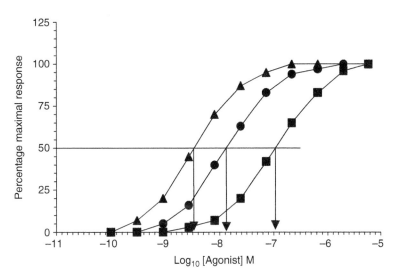

**Figure 9.4  Concentration-effect curves for a muscarinic receptor agonist on three different sections of Guinea Pig ileum.** Estimated Log$_{10}$ EC$_{50}$ values are for tissue 1 (solid triangles) = −8.47, tissue 2 (solid circles) = −7.89, and tissue 3 (solid squares) = −6.97, as indicated by the vertical arrows extrapolated from the horizontal line indicating 50% maximal response.

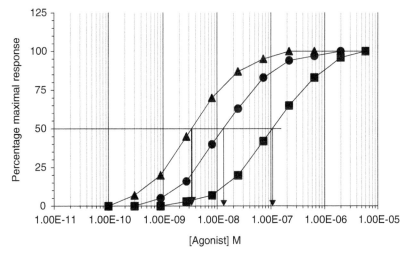

**Figure 9.5  Concentration-effect curves for a muscarinic receptor agonist on three different sections of Guinea Pig ileum.** Estimated EC$_{50}$ values are for tissue 1 (solid triangles) = $3.388 \times 10^{-9}$ M, tissue 2 (solid circles) = $1.288 \times 10^{-8}$ M, and tissue 3 (solid squares) = $1.072 \times 10^{-7}$ M, as indicated by the vertical arrows extrapolated from the horizontal line indicating 50% maximal response.

(from Figure 9.5). Many people opt to use logarithmic scales because it is easier to plot the absolute molar concentrations on a logarithmic scale (e.g. Figure 9.5). However, any manipulation of the data must be performed on the $Log_{10}$ values (see following discussion). The third point to note is that these **single data points** for each response **must be joined dot-to-dot.** The reason for this is that there is only one response value for each drug concentration (for each tissue) and so to curve-fit these points either by eye or by a curve-fitting programme makes erroneous assumptions about the position of each point that may be unjustified.

### b Calculation of the average concentration-effect curve.

Since the percentage maximal response data are plotted on a linear axis, then the average response following addition of each drug concentration to the tissue is calculated using the **arithmetic mean of the response values** shown in Table 9.5; these mean response values are shown in Table 9.6 and were used to generate the average concentration-effect curve shown in Figure 9.6.

### c Calculation of the average $EC_{50}$ value as a measure of drug potency.

The different $EC_{50}$ values of the muscarinic receptor agonist on the three different tissues were estimated either as $Log_{10}$ $EC_{50}$ values from the X-axis in Figure 9.4, or as molar concentrations from the $Log_{10}$ scale of the actual final bath concentrations in Figure 9.5. It is vitally important that you appreciate that in both cases, therefore, the estimated $Log_{10}$ $EC_{50}$ values or the molar concentrations of the $EC_{50}$ values are related to a $Log_{10}$ scale. Consequently, we **must** work in $Log_{10}$ units when calculating the average $EC_{50}$ of the drug used. Throughout the biological sciences, you will come across data that has been determined using a logarithmic progression; without exception further calculation using such data ($pA_2$, $pEC_{50}$, $pK_A$, $pH$) should always be performed using the original $Log_{10}$ values otherwise, as you shall see later, erroneous calculated values will result.

**Table 9.6** Average concentration-effect data for a muscarinic receptor agonist to induce contractile responses of the isolated Guinea-Pig ileum.

| [Drug] M | $Log_{10}$ [Drug] | % Max response Mean | S.E.M. |
|---|---|---|---|
| $1 \times 10^{-10}$ | -10.0 | 0.0 | 0.00 |
| $3 \times 10^{-10}$ | -9.523 | 2.33 | 2.33 |
| $9 \times 10^{-10}$ | -9.046 | 8.33 | 6.01 |
| $2.7 \times 10^{-9}$ | -8.569 | 21.33 | 12.41 |
| $8.1 \times 10^{-9}$ | -8.092 | 39.00 | 18.19 |
| $2.43 \times 10^{-8}$ | -7.614 | 56.67 | 19.60 |
| $7.29 \times 10^{-8}$ | -7.137 | 73.33 | 16.05 |
| $2.19 \times 10^{-7}$ | -6.660 | 86.33 | 10.81 |
| $6.56 \times 10^{-7}$ | -6.183 | 93.33 | 5.24 |
| $1.97 \times 10^{-6}$ | -5.706 | 98.67 | 1.33 |
| $5.90 \times 10^{-6}$ | -5.229 | 100.00 | 0.00 |

Table values indicate the calculated arithmetic mean of the percentage maximal response values for each drug concentration taken from the original response data presented in Table 9.5.

Table 9.7 summarises the individual $Log_{10}$ $EC_{50}$ values and the molar $EC_{50}$ values estimated from Figures 9.4 and 9.5, respectively. Note that the $Log_{10}$ $EC_{50}$ estimates from Figure 9.4 agree exactly with the estimates of the $EC_{50}$ values in molar concentrations from Figure 9.5, e.g. the antilog of -8.47 (i.e. $10^{-8.47}$) is $3.388 \times 10^{-9}$ M. Table 9.7 also summarises the corresponding arithmetic Mean, Standard Deviation, and Standard Error of the Mean (S.E.M.)

values calculated from both the $Log_{10}$ $EC_{50}$ and the molar $EC_{50}$ values. *Note that the arithmetic mean of the $Log_{10}$ $EC_{50}$ values equates to the geometric mean of the molar $EC_{50}$ concentrations (see Chapter 5).*

**Table 9.7** Summary of $EC_{50}$ data calculations.

| | $Log_{10}$ $EC_{50}$ data (Figure 9.4) | Molar $EC_{50}$ data (Figure 9.5) |
|---|---|---|
| Tissue 1 | -8.47 | $3.388 \times 10^{-9}$ M |
| Tissue 2 | -7.89 | $1.288 \times 10^{-8}$ M |
| Tissue 3 | -6.97 | $1.072 \times 10^{-7}$ M |
| Mean | -7.78 | $4.11 \times 10^{-8}$ M |
| Standard deviation | 0.76 | $5.74 \times 10^{-8}$ M |
| S.E.M. | 0.44 | $3.31 \times 10^{-8}$ M |
| **Summary:** | | |
| Mean ± S.E.M | -7.78 ± 0.44 | $4.11 \pm 3.31 \times 10^{-8}$ M |
| **Molarity values** | | |
| Mean | $1.66 \times 10^{-8}$ M | $4.11 \times 10^{-8}$ M |
| Lower S.E.M. | $0.603 \times 10^{-8}$ M | $0.80 \times 10^{-8}$ M |
| Upper S.E.M | $4.571 \times 10^{-8}$ M | $7.42 \times 10^{-8}$ M |

Table values indicate raw $Log_{10}$ $EC_{50}$ and molar $EC_{50}$ values and calculated descriptive statistics from Figures 9.4 and 9.5. Top panel indicates values for each tissue, second panel indicates calculated values, third panel indicates standard summary of calculated values, and the bottom panel indicates the molar values for the mean, lower S.E.M, and upper S.E.M. Values in red text were calculated using the *incorrect* arithmetic method applied to the molar $EC_{50}$ concentrations; see text for further details of the correct calculations using $Log_{10}$ $EC_{50}$ values.

First, consider the calculation of the respective mean values. The mean of the three $Log_{10}$ $EC_{50}$ values from Figure 9.4 equals -7.78, the antilog of which estimates the average molar $EC_{50}$ to be $1.66 \times 10^{-8}$ M. In contrast, however, the arithmetic mean of the molar $EC_{50}$ values from Figure 9.5 equals $4.11 \times 10^{-8}$ M, which is clearly greater than the estimate based on the $Log_{10}$ $EC_{50}$ values (i.e. the geometric mean). Remember, the geometric mean is calculated by taking the $n^{th}$ root of the *product* of the individual observations; this is more easily calculated by taking the sum of the appropriate $Log_{10}$ values of the observations and dividing through by the number of observations (see below). In contrast, the second mean $EC_{50}$ value is calculated using the arithmetic mean of the molar $EC_{50}$ values. These may be summarised as follows;

**Geometric mean** (i.e. arithmetic mean of $Log_{10}$ $EC_{50}$ values)

$$\frac{(-8.47 + -7.89 + -6.97)}{3} = -7.78 \text{ (antilog} = 1.66 \times 10^{-8} \text{ M)}$$

$$\equiv \frac{(Log_{10}(3.388 \times 10^{-9}) + Log_{10}(1.288 \times 10^{-8}) + Log_{10}(1.072 \times 10^{-7}))}{3}$$

$$\equiv \sqrt[3]{(3.388 \times 10^{-9}) \times (1.288 \times 10^{-8}) \times (1.072 \times 10^{-7})} = \mathbf{1.66 \times 10^{-8} \text{ M}}$$

(9.1)

**Arithmetic mean of molar $EC_{50}$ data**

$$\frac{(3.388 \times 10^{-9}) + (1.288 \times 10^{-8}) + (1.072 \times 10^{-7})}{3} = \mathbf{4.11 \times 10^{-8} \text{ M}}$$

(9.2)

Likewise, the respective standard deviation and S.E.M. values are calculated using the $Log_{10}$ $EC_{50}$ or molar $EC_{50}$ values, as appropriate. These descriptive statistics may then be summarised as shown in the third panel of Table 9.7. It should be noted that the S.E.M. of the $Log_{10}$ $EC_{50}$ becomes a *factor* by which the molar concentration equivalent of the mean $Log_{10}$ $EC_{50}$ values is multiplied or divided by to give the lower and upper values of the S.E.M, thus;

**Lower S.E.M. range value**

Log$_{10}$ values :     $-7.78 - 0.44 = -8.22$ $\left(\text{antilog} = 0.603 \times 10^{-8}\text{M}\right)$

Molar values :     $\dfrac{1.66 \times 10^{-8}}{2.754} = 0.603 \times 10^{-8}\text{M}$

$$(9.3)$$

**Upper S.E.M. range value**

Log$_{10}$ values :     $-7.78 + 0.44 = -7.34$ $\left(\text{antilog} = 4.571 \times 10^{-8}\text{M}\right)$

Molar value :     $\left(1.66 \times 10^{-8}\right) \times 2.754 = 4.571 \times 10^{-8}\text{M}$

$$(9.4)$$

These values are summarised in the bottom panel of Table 9.7; notice that I have also included in red type the incorrectly calculated values based on the arithmetic calculations using the molar EC$_{50}$ concentrations for comparison.

- *Incorrectly calculated average EC$_{50}$ value based on original molar values.*

There are two important issues to note about the incorrectly calculated average EC$_{50}$ value and its associated S.E.M. bars (see red solid square and red S.E.M. bar lines in Figure 9.6). First, the average EC$_{50}$ lies some way to the right of the average concentration-effect curve. Second, the S.E.M. bars (and indeed the Standard Deviation bars if so calculated) are asymmetric in their length when plotted on a logarithmic scale; i.e. the lower bar is visually far longer than the upper bar. These two issues reveal immediately that the average EC$_{50}$ and S.E.M. values have been calculated incorrectly.

The summary data of the average concentration-effect curve, together with the average EC$_{50}$ and S.E.M. EC$_{50}$ values, are shown in Figure 9.6, below.

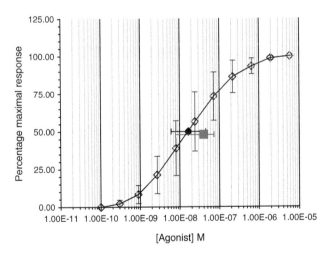

**Figure 9.6**  Average concentration-effect curve of a muscarinic receptor agonist to induce contractile responses in the Guinea-Pig ileum. Values (open diamonds) indicate average responses ($n = 3$) to increasing concentrations of a muscarinic receptor agonist. Vertical bars indicate ± S.E.M. Solid black diamond indicates the geometric mean EC$_{50}$ value calculated from the Log$_{10}$ EC$_{50}$ values (horizontal bars indicate S.E.M.). Solid red square indicates the incorrect arithmetic mean of the molar EC$_{50}$ values (horizontal bars indicate S.E.M.).

- *Correctly calculated average EC$_{50}$ value based on Log$_{10}$ EC$_{50}$ values.*

In contrast, the correctly calculated EC$_{50}$ value (and S.E.M. bars; as shown by the solid diamond and dark lines in Figure 9.6) lies exactly on the average concentration-effect curve and its S.E.M. lines are visually symmetrical. Notice also that the absolute difference between the molar values of the lower S.E.M and the mean is

different from the absolute difference between the molar values of the mean and the upper S.E.M.

Thus,

$$\text{mean} - \text{lower S.E.M.value} \neq \text{higher S.E.M.value} - \text{mean} \quad (9.5)$$

So, for this example;

$$\text{Lower S.E.M value}: 1.660 \times 10^{-8}\text{M} - 0.603 \times 10^{-8}\text{M} = 1.0576 \times 10^{-8}\text{M}$$
$$(9.6)$$

$$\text{Upper S.E.M.value}: 4.571 \times 10^{-8}\text{M} - 1.660 \times 10^{-8}\text{M} = 2.911 \times 10^{-8}\text{M}$$
$$(9.7)$$

Consequently, if we need to quote drug potency in molar values, then it is inappropriate to quote these mean and S.E.M values in the traditional format of;

Mean ± S.E.M.

(which is reserved for arithmetic, but not geometric, data sets).
$$(9.8)$$

Instead, we need to quote the lower and upper range values in parenthesis, thus;

$$\text{Mean (lower value, upper value).} \quad (9.9)$$

Consequently, for this example, these data should be reported as;

$$\text{Mean EC}_{50}(\text{S.E.M.range}) = 1.660 \,(0.603, 4.571) \times 10^{-8}\text{M}$$
$$(9.10)$$

## 3  Non-parametric data

The frequency distribution of the various behaviours exhibited by rats during periods of social interaction invariably fails to follow a normal distribution. Table 9.8 summarises the frequency of two behaviours observed following three different drug treatment schedules.

**Table 9.8**  Effect of drug treatment on the frequency of rodent Head Shake and Attempt Mounting behaviour.

|  | Head shake | | | Attempt mount | | |
|---|---|---|---|---|---|---|
|  | 1 | 2 | 3 | 1 | 2 | 3 |
|  | 10 | 3 | 20 | 11 | 44 | 6 |
|  | 12 | 3 | 18 | 23 | 37 | 9 |
|  | 12 | 3 | 23 | 23 | 33 | 7 |
|  | 12 | 3 | 20 | 13 | 31 | 8 |
|  | 13 | 4 | 24 | 16 | 32 | 5 |
|  | 15 | 3 | 20 | 11 | 28 | 5 |
|  | 16 | 2 | 22 | 19 | 28 | 5 |
|  | 15 | 4 | 27 | 20 | 40 | 9 |
|  | 13 | 4 | 21 | 19 | 40 | 11 |
|  | 10 | 4 | 20 | 21 | 31 | 8 |
|  | 12 | 3 | 20 | 25 | 43 | 9 |
|  | 11 | 2 | 22 | 17 | 42 | 6 |
|  | 15 | 2 | 25 | 19 | 53 | 7 |
|  | 11 | 4 | 21 | 20 | 38 | 11 |
|  | 16 | 4 | 21 | 20 | 39 | 10 |
| **Median** | 12 | 3 | 21 | 19 | 38 | 8 |
| **Minimum** | 10 | 2 | 18 | 11 | 28 | 5 |
| **Maximum** | 16 | 4 | 27 | 25 | 53 | 11 |
| **Range** | 6 | 2 | 9 | 14 | 25 | 6 |

Male Wistar rats were administered with three different drug treatments (Group 1 = control, Group 2 = fluoxetine, Group 3 = WAY100635 with fluoxetine), and the frequency of Head Shake and Attempt Mount behaviour exhibited during a subsequent social interaction session was recorded.

Comparison of the median and range values shows that as the **median** score of each behaviour increases so does the **range** of the values (see Figure 9.7). The frequency distributions of the data sets therefore clearly demonstrate heterogeneity of variance since the spread of the data (as shown by the range values) increases with the magnitude of the values (see also Figure 6.2). Consequently, it is inappropriate to describe such data sets using parametric descriptive statistics; such data should therefore be described using non-parametric descriptive statistics. These sets of data should therefore be best described by the Median and Interquartile range (see Table 9.9).

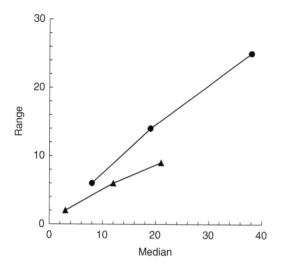

**Figure 9.7  Comparison of the median and range values for Head Shake (closed triangles) and Attempt Mount (closed circles) behaviour exhibited by male Wistar rats during social interaction.** See Table 9.8 for experimental details.

The 25th and 75th percentile values indicate the lower and upper values of the interquartile range, and the summary descriptive statistics should be quoted as the Median followed by the 25th and 75th percentile values (also known as the 1st and 3rd semi-quartile values) in parenthesis, thus;

$$\text{Median (25th, 75th percentile values).} \qquad (9.11)$$

In the example above (see Table 9.9), for animals treated with both WAY-100635 and fluoxetine, the descriptive statistics should therefore be quoted as;

**Table 9.9** Non-parametric descriptive statistics for Head shake and Attempt Mount data exhibited during social interaction.

| Behaviour | Treatment | Median | 25th percentile | 75th percentile |
|---|---|---|---|---|
| Head Shake | Control | 12 | 11.5 | 15 |
| | Fluoxetine | 3 | 3 | 4 |
| | WAY-100635 + fluoxetine | 21 | 20 | 22.5 |
| Attempt Mount | Control | 19 | 16.5 | 20.5 |
| | Fluoxetine | 38 | 31.5 | 41 |
| | WAY-100635 + fluoxetine | 8 | 6 | 9 |

$$\text{Head Shake behaviour;} \qquad 21\,(20, 22.5) \qquad (9.12)$$

$$\text{Attempt Mount behaviour;} \qquad 8\,(6, 9) \qquad (9.13)$$

Such data could be summarised as bar charts (where the error bars indicate the percentile values), but perhaps a better representation may be achieved by using Box–Whisker plots (see Figure 9.8).

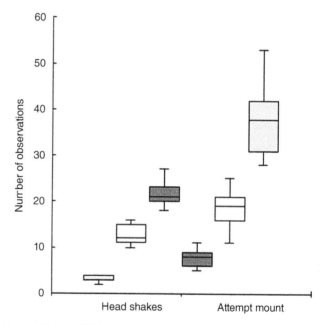

**Figure 9.8  Box–Whisker plot of Head Shake and Attempt Mount data exhibited by male Wistar rats during social interaction.** Open box indicates control subjects, while light grey fill indicates rats treated with fluoxetine, and dark grey fill indicates rats treated with WAY-100635 and fluoxetine.

# Example output from statistical software

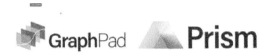

**A**

| | A HS1 | B HS2 | C HS3 |
|---|---|---|---|
| 1 Number of values | 15 | 15 | 15 |
| 2 | | | |
| 3 25% Percentile | 11.00 | 3.000 | 20.00 |
| 4 Median | 12.00 | 3.000 | 21.00 |
| 5 75% Percentile | 15.00 | 4.000 | 23.00 |
| 6 | | | |
| 7 Mean | 12.87 | 3.200 | 21.60 |
| 8 Std. Deviation | 2.066 | 0.7746 | 2.324 |
| 9 Std. Error of Mean | 0.5333 | 0.2000 | 0.6000 |
| 10 | | | |

| | | |
|---|---|---|
| 10 | | |
| 11 **Brown-Forsythe test** | | |
| 12 F (DFn, DFd) | | 3.306 (2, 42) |
| 13 P value | | 0.0464 |
| 14 P value summary | | * |
| 15 Are SDs significantly different (P < 0.05)? | | Yes |
| 16 | | |
| 17 **Bartlett's test** | | |
| 18 Bartlett's statistic (corrected) | | 14.44 |
| 19 P value | | 0.0007 |
| 20 P value summary | | *** |
| 21 Are SDs significantly different (P < 0.05)? | | Yes |

**B**

| | A AM1 | B AM2 | C AM3 |
|---|---|---|---|
| 1 Number of values | 15 | 15 | 15 |
| 2 | | | |
| 3 Minimum | 11.00 | 28.00 | 5.000 |
| 4 25% Percentile | 16.00 | 31.00 | 6.000 |
| 5 Median | 19.00 | 38.00 | 8.000 |
| 6 75% Percentile | 21.00 | 42.00 | 9.000 |
| 7 Maximum | 25.00 | 53.00 | 11.00 |
| 8 Range | 14.00 | 25.00 | 6.000 |
| 9 | | | |
| 10 Mean | 18.47 | 37.27 | 7.733 |
| 11 Std. Deviation | 4.207 | 6.881 | 2.086 |
| 12 Std. Error of Mean | 1.086 | 1.777 | 0.5387 |

| | | |
|---|---|---|
| 10 | | |
| 11 **Brown-Forsythe test** | | |
| 12 F (DFn, DFd) | | 6.003 (2, 42) |
| 13 P value | | 0.0051 |
| 14 P value summary | | ** |
| 15 Are SDs significantly different (P < 0.05)? | | Yes |
| 16 | | |
| 17 **Bartlett's test** | | |
| 18 Bartlett's statistic (corrected) | | 16.58 |
| 19 P value | | 0.0003 |
| 20 P value summary | | *** |
| 21 Are SDs significantly different (P < 0.05)? | | Yes |
| 22 | | |

**C**

| Identify outliers Summary | A HS1 | B HS2 | C HS3 | D AM1 | E AM2 | F AM3 |
|---|---|---|---|---|---|---|
| 1 **Method** | | | | | | |
| 2 Grubbs (Alpha = 0.05) | G = 1.517 | G = 1.549 | G = 2.324 | G = 1.775 | G = 2.286 | G = 1.566 |
| 3 | | | | | | |
| 4 **Number of points** | | | | | | |
| 5 # Y values analyzed | 15 | 15 | 15 | 15 | 15 | 15 |
| 6 Outliers | 0 | 0 | 0 | 0 | 0 | 0 |
| 7 | | | | | | |

Summary descriptive statistics from GraphPad Prism, v8. Panels A and B show the summary descriptive statistics for the Head Shake and Attempt Mount data from Table 9.8, respectively, together with the respective results of the Brown–Forsythe and Bartlett's tests for homogeneity of variance. Panel C summarises the results of Grubb's test for outliers.

*Source*: GraphPad Software.

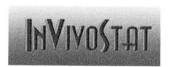

A

## InVivoStat Summary Statistics

### Variable selection

Responses HS1,HS2,HS3 are analysed in this module.

### Summary statistics

#### Summary statistics for HS1

| Response | Mean | N | Variance | Std dev | Median | Lower quartile | Upper quartile |
|---|---|---|---|---|---|---|---|
| HS1 | 12.8667 | 15 | 4.2667 | 2.0656 | 12.0000 | 11.0000 | 15.0000 |

#### Summary statistics for HS2

| Response | Mean | N | Variance | Std dev | Median | Lower quartile | Upper quartile |
|---|---|---|---|---|---|---|---|
| HS2 | 3.2000 | 15 | 0.6000 | 0.7746 | 3.0000 | 3.0000 | 4.0000 |

#### Summary statistics for HS3

| Response | Mean | N | Variance | Std dev | Median | Lower quartile | Upper quartile |
|---|---|---|---|---|---|---|---|
| HS3 | 21.6000 | 15 | 5.4000 | 2.3238 | 21.0000 | 20.0000 | 23.0000 |

B

#### Summary statistics for AM1

| Response | Mean | N | Variance | Std dev | Median | Lower quartile | Upper quartile |
|---|---|---|---|---|---|---|---|
| AM1 | 18.4667 | 15 | 17.6952 | 4.2066 | 19.0000 | 16.0000 | 21.0000 |

#### Summary statistics for AM2

| Response | Mean | N | Variance | Std dev | Median | Lower quartile | Upper quartile |
|---|---|---|---|---|---|---|---|
| AM2 | 37.2667 | 15 | 47.3524 | 6.8813 | 38.0000 | 31.0000 | 42.0000 |

#### Summary statistics for AM3

| Response | Mean | N | Variance | Std dev | Median | Lower quartile | Upper quartile |
|---|---|---|---|---|---|---|---|
| AM3 | 7.7333 | 15 | 4.3524 | 2.0862 | 6.0000 | 6.0000 | 9.0000 |

Summary descriptive statistics from InVivoStat, v4.0.2. Panels A and B show the summary descriptive statistics for the Head Shake and Attempt Mount data from Table 9.8, respectively.

*Source*: InVivoStat.

## Minitab

**A**

| Variable | Mean | St Dev | Variance | Q1 | Median | Q3 | IQR | Mode | N for Mode |
|---|---|---|---|---|---|---|---|---|---|
| HS1 | 12.867 | 2.066 | 4.267 | 11.000 | 12.000 | 15.000 | 4.000 | 12 | 4 |
| HS2 | 3.200 | 0.775 | 0.600 | 3.000 | 3.000 | 4.000 | 1.000 | 3, 4 | 6 |
| HS3 | 21.600 | 2.324 | 5.400 | 20.000 | 21.000 | 23.000 | 3.000 | 20 | 5 |
| AM1 | 18.47 | 4.21 | 17.70 | 16.00 | 19.00 | 21.00 | 5.00 | 19, 20 | 3 |
| AM2 | 37.27 | 6.88 | 47.35 | 31.00 | 38.00 | 42.00 | 11.00 | 28, 31, 40 | 2 |
| AM3 | 7.733 | 2.086 | 4.352 | 6.000 | 8.000 | 9.000 | 3.000 | 5, 9 | 3 |

**B**

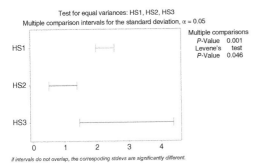

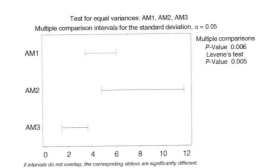

| Method | Test Statistic | P-Value |
|---|---|---|
| Multiple comparisons | — | 0.001 |
| Levene | 3.31 | 0.046 |

| Method | Test Statistic | P-Value |
|---|---|---|
| Multiple comparisons | — | 0.006 |
| Levene | 6.00 | 0.005 |

**C**

| Variable | N | Mean | St Dev | Min | Max | G | P |
|---|---|---|---|---|---|---|---|
| Female | 40 | 1.6511 | 0.0701 | 1.4820 | 1.7940 | 2.41 | 0.499 |
| Male | 33 | 1.8076 | 0.0583 | 1.6700 | 1.9200 | 2.36 | 0.459 |

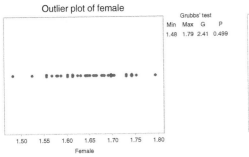

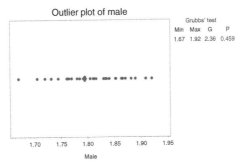

Summary descriptive statistics from MiniTab, v19. Panel A shows the summary descriptive statistics for the Head Shake and Attempt Mount data from Table 9.8, together with the results from Levene's test shown in Panel B. Panel C shows the descriptive statistics for the female and male height data from Tables 5.1 and 5.2, respectively, together with the corresponding results from Grubb's test for outliers.

*Source*: Minitab, LLC.

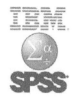

**A**

**Statistics**

| | | HS1 | HS2 | HS3 |
|---|---|---|---|---|
| N | Valid | 15 | 15 | 15 |
| | Missing | 113 | 113 | 113 |
| Mean | | 12.8667 | 3.2000 | 21.6000 |
| Median | | 12.0000 | 3.0000 | 21.0000 |
| Std. Deviation | | 2.06559 | .77460 | 2.32379 |
| Variance | | 4.267 | .600 | 5.400 |
| Percentiles | 25 | 11.0000 | 3.0000 | 20.0000 |
| | 50 | 12.0000 | 3.0000 | 21.0000 |
| | 75 | 15.0000 | 4.0000 | 23.0000 |

**Test of Homogeneity of Variances**

| | | Levene Statistic | df1 | df2 | Sig. |
|---|---|---|---|---|---|
| HeadShake | Based on Mean | 5.808 | 2 | 42 | .006 |
| | Based on Median | 3.306 | 2 | 42 | .046 |
| | Based on Median and with adjusted df | 3.306 | 2 | 30.206 | .050 |
| | Based on trimmed mean | 5.501 | 2 | 42 | .008 |

**Robust Tests of Equality of Means**

HeadShake

| | Statistic[a] | df1 | df2 | Sig. |
|---|---|---|---|---|
| Welch | 503.857 | 2 | 22.507 | .000 |
| Brown-Forsythe | 371.305 | 2 | 30.920 | .000 |

a. Asymptotically F distributed.

**B**

**Statistics**

| | | AM1 | AM2 | AM3 |
|---|---|---|---|---|
| N | Valid | 15 | 15 | 15 |
| | Missing | 113 | 113 | 113 |
| Mean | | 18.4667 | 37.2667 | 7.7333 |
| Median | | 19.0000 | 38.0000 | 8.0000 |
| Std. Deviation | | 4.20657 | 6.88131 | 2.08624 |
| Variance | | 17.695 | 47.352 | 4.352 |
| Percentiles | 25 | 16.0000 | 31.0000 | 6.0000 |
| | 50 | 19.0000 | 38.0000 | 8.0000 |
| | 75 | 21.0000 | 42.0000 | 9.0000 |

**Test of Homogeneity of Variances**

| | | Levene Statistic | df1 | df2 | Sig. |
|---|---|---|---|---|---|
| AttempMount | Based on Mean | 6.763 | 2 | 42 | .003 |
| | Based on Median | 6.003 | 2 | 42 | .005 |
| | Based on Median and with adjusted df | 6.003 | 2 | 27.236 | .007 |
| | Based on trimmed mean | 6.957 | 2 | 42 | .002 |

**Robust Tests of Equality of Means**

AttempMount

| | Statistic[a] | df1 | df2 | Sig. |
|---|---|---|---|---|
| Welch | 145.887 | 2 | 23.374 | .000 |
| Brown-Forsythe | 144.906 | 2 | 26.193 | .000 |

a. Asymptotically F distributed.

Summary descriptive statistics from SPSS, v27. Panel A shows the summary descriptive statistics for the Head Shake data from Table 9.8, together with the results from Levene's test for homogeneity of variance and from the Welch and Brown–Forsythe tests for the equality of the means. Similarly, Panel B shows the summary descriptive statistics for the Attempt Mount data from Table 9.8 together with the results from Levene's test for homogeneity of variance and from the Welch and Brown–Forsythe tests for the equality of the means.

*Source*: IBM Corporation.

# Decision Flowchart 1: Descriptive Statistics – Parametric v Non-Parametric data

| If your data sets meet the following criteria: | |
| --- | --- |
| **Data type:** | Measurement |
| **Form:** | Continuos |
| **Scale:** | Interval<br>Ratio |
| **Spread:** | Homogeneity of variance.<br>Levene's test: $p > 0.05$ |
| **Distribution:** | Approximately normally distributed.<br>Kolmogorov–Smirnov (D): $p > 0.05$<br>Shapiro–Wilk (W): $p > 0.05$ |
| **Skewness:** | Fisher–Pearson skewness coefficient<br>F–P: $< \pm2$. z-score: $<1.96$, $p > 0.05$ |
| **Kurtosis:** | Kurtosis: $< 5$. z-score: $<1.96$, $p > 0.05$ |

| **Descriptive measures**<br>**Parametric data**<br>**(raw or transformed)** | |
| --- | --- |
| **Central tendency** | Mean |
| **Spread** | Sum of squares<br><br>Variance<br><br>Standard deviation<br><br>Standard Error of the Mean |

Data transformation
(to approximate a normal distribution)

| If your data sets meet the following criteria: | |
| --- | --- |
| **Data type:** | Nominal (Categories)<br>Ordinal (Ranks) |
| **Form:** | Discrete |
| **Scale:** | Limited: defined maximum and minimum scores |
| **Spread:** | Heterogeneity of variance.<br>Levene's test: $p < 0.05$ |
| **Distribution:** | Non-normal distribution.<br>Kolmogorov–Smirnov (D): $p > 0.05$<br>Shapiro–Wilk (W): $p < 0.05$ |
| **Skewness:** | Fisher–Pearson skewness coefficient<br>F-P: $> \pm2$. z-score: $>1.96$, $p < 0.05$ |
| **Kurtosis:** | Kurtosis: $> 5$. z-score: $>1.96$, $p < 0.05$ |

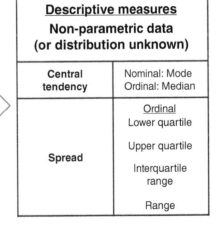

| **Descriptive measures**<br>**Non-parametric data**<br>**(or distribution unknown)** | |
| --- | --- |
| **Central tendency** | Nominal: Mode<br>Ordinal: Median |
| **Spread** | Ordinal<br>Lower quartile<br><br>Upper quartile<br><br>Interquartile range<br><br>Range |

# 10 Introduction to inferential statistics

## Overview

Inferential Statistics is the branch of statistical analysis that applies statistical techniques on a random sample of data drawn from a population to make inferences about that population. As we have already seen in the previous chapters, Descriptive Statistical techniques provide a concise summary of the sampled data that allow us to describe the profile of the data set which is assumed to represent the parent population. In contrast, Inferential Statistics allow conclusions to be reached that extend beyond the immediate data alone. This is especially important when judgements about the relationship between different groups of data are required, and such statistical analysis provides support in answering questions such as,

- What is the probability that the different groups of data are similar,.....or different?
- If there is a difference between the groups of data, then is that difference dependable (is it real?), or is it a difference that happened purely by chance?
- What is the probability of a direct correlative relationship or association between the groups of data?

The techniques employed in Inferential Statistical analysis have been developed to answer these rather specific questions about the data we wish to analyse. So, the correct statistical test to apply to a set data depends on the question being asked (see above) together with the following:

- What type of data we wish to analyse (is it normally distributed or not; see Chapters 5–9)?
- How many groups of data are there?
- Are these groups of data related in some way (i.e. are the data generated by independent groups or are repeated measurements taken from the same subjects)?

These latter questions are a consequence of the experimental design (see below) employed to satisfy the aim(s) of your experiment, but the answers to these, as we shall see, are absolutely critical in defining the correct strategy to analyse experimental data.

## Hypothesis testing

The most common approach to analysing experimental data with statistical models is the **Null Hypothesis significance testing** process which arose from the amalgamation of two different approaches of how to use data to test theories. **Fisher** argued that the calculated probability, $p$, of an event occurring by chance (e.g. a meaningful effect of a drug) should be evaluated within the context of research, such that if $p < 0.01$ (i.e. <1/100), then this would be accepted as strong evidence of the event, while $p > 0.2$ (>1/5) would be considered weak evidence of the event. In contrast, **Neyman and Pearson** argued that scientific statements should be aligned with hypotheses which could be tested experimentally.

In any scientific experiment, you generally have an idea of how the measured data (the experimental output) may change according to how you modify the experimental conditions between the groups of subjects (drug, dose, time lapse between treatment and measurement, etc.). These ideas reflect two opposing hypotheses:

**1** There is no effect of the change in the experimental condition; this is known as the **Null Hypothesis,** denoted by $H_0$.
**2** There is an effect of the change in the experimental condition; this is known as the **Alternate Hypothesis,** denoted by $H_1$.

Whenever we draw conclusions about our experimental theories, we do so in relation to these hypotheses blended with Fisher's use of probability. So,

**1** We always start from the basic assumption or premise that the **Null Hypothesis is true** (i.e. whatever experimental manipulation we have applied to our groups of subjects has had no effect on the experimental output).
**2** We then examine our data with a statistical model (i.e. the statistical test) and calculate the probability that the model fits the data if the Null Hypothesis was true.
**3** If the resulting probability in support of the Null Hypothesis is very small (i.e. $p < 0.05$), then we gain confidence in the Alternate Hypothesis, so much so that we become convinced that the Alternate Hypothesis is closer to the truth than the Null Hypothesis.

It is important to note that as we are dealing with probabilities, we can never be sure which of these hypotheses is correct, and so inferential statistics *never prove* differences between two or more groups of data. As the probability of an event happening by chance decreases, we gain even more confidence that the Alternative Hypothesis is correct and so we can justify rejecting the Null Hypothesis. Finally, we should also note that the $p$ value from any statistical test reflects the calculated probability that the data sets are the same, and **not** that they are different! Students often ask me why 5% (i.e. $p = 0.05$) is chosen as the threshold to decide whether to accept the Null or Alternate Hypothesis. The answer is I have no idea, and indeed, Fisher never claimed that $p = 0.05$ was a special value with mythical properties! I guess this is just a probability value that the general scientific community has chosen to accept as being a suitable threshold to allow acceptable objective conclusions to be drawn from scientific data.

## Experimental design

The fact that so much store is placed on the resulting probability calculated from inferential statistical tests demands that the design of any experiment is critical if the resulting data are to provide information that allows suitable conclusions to be drawn; any badly designed experiment will only produce unusable data or allow erroneous, inaccurate, conclusions to be drawn. There is a huge literature devoted to various aspects of experimental design, and this publication is not the place for an in-depth appraisal or guide to robust experimental design. Throughout the remaining chapters I will, however, demonstrate how experimental design informs our choice of appropriate inferential statistics that we subsequently employ to analyse experimental data.

## One-tailed or two-tailed, that is the question!

Consider the situation where we have an idea that a drug may induce a change in the heart rate. We design an experiment where the aim is to examine the effect of this drug (Drug A) on the resting heart rate of a group of rats. There are four hypotheses related to the possible outcomes of the experiment:

**1** Drug A induces *no change* in heart rate (Null Hypothesis)
**2** Drug A induces a *reduction* in heart rate (Alternate Hypothesis 1). *The correct Null Hypothesis here would be Drug A does not reduce heart rate.*
**3** Drug A induces an *increase* in heart rate (Alternate Hypothesis 2). *The correct Null Hypothesis here would be Drug A does not increase heart rate.*
**4** Drug A induces a *change* in heart rate (Alternate Hypothesis 3).

The first three items in the list are logical because these are the only possible outcomes of the experiment. Some may argue that item four is superfluous since surely this covers both outcomes described in items two and three. From a statistical viewpoint, however, item four (Alternate Hypothesis 3) is very different from item two (Alternate Hypothesis 1) and item three (Alternate Hypothesis 2) because the direction of change in heart rate (i.e. a decrease or an increase in heart rate, respectively) is *not specified*.

Chapter 7 discussed in detail the Standard Normal Distribution. In particular, look closely at Figure 7.5 which is also reproduced here so you do not have to flick back and forth (see Figure 10.1). I previously argued that the relationship between $z$-scores and probability is very important as it allows us to determine areas under the curve (AUC) related to specific proportions of the data set according to the $z$-score. Thus, the top 5% of the data set lies above a $z$-score of +1.64, while the bottom 5% lies below a $z$-score of −1.64 (note that the sign of a $z$-score is critical; see Figure 10.1). Furthermore, 2.5% of the data lies either above or below $z$-scores of +1.96 and −1.96, respectively, while 1% of the data lies either above or below $z$-scores of +2.33 and −2.33, respectively.

These $z$-score values are really very important when we consider the three different Alternate Hypotheses indicated above.

**1** *Drug A induces a reduction in heart rate (Alternate Hypothesis 1)*
Let us assume that the experiment revealed that Drug A **reduced** heart rate to such an extent that the result of a statistical test showed the probability in support of the Null Hypothesis was less than 5% (i.e. $p < 0.05$). This would mean that the probability that the heart rate values before and following treatment with Drug A were the same was less than 5%, thereby allowing us to reject the Null Hypothesis. According to the Standard Normal Distribution curve (Figure 10.1), this would mean that the calculated probability value would lie in the small **left-hand** section of the Standard Normal Distribution where the $z$-score was <−1.64. In contrast, if the calculated probability lays anywhere in the large **right**-hand section of the curve such that the $z$-score was > −1.64, then the probability of the pre- and post-treatment heart rate values being the same would be greater than 5%, and so the Null Hypothesis would be accepted.

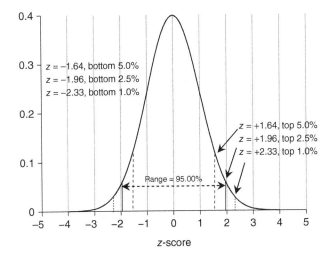

**Figure 10.1** Areas under the curve of the standard normal distribution corresponding to the top and bottom 5% (dashed line), 2.5% (solid line), and 1% (dotted line) of the sample population.

**2** *Drug A induces an increase in heart rate (Alternate Hypothesis 2)*
Let us now assume that the experiment revealed that Drug A **increased** heart rate to such an extent that the result of a statistical test again showed the probability in support of the Null Hypothesis was less than 5% (i.e. $p < 0.05$). This would mean that the probability that the heart rate values before and following treatment with Drug A were the same was less than 5%, thereby allowing us to (again!) reject the Null Hypothesis. According to the Standard Normal Distribution curve (Figure 10.1), this would mean that the calculated probability value would lie in the small **right-hand** section of the Standard Normal Distribution where the $z$-score was >+1.64. In contrast, if the calculated probability lays anywhere in the large **left**-hand section of the curve such that the $z$-score was <+1.64, then the probability of the pre- and post-treatment heart rate values being the same would be greater than 5% and so the Null Hypothesis would be accepted.

It is important to notice that in both cases 1 and 2, we have concentrated on the $z$-scores located at one end (left or right) of the Standard Normal Distribution curve. These sections of the curve are known as the **tails** of the Standard Normal Distribution and come into play when the direction of change in the data according to your hypothesis is **specified**. A statistical model that examines a hypothesis where the direction is specified is called a **one-tailed test**. The problem with experiments where the direction of change is specified is that we are essentially putting all our eggs in one basket and are only looking for a decrease **or** an increase in the values of our data, **but not both!** Consequently, only where the calculated probability equates to $z$-scores that are either less than −1.64 or greater than +1.64 allow us to reject the Null Hypothesis and accept the appropriate Alternate Hypothesis. As an example, let us assume a Null Hypothesis that *Drug A does not decrease heart rate*. Let us further assume that the calculated probability from the appropriate one-tailed test indicates that probability lies in the top 5% of the Standard Normal Distribution curve such that the $z$-score was greater than +1.64. You may argue that such a result suggests that Drug A significantly **elevates** heart rate. However, this result is still in agreement with the Null Hypothesis (which specifically states that *Drug A does not decrease heart rate*) because the direction of change (a reduction) is specified.

One way around this dilemma is to examine both ends of the Standard Normal Distribution curve, but this comes at a price since we need to keep the overall probability of the statistical test at 5%. To do this, we split the 5% between the two ends of the Standard Normal Distribution curve and subsequently have 2.5% in the left tail (where the corresponding $z$-score = $-1.96$) and 2.5% in the right tail (where the corresponding $z$-score = $+1.96$) with 95% of the probability split equally between these two extremes. This approach is very useful when testing a Null Hypothesis where the direction of change in the data is not specified (see hypothesis 1 in the list above) and is discussed in the following section. A statistical model that examines a hypothesis where the direction is not specified is called a **two-tailed test**.

**3** *Drug A induces a change in heart rate (Alternate Hypothesis 3).* Let us assume that the experiment revealed that Drug A **changed** heart rate to such an extent that the result of a statistical test showed that the probability in support of the Null Hypothesis was less than 5% (i.e. $p < 0.05$). This would mean that the probability that the heart rate values before and following treatment with Drug A were the same was less than 5%, thereby allowing us to reject the Null Hypothesis. According to the Standard Normal Distribution curve (Figure 10.1), this would mean that the calculated probability value would lie *either* in the small **left-hand** section of the Standard Normal Distribution where the $z$-score was $<-1.96$ or in the small **right**-hand section of the curve such that the $z$-score was $>+1.96$. In contrast, if the calculated probability of the pre- and post-treatment heart rate values being the same laying **between** $z$-scores of $-1.96$ and $+1.96$, then the probability would be greater than 5% and so the Null Hypothesis would be accepted.

There is one very important point to note from consideration of these three hypotheses. When the direction of change is specified, then the $z$-score required to reach our criterion of 5% (i.e. $-1.64$ or $+1.64$) is smaller than the $z$-score (in absolute terms) required to reach the criterion of 2.5% in either tail when the direction of change is not specified (i.e. $-1.96$ or $+1.96$); this is sometimes referred to as **increasing the burden of proof** where we essentially require a greater difference between our groups thereby making it more difficult to reject the Null Hypothesis. Consequently, if a specific hypothesis is made, then a smaller test statistic is required to reject the Null Hypothesis and achieve a significant result. However, if our hypothesis is in the wrong direction, then we may miss out on identifying a change in the data that does exist. If this happens and you perform a one-tailed test but the change in the data is opposite to what was expected, then it becomes very tempting to ignore the fact that you performed a one-tailed test and interpret the results as if you had performed a two-tailed test. However, at this point, you are essentially examining the data with 5% in each tail of the Standard Normal Distribution curve, such that the overall probability level is now 10% and is very different from your original intention to set the threshold for making a decision about the Null Hypothesis at a probability of 5%. Consequently, if the result of a one-tailed test is in the opposite direction to your Alternate Hypothesis, then *you must accept the Null Hypothesis.*

It could be argued that the use of *one-tailed tests promotes cheating.* If the probability following a two-tailed test = 0.078, then you would accept the Null Hypothesis and conclude that there was no difference between your two groups of data. However, had you performed a one-tailed test on the same data (and the change in the data values was in the right direction!), then the probability value determined would be half that of the two-tailed result (i.e. $p = 0.039$), whereupon you would be persuaded to reject the Null

Hypothesis (since 0.038 is less than the critical value of 0.05) and erroneously accept the Alternate Hypothesis.

This raises one very important fundamental issue regarding robust Experimental Design; the Null Hypothesis Significance Testing process only works if your hypothesis and criterion for concluding whether an effect is significant (or not!) are identified **before** you perform your experiment and collect your data. Consequently, it is totally unacceptable and indicative of poor experimental technique to design an experiment and collect your data and then think to yourself, 'Now, what is the best way to analyse these results?' (see Foreword, Example 1). The bottom line is that the strategy of your statistical analysis (both Descriptive and Inferential) must be decided *before* you perform the experiment and, furthermore, you must **not** change the goalposts (i.e. change the statistical tests you have decided to use) once you have collected your data.

## Type 1 and Type 2 errors

Whenever we apply inferential statistical techniques to our data to test our hypotheses, we are essentially using sample groups of data to inform us about the larger population as a whole (see Chapter 4) and to determine whether our experimental changes (drug, concentration, dose etc.) have an effect on that population. There are only two possibilities here: either there really is an effect on the population (in agreement with our Alternate Hypothesis) or there really is not (in agreement with the Null Hypothesis), and we use the probability determined by inferential statistical tests to inform us which of these two possibilities is more likely. Because we are relying on probability values, then this raises the problem that we cannot be absolutely certain which of these possibilities is true! Consequently, whenever we draw conclusions from the results of statistical tests performed on experimental data, then we are always at risk of making one of two errors and drawing the wrong conclusion; these are known as Type 1 and Type 2 errors.

The **Type 1 error** is where we conclude that there is a real effect on our data when really there is not one! I argued above that if the resulting probability in support of the Null Hypothesis is very small (i.e. $p < 0.05$), then we generally reject the Null Hypothesis and are persuaded to accept the Alternate Hypothesis. This also means that where there is no effect on the population, then there is a probability of 5% of making a Type 1 error. This value is often referred to as the **α value**. This means that if we repeat an experiment where we assume there is no effect on the population a number of times, then in 5% of those experiments (i.e. 1 in 20), we would expect to determine a statistical result large enough to persuade us that there was a real effect even though there was not; those 5% of occasions would be associated with a Type 1 error.

In contrast, a **Type 2 error** is where we conclude that there is not a real effect on our population when really there is one! Such an error may occur where we obtain a small test statistic, perhaps because there is a lot of experimental noise in our data in relationship to the effect size such that the true effect of our experimental change becomes masked. It has been argued that the maximum acceptable probability of a Type 2 error is 20% (i.e. 1 in 5); this is known as the **β value**.

I am often asked, by students and academic staff alike, '*what is the purpose of the statistical tests? Why bother? After all, I can see whether 2 (or more) groups of data are similar (or different), so why waste my time?*' Well, apart from allowing me to show-off my knowledge of (or lack of) statistical theory and application, inferential statistical tests are simply there to stop us making complete idiots of ourselves by misinterpreting our experimental data (or changes in our data) and making erroneous/false conclusions. To put this in statistical terms, the application of inferential statistical tests is to prevent us making a Type 1 or Type 2 error!

## Power analysis calculations and sample size

The ability of an inferential statistical test to determine a significant difference between groups of data when a real difference exists (i.e. when the Null Hypothesis really is in fact false) is known as the **statistical power** of the test. This is therefore the opposite of the probability that the test will be unable to identify a real effect in a population which, as seen in the previous paragraph, is the Type 2 error rate known as the $\beta$-value. Consequently, statistical power may be expressed as $1 - \beta$. So, if the acceptable probability of a Type 2 error is set to 20% (i.e. 0.2, see above), then the corresponding power of the test will be 0.8, which means the test will have an 80% chance of detecting an effect if that effect really exists.

The power of a statistical test $(1 - \beta)$ is determined by three factors:

**1 The $\alpha$-value** (the Type 1 error rate). By convention, the $\alpha$-value is set to 0.05. However, as shall be described later (see multiple pairwise *post hoc* tests following ANOVA in Chapter 15), there are circumstances when the Type 1 error rate for each individual test must be reduced, the consequence of which is to reduce the power of the test being used.
**2 The effect size.** As the name indicates, this is the size of the effect observed in the data that is required in order to identify a real significant difference between the two sets of data. The larger the difference between the data sets, then the easier it is to see.
**3 The sample size.** I argued earlier that larger sample sets provide a closer approximation of the overall population than smaller samples taken from the same population. Consequently, larger sample sizes have less sampling error and therefore less 'noise' within the sample.

Researchers are generally concerned about the power of a statistical test when a study is proposed prior to data collection (e.g. application for a Project Licence to perform experiments on living animals, submission of grant applications to charitable funding sources). In such cases, the researcher may have to justify a proposed sample size in order that the statistical test(s) used to analyse the data has sufficient power to identify a significant change in the data should that effect really exist. By knowing an acceptable power value (i.e. $1 - \beta > 0.8$) and the $\alpha$-value (0.05), then estimates of the sample size may be determined by due consideration of the likely effect size using data from previous experiments. Generally, there are three points to note here:

**1** A reduction in the $\alpha$-value will increase the necessary sample size for a given effect size and statistical power.
**2** An increase in the effect size will reduce the necessary sample size for a given $\alpha$-value and statistical power.
**3** A reduction in statistical power will reduce the necessary sample size for a given effect size and $\alpha$-value.

## Single comparison between 2 groups

The simplest experimental design is composed of just 2 groups of data which differ in one aspect, the effect of which on an experimental measurement (the experimental output) we wish to identify. In most cases, this will be a comparison between a **control** group and a **test** group. In pharmacology, this may be an experiment to examine the effect of a drug administered in an excipient (drug-vehicle) to a group of subjects; this is the test group, compared to another group of subjects treated with the drug-vehicle alone (i.e. without the drug); this is the control group. Note that in this example there are two groups of subjects, and these are said to be **independent** from each other because each of the two groups are composed of entirely different individual subjects. In this example, the treatment schedule is said to be an **independent variable** and represents a single **Between-Group Factor**. Consequently, the experimenter is interested in the absolute scores obtained from the two groups. In contrast, another experimental design may examine the effect of a drug on an experimental output from the *same* subjects. For example, an experimenter may wish to examine the effect of a drug on the heart rate of a group of subjects. Here, the heart rates of the subjects are recorded before and after treatment (control and test recordings, respectively) with the drug. Consequently, the experimenter is not so much interested in the absolute heart rate measurements obtained in each part of the experiment, but in the *differences* between the pre- and post-treatment heart rate measurements obtained from each of the subjects. Note that here there is only one group of subjects from which repeated measurements of heart rate are obtained. These data sets are said to be **paired** because the two sets of data are linked as they are generated by the same individuals. Here, the treatment is said to be a **paired variable** and represents a single **Within-Group Factor**.

So, in general terms, the basic experimental design will have either an independent variable or a paired variable. In addition, the data generated by the experiment will have a normal or non-normal distribution depending on the experimental data. These factors determine the type of statistical test appropriate to compare the two groups of data, known as a pairwise comparison test. The statistical tests that are used to compare such experimental data are summarized in Table 10.1.

Table 10.1 Summary of pairwise comparison tests for 2 groups only.

| Data distribution | Number of groups | Group type | Type of statistical test | Statistical test |
|---|---|---|---|---|
| Normal | 2 | Independent | Parametric | Independent 'Student's' *t*-test *See Chapter 11* |
| Normal | 2 | Paired | Parametric | Paired *t*-test *See Chapter 12* |
| Non-normal | 2 | Independent | Non-parametric | Wilcoxon rank sum test **Or** Mann–Whitney *U*-test *See Chapter 13* |
| Non-normal | 2 | Paired | Non-parametric | Wilcoxon Signed-Rank test *See Chapter 14* |

Consider the experiment where two groups of subjects are independent from each other. The Null Hypothesis (see above) for this experiment is that there is no effect of the experimental manipulation on the resulting sample data. If this statement is most likely to be true (i.e. $p > 0.05$), then one may conclude that the two sets of samples are drawn from the same population, and so their mean values would be expected to be approximately equal. In contrast, if the two sample means are very different, then the Null Hypothesis is unlikely to be true and thus we may conclude that the two sets of samples arise from different populations (in which case the Alternate Hypothesis is most likely to be true; i.e. $p < 0.05$). Furthermore, the larger the difference in the sample means, then the greater our confidence that the two sample means are truly different due to the effect of the experimental manipulation.

So, the basic premise for an experiment composed of just two independent groups, in accordance with the Null Hypothesis, is that the two sets of sample data arise from the *same* population. In essence, this is exactly what the independent Student's *t*-test assesses (see Chapter 11).

## Comparing several groups of data

Most pharmacological experiments, however, contain more than just two groups of data, and thus the number of pairwise comparisons you wish to make increases. For example, you may wish to determine the effect of different diets on weight gain, examine the effect of a range of drugs or doses on an experimental output, or determine the ability of a receptor antagonist to block the response to a receptor agonist drug acting at the same receptor. Each of these experimental scenarios will result in more than two sample sets of data at the end of the experiment which you may wish to compare. However, the basic general Null Hypothesis will still apply. Therefore, no matter how many different sample groups there are in our experiment, the Null Hypothesis will *always* state; there is no effect of the change in experimental condition on any of the sample groups. In other words, the basic premise of an experiment, regardless of how many sample groups are involved, is that all sample groups arise from the *same* population.

We saw earlier that the probability of making a Type 1 error when comparing just two sample sets of data is 5% (i.e. the α-value, $p < 0.05$). Consequently, the probability of not making a Type 1 error is 95% (i.e. $1 - 0.05 = 0.95$). It is clear from the examples of typical pharmacological experiments in the previous paragraph that there may be numerous occasions when we wish to compare more than just two groups, and so we would often need to perform multiple pairwise comparison tests.

In some cases, e.g. comparison of different diets on weight gain, there may not be an obvious control group and so we may wish to

compare all groups against all the others; these are known as **All Means multiple pairwise comparisons**. In other experiments, an obvious control group may be integral to the experimental design and which we wish to compare to a number of test groups, e.g. the effect of a range of drugs or doses on an experimental output; these are known as **Control Means multiple pairwise comparisons**. If we assume in both cases that all the required comparison tests are independent, then the *overall* level of probability of no Type 1 error occurring is $(0.95)^n$, where $n$ is the number of comparisons we wish to make. At this point, our experimental design question over whether we wish to compare all groups against each other or whether our experiment includes a control group is critical.

In an All Means situation, the total number of comparisons is determined by the equation,

$$\frac{N(N-1)}{2} \tag{10.1}$$

where $N$ is the number of groups in our experiment. In a Control Means situation, however, the total number of comparisons is $N - 1$.

Consider the experiment where four groups of mice are fed different diets over a two-week period and their total weight gain during this time was recorded. There is no obvious control group and so if we wish to compare the effect of each diet against all the other diets, then the total number of comparisons required is,

$$\frac{4(3)}{2} = 6 \tag{10.2}$$

Consequently, the probability of no Type 1 errors occurring is $(0.95)^6 = 0.735$. This means that the probability of a Type 1 error occurring across the whole data set has increased from α = 0.05 to $(1 - 0.735) = 0.265$; i.e. from 5 to 26.5%! This inflationary creep in the Type 1 error rate performed on a single group of data sets is known as the **Family Error Rate** (also known as familywise or experimental-wise error rate).

In contrast, consider an experimental situation where a control group is one of four independent sample groups. Here, the total number of comparisons required is $4 - 1 = 3$, and consequently the probability of no Type 1 error occurring is $(0.95)^3 = 0.857$. In this case, therefore, the probability of a Type 1 error occurring is $(1 - 0.857) = 0.143$ (or 14.3%). Inflationary creep in the Type 1 error rate has still occurred due to the multiple comparisons, but the effect of the Control Means comparison strategy is not nearly as detrimental on the *p* value as that seen with All Means multiple comparisons. Table 10.2 summarises the effect of these different

Table 10.2 Summary of effect of multiple comparisons on the probability of Type 1 errors.

| | | All Means multiple pairwise comparisons | | | Control Means multiple pairwise comparisons | | |
|---|---|---|---|---|---|---|---|
| | | | Probability | | | Probability | |
| No of groups | No of comparisons | No Type 1 error | Type 1 error | No of comparisons | No Type 1 error | Type 1 error |
| 2 | 1 | 0.95 | 0.05 | 1 | 0.95 | 0.05 |
| 3 | 3 | 0.857 | 0.143 | 2 | 0.903 | 0.097 |
| 4 | 6 | 0.735 | 0.265 | 3 | 0.857 | 0.143 |
| 5 | 10 | 0.599 | 0.401 | 4 | 0.815 | 0.185 |
| 6 | 15 | 0.463 | 0.537 | 5 | 0.774 | 0.226 |
| 7 | 21 | 0.341 | 0.659 | 6 | 0.735 | 0.265 |
| 8 | 28 | 0.238 | 0.762 | 7 | 0.698 | 0.302 |
| 9 | 36 | 0.158 | 0.842 | 8 | 0.663 | 0.337 |
| 10 | 45 | 0.099 | 0.901 | 9 | 0.630 | 0.370 |

multiple comparison strategies on the probability of Type 1 errors occurring and clearly illustrates the need for the careful robust design of our experiments in terms of both the number of groups used and the subsequent strategy of statistical analysis to analyse the resulting data sets.

There are ways of controlling the build-up of errors due to the experimental need for multiple comparisons of our data sets. The general approach is to adjust the level of significance for each individual test to ensure that the overall Type 1 error rate across all the comparisons required remains at $p < 0.05$. The most accurate way to calculate the new threshold for accepting/rejecting the Null Hypothesis for each comparison is to first adjust the probability of no Type 1 error occurring by calculating the $n$th root of 0.95, where $n$ is the total number of comparisons required. The adjusted threshold for a Type 1 error occurring for each comparison is then $(1 - \sqrt[n]{0.95})$. In practical terms, this is somewhat cumbersome and so the most common method to control the Family Error Rate is to apply the **Bonferroni correction**, where the α-value is divided by the number of comparisons required.

So, if our experiment requires six comparisons, then the $p$ value is adjusted to $0.05/6 = 0.00833$ which now becomes our new threshold for accepting/rejecting the Null Hypothesis. In comparison, the accurate adjustment to the $p$ value $(1 - \sqrt[6]{0.95}) = 0.00851$. Table 10.3 compares the calculated accurate thresholds to those estimated by the Bonferroni correction. It is worth noting that the Bonferroni procedure always results in an adjusted $p$ value that is slightly less than that resulting from the more-formal calculation; this is rather beneficial as it adds extra protection against making erroneous conclusions based on a Type 1 error. While such an adjustment to the $p$ value is acceptable where only a small number of multiple comparisons are required, the effect is severe where a large number of comparisons are required. One further important point to note is that by controlling the Family Error Rate, there is a loss of statistical power (see discussion above) which may even result in an increase in the Type 2 error rate where real differences between groups are missed entirely.

Table 10.3 Comparison of adjustment to Type 1 error rate.

| Number of comparisons | No Type 1 error | Type 1 error | Bonferroni correction |
|---|---|---|---|
| 1 | $\sqrt[1]{0.95} = 0.95$ | 0.05 | |
| 2 | $\sqrt[2]{0.95} = 0.97468$ | 0.02532 | 0.02500 |
| 3 | $\sqrt[3]{0.95} = 0.98305$ | 0.01695 | 0.01667 |
| 4 | $\sqrt[4]{0.95} = 0.98726$ | 0.01274 | 0.01250 |
| 5 | $\sqrt[5]{0.95} = 0.98979$ | 0.01021 | 0.01000 |
| 6 | $\sqrt[6]{0.95} = 0.99149$ | 0.00851 | 0.00833 |
| 7 | $\sqrt[7]{0.95} = 0.99270$ | 0.00730 | 0.00714 |
| 8 | $\sqrt[8]{0.95} = 0.99361$ | 0.00639 | 0.00625 |
| 9 | $\sqrt[9]{0.95} = 0.99432$ | 0.00568 | 0.00556 |
| 10 | $\sqrt[10]{0.95} = 0.99488$ | 0.00512 | 0.00500 |
| 15 | $\sqrt[15]{0.95} = 0.99659$ | 0.00341 | 0.00333 |
| 20 | $\sqrt[20]{0.95} = 0.99744$ | 0.00256 | 0.00250 |
| 30 | $\sqrt[30]{0.95} = 0.99829$ | 0.00171 | 0.00167 |
| 40 | $\sqrt[40]{0.95} = 0.99872$ | 0.00128 | 0.00125 |

I argued above that regardless of how many groups of data arise from our experiment, the basic general Null Hypothesis will *always* state that there is no effect of the change in experimental condition on any of the sample groups such that all sample groups arise from the *same* population. When we have only two groups of data in our experiment which we wish to compare, then for normally distributed data sets, an independent or paired *t*-test will suffice. However, this is not the case where we have more than two groups to compare. In such situations, we need to employ a method of inferential statistical analysis that examines the whole data set to determine the probability that all the sample data sets come from the same population (i.e. consistent with the Null Hypothesis) or whether one or more of the sample data sets are more likely to come from a different population(s) (i.e. in accordance with the Alternate Hypothesis). The **Analysis of Variance (ANOVA)** provides a statistical test that examines whether the different sample means (which are argued to represent the population means) of several groups are equal, and as such, for normally distributed independent data sets at least, generalizes the premise of the independent *t*-test to more than two groups, but results in fewer Type 1 errors. However, the ANOVA is not a single test, but a series of statistical models are dependent on the number of **Between- and Within-Group Factors**.

*Between-Group Factors* reflect the number of variables (different factors) in the experiment that differentiate one group from another and include, for example,

- Acute treatment: reflects a single treatment, e.g. receptor agonists.
- Chronic treatment: reflects a treatment given repeatedly over days/weeks/months etc.
- Single pre-treatment: where a pre-treatment is administered before a subsequent acute treatment, e.g. Antagonist/agonist interaction.
- Differences in cell media.
- Gender.
- Diet.
- Single circadian time point

In all cases, there is only a single measured output obtained at the end of the experiment. If there is only a single Between-Group Factor (a variable factor) that differentiates the groups, then the simplest form of parametric ANOVA, a one-way ANOVA, is required and will be discussed in detail in Chapter 15, with the non-parametric equivalent ANOVA models discussed in Chapter 18. However, if there is more than one factor involved, then a more complex ANOVA model is required. For example,

- the effect of pre-treatment with a receptor antagonist on the response to a receptor agonist and
- the effect of chronic treatment on the response to a receptor agonist

are both experimental designs with two Between-Group Factors and consequently require a two-way ANOVA to analyse the data sets. Adding an additional Between-Group Factor into the experimental design (e.g. Gender) will consequently require initial analysis by a three-way ANOVA; more complex ANOVA models are discussed in Chapter 17.

*The* **Within-Group Factor** reflects the situation where repeated measurements are taken from the same group, regardless of whether the experimental design includes one or more Between-Group Factors or not. This invariably involves a *Time* variable in the experiment. Such an experiment may simply involve a single group examined repeatedly on more than two occasions – these data should be analysed by a Repeated Measure ANOVA (sometimes referred to as a one-way Repeated Measures ANOVA) and will be discussed in Chapter 16. For example, the ability of the same sequence of concentrations of acetylcholine to induce contractions of a number of sections of isolated guinea-pig ileum would be suitably analysed by a Repeated Measure ANOVA. If an experiment involves a number of different treatment groups (1 Between-Group Factor) examined over a series of time points, then such data should be analysed by a one-way ANOVA with Repeated Measures to take account of the Between-Group Factors. More complicated ANOVA models will be required with the addition of further Between- and Within-Group Factors.

The more complicated ANOVA models alluded to here, and how to choose the correct ANOVA model, will be discussed in Chapter 17.

In the same way that a *t*-test reveals whether two groups arise from the same population (or not), so the ANOVA tests reveal whether all the sample sets of data come from the same population (or not). The result of an ANOVA test that allows the Null Hypothesis to be rejected in favour of accepting the Alternate Hypothesis, however, **does not** identify which groups from the sample data sets are different. Consequently, the inferential statistical analysis of more than two groups of data is a two-stage process, where analysis by the appropriate ANOVA model is followed by subsequent *post hoc* analysis, but only if justified by the former.

## Association between 2 groups of data

In some cases, we are not interested in whether there are differences between 2 or more groups of data but whether there is a relationship or association between two random variables. For example, we may be interested in the plasma concentration of two enzymes; if the concentration of one enzyme changes, is this reflected by a similar or opposite change in the concentration of the second enzyme? To understand the strength of the relationship between two variables, we need to analyse the data by **correlation analysis** which will be discussed in detail in Chapter 19.

In some cases, we may wish to examine the influence of an independent variable on the value of a dependent variable. The **dependent variable** represents the output of our experiment the value of which is dependent on the value of the **independent variable** which is manipulated (controlled) by the experimenter. To understand the strength of the relationship between the independent and dependent variables, we need to analyse the data by **regression analysis** which will be discussed in detail in Chapter 20.

## Relationship between categorical variables

Back in Chapter 4, I discussed different types of data and introduced the idea of Nominal data where scales are used to label variables (categorise) without any quantitative value (e.g. gender, hair colour). The association or relationship between 2 categorical variables is analysed by the **chi-square test** and will be discussed in detail in Chapter 21.

Additional chapters will discuss the use of **Confidence Intervals** (see Chapter 22), the **Permutation Test of Exact Inference** (discussed in Chapter 23), and the **General Linear Model** (Chapter 24) to compare 2 or more groups of data.

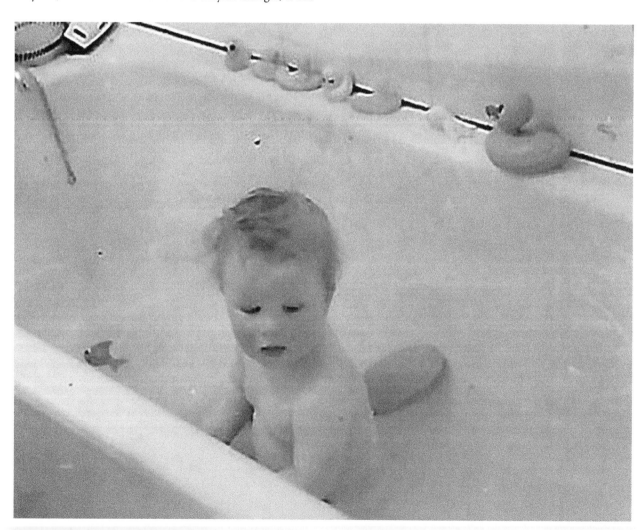

Mummy! Think I misunderstood what you meant by 'p'!
My first stats lesson, circa early 1958.

**Write Your Own Notes**

# 11 Comparing two sets of data – Independent *t*-test

## The Independent *t*-test

The **Independent *t*-test** is a parametric test based on the normal distribution that is used to examine the effect of a single experimental manipulation (e.g. drug treatment) on two *separate* groups of subjects.

Under the Null Hypothesis, we assume that the experimental manipulation has no effect on the experimental output measurement such that the sample means, and their respective variances, of the two sets of data are very similar and, therefore, come from the same population.

It therefore follows that for an independent *t*-test, the following assumptions should be met:

- The data should be a continuous measurement in form and type, respectively, and theoretically without limit (see Chapter 9).
- The data sets and their respective mean values should be normally distributed (see Chapter 6);
- The data sets should have similar variances (see Chapter 6).
- The data should be sampled independently (i.e. different subjects in each group).

In simple terms, the *t*-test results in a *t* statistic which reflects the signal-to-noise ratio of the data produced by the experiment. As you will see later, and as I stated towards the end of the last chapter, a very similar approach is used by ANOVA models when analysing more than two groups of data. The signal-to-noise ratio is really the effect observed between the two groups (here provided by the difference between the two sample mean values) divided by the error in the data that we cannot explain by differences in the sample mean values alone (here provided by an estimate of the standard error of the differences between the two sample means). Thus,

$$t = \frac{\overline{x}_1 - \overline{x}_2}{\text{estimate of the standard error of the difference between two sample means}} \quad (11.1)$$

The standard error of the difference in the sample means may be calculated by adding the variances of the two sample means (to calculate the variance of a set of data see Chapter 5) and taking the square root. At this point it is necessary to consider when there are equal number of observations in each group compared with when the group sizes are unequal.

## Equal group sizes

Here we take the standard error of the sampling distribution for each group of data and square that value to produce the variance of the sampling distribution (since we already know that the variance is simply the standard deviation squared). Thus, for the first group of data,

$$\text{standard error of the sampling distibution} = \frac{s_1}{\sqrt{n_1}} \quad (11.2)$$

$$\text{variance of the sampling distribution} = \left[\frac{s_1}{\sqrt{n_1}}\right]^2 = \frac{s_1^2}{n_1} \quad (11.3)$$

where $s_1$ and $n_1$ are the standard deviation and group size for group 1, respectively.

Interestingly, the variance of a difference between two independent sample groups of data is equal to the sum of their respective variances; this is known as the **variance sum law**. So here we simply add the variances of the respective sampling distributions for the two groups of data together. Thus,

$$\text{variance of the sampling distribution of the differeces} = \frac{s_1^2}{n_1} + \frac{s_2^2}{n_2} \quad (11.4)$$

Notice that here the relative equal weighting of these two components to the variance of the sampling distribution of the differences is the same since the group sizes ($n_1$ and $n_2$) are the same. We now simply take the square root of this variance value to determine the standard error (SE) of the sampling distribution of the differences in sample means. Thus,

$$\text{SE of the sampling distribution of the differences} = \sqrt{\frac{s_1^2}{n_1} + \frac{s_2^2}{n_2}} \quad (11.5)$$

Consequently, the calculation of the *t* statistic becomes,

$$t = \frac{\overline{x}_1 - \overline{x}_2}{\sqrt{\dfrac{s_1^2}{n_1} + \dfrac{s_2^2}{n_2}}} \quad (11.6)$$

## Unequal group sizes

In contrast, where we want to compare two groups where the respective group sizes are different, then the equation above is not appropriate since this would produce different weighting to the variance of each data sample. Instead we pool the variance of the two sample groups to circumvent this problem. The **pooled variance estimate** is given by,

$$s_p^2 = \frac{(n_1 - 1)s_1^2 + (n_2 - 1)s_2^2}{n_1 + n_2 - 2} \quad (11.7)$$

where each variance is weighted by the respective degrees of freedom of each group (given by $n_1 - 1$ and $n_2 - 1$, respectively; see chapter 5). The weighted average (pooled) variance is then substituted into the equation for *t* above.

*Experimental Design and Statistical Analysis for Pharmacology and the Biomedical Sciences*, First Edition. Paul J. Mitchell.
© 2022 John Wiley & Sons Ltd. Published 2022 by John Wiley & Sons Ltd.

Thus,

$$t = \frac{\overline{x}_1 - \overline{x}_2}{\sqrt{\dfrac{s_p^2}{n_1} + \dfrac{s_p^2}{n_2}}} \qquad (11.8)$$

## Interpretation of the *t* statistic

Regardless of whether we have equal or unequal group sizes in our experiment, we then compare the calculated value of *t* against the critical values of *t* provided in tables of the *t*-distribution (see Appendix C). These tables list the maximum value of *t* if the Null Hypothesis was true with the same degrees of freedom (for an explanation of the degrees of freedom, see Chapter 5). For the independent *t*-test, the degrees of freedom are calculated as follows,

$$df = (n_1 - 1) + (n_2 - 1) = (n_1 + n_2) - 2 \qquad (11.9)$$

The value of *t* determined from our data allows us to determine the probability that the Null Hypothesis is true, and if that calculated *t* value **exceeds** the critical *t* value listed in the table for a probability of 0.05, then we can be confident that there is little support in favour of the Null Hypothesis; consequently, we may conclude that our experimental intervention had an effect (i.e. $p < 0.05$). The table of critical values for *t* also allows us to determine the critical value

of *t* at other probability values that the Null Hypothesis is true, e.g. 0.01 (1/100) and 0.001 (1/1000). The critical values of the *t*-distribution for both one- and two-tailed tests (see Chapter 10) are summarised in Appendix C. Of course, if the calculated value of *t* from our data exceeds the appropriate critical *t* value indicating the probability that the Null Hypothesis is true is $p < 0.001$, then this indicates a greater relative difference in the respective mean values of our sample groups of data than if $p < 0.05$ (and so we have even greater confidence in rejecting the Null Hypothesis in favour of the Alternate Hypothesis). However, because the respective variance values of the two groups of data have a large effect on the calculated value of *t*, then such a result may simply reflect less variance of the individual values within each data set (i.e. the data distribution is tighter around each respective mean value) rather than a greater absolute difference between the respective mean values.

Whenever the result of an independent *t*-test is reported the *t* value, degrees of freedom and *p* value should always be quoted as follows (this allows your reader to double-check your result in published tables of the *t*-distribution):

$$t(df) = t \text{ value}, p = p \text{ value} \qquad (11.10)$$

Of course, as we shall see below, modern statistical software packages provide the resulting *p* value for you so that you do not have to resort to looking up such values in tables of the *t*-distribution!

## Example 11.1 Equal group sizes

Consider the experiment where we wish to examine the effect of Drug A at a single dose on the exploratory locomotor activity of a group of rats in a novel environment. Such an experiment requires a suitable control group of rats since all subjects in the experiment need to be naïve to the experimental conditions. Also, the Null Hypothesis for the experiment would be that treatment with Drug A has no effect on the locomotor activity of rats. The table below (Table 11.1) summarises the locomotor activity counts for each subject in the experiment according to treatment group.

Table 11.1 Rodent locomotor activity data.

| | Treatment group | |
|---|---|---|
| | **Control** | **Drug A** |
| 1 | 583 | 347 |
| 2 | 654 | 475 |
| 3 | 555 | 333 |
| 4 | 590 | 354 |
| 5 | 727 | 462 |
| 6 | 479 | 250 |
| 7 | 614 | 370 |
| 8 | 622 | 357 |

Before we identify which inferential statistical test to analyse the two data sets, we need to obtain further information about the distribution of each set of data. Table 11.2 (below) summarises such information for the two sets of data.

Table 11.2 Summary descriptive statistics for control and Drug A data.

| | Treatment group | |
|---|---|---|
| | **Control** | **Drug A** |
| **Median** | 602.0 | 355.5 |
| **Mean** | 603.0 | 368.5 |
| **Variance** | 5244.00 | 5170.57 |
| **Standard Deviation** | 72.42 | 71.91 |
| **Standard Error of the Mean** | 25.60 | 25.42 |
| **F–P Skew** | 0.010 | 0.155 |
| Std Error | 0.752 | 0.752 |
| *z*-score | 0.0133 | 0.206 |
| *p* value | $p > 0.05$ | $p > 0.05$ |
| **Kurtosis** | 1.150 | 0.283 |
| Std Error | 1.481 | 1.481 |
| *z*-score | 0.7765 | 0.191 |
| *p* value | $p > 0.05$ | $p > 0.05$ |
| **K–S test; D** | 0.147 | 0.242 |
| Df | 8 | 8 |
| *p* value | $p = 0.200$ | $p = 0.188$ |
| **S–W test; W** | 0.979 | 0.907 |
| Df | 8 | 8 |
| *p* value | $p = 0.957$ | $p = 0.330$ |

Summary values were calculated using SPSS v26 software. *z*-scores for both Fisher–Pearson skewness and kurtosis were calculated by dividing the coefficient values by respective standard error values. Threshold values for *z* (irrespective of sign); if $z > 1.96$, then $p < 0.05$, if $z > 2.58$, then $p < 0.01$, if $z > 3.29$, then $p < 0.001$ (for further explanation of *z* scores see Chapter 7). K–S and S–W indicate Kolmogorov–Smirnov (D) and Shapiro–Wilk (W) test statistics, respectively, for normality.

The results of the Kolmogorov–Smirnov and Shapiro-Wilk tests strongly indicate that the data sets are normally distributed ($p > 0.05$ in all cases), while the Fisher–Pearson coefficient indicates no significant skew in the distribution of either data set ($p > 0.05$ in both cases); for a description of these tests, see Chapter 6. The descriptive statistics above therefore show the two data sets to be closely normally distributed and as a different group of rats were used for each treatment, they are independent. Such data may therefore be compared using the Independent $t$-test for equal group sizes, where the Null Hypothesis is that there is no difference in the mean of the two data sets. Now we simply substitute the correct values for each mean, variance, and number of animals in each group into the equation above in order to calculate the value of $t$.

Thus,

$$t = \frac{603.0 - 368.5}{\sqrt{\dfrac{5244.00}{8} + \dfrac{5170.57}{8}}}$$

$$t = \frac{234.5}{\sqrt{655.5 + 646.32}} = \frac{234.5}{\sqrt{1301.82}} \qquad (11.11)$$

$$t = \frac{234.5}{36.08} = 6.499$$

The estimate of $t$ is therefore 6.499 with 14 degrees of freedom. This is a two-tailed test since we only asked whether the two sets of locomotor activity data differed without specifying the direction of change. If we now refer to the table of critical values of $t$ (see Appendix C) with 14 degrees of freedom, then $p < 0.05$ when $t_{crit} > 2.145$, $p < 0.01$ when $t_{crit} > 2.977$, and $p < 0.001$ when $t_{crit} > 4.140$. The calculated estimate of $t$, 6.499, therefore clearly exceeds the $t_{crit}$ with 14 degrees of freedom when $p = 0.001$. Consequently, the probability that the mean values for the two sets of height data are the same is markedly less than 1/1000, i.e. $p < 0.001$. We may therefore reject the Null Hypothesis and conclude that there is a significant difference between the sample mean values for the two groups of locomotor activity data. This result may be summarised as follows:

$$t(14) = 6.499, p < 0.001 \qquad (11.12)$$

To decide whether the difference in locomotion is due to Drug A increasing or decreasing locomotion, we need to inspect the descriptive statistics for the two sets of data (see Table 11.2). Since the mean locomotor activity for subjects treated with Drug A is less than the locomotor activity shown by control subjects, we may therefore conclude that Drug A significantly reduces locomotor activity.

## Example 11.2 Unequal group sizes

Earlier in Chapter 5, I introduced two sets of height data for female and male students (see Tables 5.1 and 5.2 respectively) from which I calculated the respective sample group means, standard deviations, and standard error of the means (S.E.M.). I further posed the question (see Figure 5.2) whether the female heights differed from the male heights. Before we identify which inferential statistical test to analyse the data sets, we need to obtain further information about the distribution of each set of data. Table 11.3 summarises such information for the sets of both female and male data.

The descriptive statistics above show the two data sets to be normally distributed and clearly, due to differences in gender, they are independent. Such data may therefore be compared using the Independent $t$-test, where the Null Hypothesis is that there is no difference in the mean of the two data sets. However, because there are a different number of subjects in each set, we need to use the pooled variance estimate, as described above. Thus,

$$s_p^2 = \frac{(39 \times 0.004897) + (32 \times 0.003406)}{(40 + 33) - 2}$$

$$s_p^2 = \frac{0.190983 + 0.108992}{71} \qquad (11.13)$$

$$s_p^2 = \frac{0.299975}{71} = 0.004225$$

**Table 11.3** Summary descriptive statistics for female and height data.

| | Height data | |
|---|---|---|
| | **Female** | **Male** |
| | (Table 5.1) | (Table 5.2) |
| **Median** | 1.650 | 1.805 |
| **Mean** | 1.651 | 1.808 |
| **Variance** | 0.004897 | 0.003406 |
| **Standard Deviation** | 0.06999 | 0.05836 |
| **Standard Error of the Mean** | 0.0111 | 0.0102 |
| **F–P Skew** | −0.176 | −0.194 |
| Std Error | 0.374 | 0.409 |
| $z$-score | −0.471 | −0.474 |
| $p$ value | $p > 0.05$ | $p > 0.05$ |
| **Kurtosis** | −0.359 | −0.112 |
| Std Error | 0.733 | 0.798 |
| $z$-score | −0.490 | −0.140 |
| $p$ value | $p > 0.05$ | $p > 0.05$ |
| **K–S test; D** | 0.073 | 0.064 |
| Df | 40 | 33 |
| $p$ value | $p = 0.200$ | $p = 0.200$ |
| **S–W test; W** | 0.986 | 0.991 |
| Df | 40 | 33 |
| $p$ value | $p = 0.906$ | $p = 0.992$ |

Summary values were calculated using SPSS v26 software. $z$-scores for both Fisher-Pearson skewness and kurtosis were calculated by dividing the coefficient values by respective standard error values. Threshold values for $z$ (irrespective of sign); if $z > 1.96$, then $p < 0.05$, if $z > 2.58$, then $p < 0.01$, if $z > 3.29$, then $p < 0.001$ (for further explanation of $z$ scores see Chapter 7). K–S and S–W indicate Kolmogorov–Smirnov (D) and Shapiro–Wilk (W) test statistics, respectively for normality.

Therefore, the estimate of $t$ equals,

$$t = \frac{1.651 - 1.808}{\sqrt{\dfrac{0.004225}{40} + \dfrac{0.004225}{33}}}$$

$$t = \frac{-0.157}{\sqrt{0.0001015625 + 0.0001280303}} \qquad (11.14)$$

$$t = \frac{-0.157}{\sqrt{0.00022959}} = \frac{-0.157}{0.01515} = -10.363$$

The estimate of $t$ is therefore $-10.363$ with 71 degrees of freedom. This is a two-tailed test since we only asked whether the two sets of height data differed without specifying the direction of change. If we now refer to the table of critical values of $t$ (see Appendix C) with 71 degrees of freedom, then $p < 0.05$ when $t_{crit}$ lies between 2.009 (for 50 degrees of freedom) and 1.984 (for 100 degrees of freedom), $p < 0.01$ when $t_{crit}$ lies between

2.678 (for df = 50) and 2.626 (for df = 100), and $p < 0.001$ when $t_{crit}$ lies between 3.496 (for df = 50) and 3.390 (for df = 100).

The calculated estimate of $t$, 10.363 (we can drop the sign because, as this is a two-tailed test, we are only interested in the absolute magnitude of $t$), therefore clearly exceeds the $t_{crit}$ with 71 degrees of freedom for $p < 0.001$ (the appropriate $t_{crit}$ value actually lies between 3.390 and 3.496). Consequently, the probability that the mean values for the two sets of height data are the same is markedly less than 1/1000. This result may be summarised as follows:

$$t(71) = -10.363, p < 0.001 \qquad (11.15)$$

We may therefore reject the Null Hypothesis and conclude that the sample mean values for the female and male height data are markedly different, i.e. the male students are generally significantly taller than the female students (see summary of descriptive statistics in Table 11.3).

# Example output from statistical software

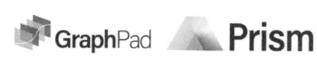

## A

| Unpaired t test Descriptive statistics | Loco C | Loco DgA |
|---|---|---|
| 1 Number of values | 8 | 8 |
| 2 | | |
| 3 Minimum | 479.0 | 250.0 |
| 4 25% Percentile | 562.0 | 336.5 |
| 5 Median | 602.0 | 355.5 |
| 6 75% Percentile | 646.0 | 439.0 |
| 7 Maximum | 727.0 | 475.0 |
| 8 | | |
| 9 Mean | 603.0 | 368.5 |
| 10 Std. Deviation | 72.42 | 71.91 |
| 11 Std. Error of Mean | 25.60 | 25.42 |
| 12 | | |
| 13 Lower 95% CI | 542.5 | 308.4 |
| 14 Upper 95% CI | 663.5 | 428.6 |

| Unpaired t test Tabular results | |
|---|---|
| 1 Table Analyzed | Complete data set for stats analysis |
| 2 | |
| 3 Column W | Loco DgA |
| 4 vs. | vs. |
| 5 Column V | Loco C |
| 6 | |
| 7 Unpaired t test | |
| 8 P value | <0.0001 |
| 9 P value summary | **** |
| 10 Significantly different (P < 0.05)? | Yes |
| 11 One- or two-tailed P value? | Two-tailed |
| 12 t, df | t=6.499, df=14 |

## B

| Unpaired t test Descriptive statistics | Female | Male |
|---|---|---|
| 1 Number of values | 40 | 33 |
| 2 | | |
| 3 Minimum | 1.482 | 1.670 |
| 4 25% Percentile | 1.602 | 1.768 |
| 5 Median | 1.650 | 1.805 |
| 6 75% Percentile | 1.701 | 1.853 |
| 7 Maximum | 1.794 | 1.920 |
| 8 | | |
| 9 Mean | 1.651 | 1.808 |
| 10 Std. Deviation | 0.07006 | 0.05827 |
| 11 Std. Error of Mean | 0.01108 | 0.01014 |
| 12 | | |
| 13 Lower 95% CI | 1.629 | 1.787 |
| 14 Upper 95% CI | 1.674 | 1.828 |
| 15 | | |

| Unpaired t test Tabular results | |
|---|---|
| 1 Table Analyzed | Complete data set for stats analysis |
| 2 | |
| 3 Column B | Male |
| 4 vs. | vs. |
| 5 Column A | Female |
| 6 | |
| 7 Unpaired t test | |
| 8 P value | <0.0001 |
| 9 P value summary | **** |
| 10 Significantly different (P < 0.05)? | Yes |
| 11 One- or two-tailed P value? | Two-tailed |
| 12 t, df | t=10.24, df=71 |

Summary statistical analysis from GraphPad Prism, v8. Panels A and B show the summary descriptive statistics together with the independent $t$-test analysis of the locomotor activity data (Table 11.1, equal group numbers) and female and male height data (Tables 5.1 and 5.2, unequal group numbers), respectively.

*Source*: GraphPad Software.

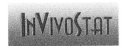

**A**

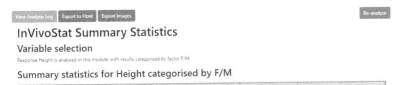

**InVivoStat Summary Statistics**

Variable selection

Response Loco C is analysed in this module, with results categorised by factor Treatment.

Summary statistics for Loco C categorised by Treatment

| Categorisation Factor levels | Mean | N | Std dev | Std error | Lower 95% CI | Upper 95% CI | Median | Lower quartile | Upper quartile |
|---|---|---|---|---|---|---|---|---|---|
| 1 | 603.0000 | 8 | 72.4155 | 25.6027 | 542.4592 | 663.5408 | 602.0000 | 569.0000 | 638.0000 |
| 2 | 368.5000 | 8 | 71.9067 | 25.4229 | 308.3845 | 428.6155 | 355.5000 | 340.0000 | 416.0000 |

Statistical analysis results assuming equal variances
Unpaired t-test result

| | t-statistic | Degrees of freedom | p-value |
|---|---|---|---|
| Equal variance unpaired t-test | 6.499 | 14 | < 0.0001 |

Conclusion: There is a statistically significant difference between the levels of Loco C at the 5% level.

**B**

**InVivoStat Summary Statistics**

Variable selection

Response Height is analysed in this module, with results categorised by factor F/M.

Summary statistics for Height categorised by F/M

| Categorisation Factor levels | Mean | N | Std dev | Std error | Lower 95% CI | Upper 95% CI | Median | Lower quartile | Upper quartile |
|---|---|---|---|---|---|---|---|---|---|
| 1 | 1.6512 | 40 | 0.0701 | 0.0111 | 1.6287 | 1.6736 | 1.6493 | 1.6000 | 1.7000 |
| 2 | 1.8076 | 33 | 0.0583 | 0.0101 | 1.7870 | 1.8283 | 1.8050 | 1.7700 | 1.8520 |

Statistical analysis results assuming equal variances
Unpaired t-test result

| | t-statistic | Degrees of freedom | p-value |
|---|---|---|---|
| Equal variance unpaired t-test | -10.236 | 71 | < 0.0001 |

Conclusion: There is a statistically significant difference between the levels of Height at the 5% level.

Summary statistical analysis from InVivoStat, v4.0.2. Panels A and B show the summary descriptive statistics together with the independent *t*-test analysis of the locomotor activity data (Table 11.1, equal group numbers) and female and male height data (Tables 5.1 and 5.2, unequal group numbers), respectively.
*Source*: InVivoStat.

 Minitab

**A**

**Descriptive statistics**

| Sample | N | Mean | St Dev | SE mean |
|---|---|---|---|---|
| Loco C | 8 | 603.0 | 72.4 | 26 |
| Loco DgA | 8 | 368.5 | 71.9 | 25 |

**Test**

| Null hypothesis | $H_0: \mu_1 - \mu_2 = 0$ |
|---|---|
| Alternative hypothesis | $H_1: \mu_1 - \mu_2 \neq 0$ |

| T-Value | DF | P-Value |
|---|---|---|
| 6.50 | 14 | 0.000 |

**B**

**Descriptive statistics**

| Sample | N | Mean | St Dev | SE mean |
|---|---|---|---|---|
| Female | 40 | 1.6511 | 0.0701 | 0.011 |
| Male | 33 | 1.8076 | 0.0583 | 0.010 |

**Test**

| Null hypothesis | $H_0: \mu_1 - \mu_2 = 0$ |
|---|---|
| Alternative hypothesis | $H_1: \mu_1 - \mu_2 \neq 0$ |

| T-Value | DF | P-Value |
|---|---|---|
| −10.24 | 71 | 0.000 |

Summary statistical analysis from MiniTab, v19. Panels A and B show the summary descriptive statistics together with the independent *t*-test analysis of the locomotor activity data (Table 11.1, equal group numbers) and female and male height data (Tables 5.1 and 5.2, unequal group numbers), respectively.
*Source*: Minitab, LLC.

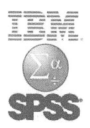

## A

**T-Test**

**Group Statistics**

| | Locofactor | N | Mean | Std. Deviation | Std. Error Mean |
|---|---|---|---|---|---|
| Loco_C | 1.00 | 8 | 603.0000 | 72.41547 | 25.60273 |
| | 2.00 | 8 | 368.5000 | 71.90669 | 25.42285 |

**Independent Samples Test**

| | | Levene's Test for Equality of Variances | | t-test for Equality of Means | | | | | 95% Confidence Interval of the Difference | |
|---|---|---|---|---|---|---|---|---|---|---|
| | | F | Sig. | t | df | Sig. (2-tailed) | Mean Difference | Std. Error Difference | Lower | Upper |
| Loco_C | Equal variances assumed | .001 | .971 | 6.499 | 14 | .000 | 234.50000 | 36.08076 | 157.11446 | 311.88554 |
| | Equal variances not assumed | | | 6.499 | 13.999 | .000 | 234.50000 | 36.08076 | 157.11410 | 311.88590 |

## B

**T-Test**

**Group Statistics**

| | FMfactor | N | Mean | Std. Deviation | Std. Error Mean |
|---|---|---|---|---|---|
| FMwhts | 1.00 | 40 | 1.6512 | .07006 | .01108 |
| | 2.00 | 33 | 1.8076 | .05827 | .01014 |

**Independent Samples Test**

| | | Levene's Test for Equality of Variances | | t-test for Equality of Means | | | | | 95% Confidence Interval of the Difference | |
|---|---|---|---|---|---|---|---|---|---|---|
| | | F | Sig. | t | df | Sig. (2-tailed) | Mean Difference | Std. Error Difference | Lower | Upper |
| FMwhts | Equal variances assumed | 1.476 | .228 | -10.236 | 71 | .000 | -.15649 | .01529 | -.18697 | -.12600 |
| | Equal variances not assumed | | | -10.419 | 70.992 | .000 | -.15649 | .01502 | -.18643 | -.12654 |

Summary statistical analysis from SPSS, v27. Panels A and B show the summary descriptive statistics together with the independent *t*-test analysis of the locomotor activity data (Table 11.1, equal group numbers) and female and male height data (Tables 5.1 and 5.2, unequal group numbers), respectively.

*Source*: IBM Corporation.

# Write Your Own Notes

# 12 Comparing two sets of data – Paired *t*-test

## The Paired *t*-test

In contrast to the independent *t*-test described in the previous chapter, the **Paired *t*-test** is a parametric test that is used to examine the effect of a single experimental manipulation (e.g. drug treatment) on two sets of observations taken from the *same* group of subjects. So, rather than examining for differences in the *absolute* scores of the observations from two groups of subjects (by comparing the two sample means from these groups), when we examine paired data sets, we are interested in the **difference** in the magnitude of the observations obtained from each subject in a single group.

Under the Null Hypothesis, we assume that the experimental manipulation has no effect on the experimental output measurement such that the mean difference between the two sets of observations is zero. The paired *t*-test (sometimes called the dependent sample *t*-test) therefore determines the probability that the Null Hypothesis is true.

It therefore follows that for a paired *t*-test the following assumptions should be met:

- The data should be a continuous measurement in form and type, respectively, and theoretically without limit (see Chapter 9),
- The values of the differences between the observations for each subject should be normally distributed (see Chapter 6),
- The two sets of data sets from the individual subjects should have similar variances without any outliers (see Chapter 6),
- The data should be sampled independently (i.e. different timepoints for each observation).

In the independent *t*-test, we were interested in the difference between the two mean values of the two sets of data we wished to compare (see Chapter 11). A similar approach is taken in the paired *t*-test, except that here we are interested in the mean difference of our test data, denoted by $\overline{D}$, compared to the mean difference in observations taken from the general population, $\mu_D$. Consequently, the equation to calculate the value of *t* for paired data is

$$t = \frac{\overline{D} - \mu_D}{S_D / \sqrt{N}} \tag{12.1}$$

where $S_D / \sqrt{N}$ is the standard error of the differences (i.e. standard deviation of the differences divided by the square root of the number of subjects).

If the Null Hypothesis is true, then there should be no difference between two consecutive measurements taken from a subject in the general population. Consequently, the mean of the differences for the subjects taken from the general population should also be zero, i.e. $\mu_D = 0$.

The equation for *t* for a paired *t*-test therefore reduces to

$$t = \frac{\overline{D}}{S_D / \sqrt{N}} \tag{12.2}$$

## Interpretation of the *t* statistic

Of course, because we have paired data, there will always be an equal number of first and second observations for each subject and so the issue of whether there are equal or unequal group sizes does not arise. As we saw for the result of the independent *t* test, we now compare the calculated value of the paired *t* statistic against the critical values of *t* provided in tables of the *t*-distribution (see Appendix C). For the paired *t*-test, the degrees of freedom are calculated as follows:

$$\text{df} = N - 1, \text{where } N \text{ is the number of subjects} \tag{12.3}$$

As before, the value of *t* determined from our data allows us to determine the probability that the Null Hypothesis is true, and if that calculated *t* value **exceeds** the critical *t* value listed in the table for a probability of 0.05, then we can be confident that there is little support in favour of the Null Hypothesis; consequently, we may conclude that our experimental intervention had an effect (i.e. $p < 0.05$). Similarly, the table of critical values for *t* also allows us to determine the critical value of *t* at other probability values that the Null Hypothesis is true, e.g. 0.01 (1/100) and 0.001 (1/1000). The critical values of the *t*-distribution for both one- and two-tailed tests (see Chapter 10) are summarised in Appendix C.

Whenever the result of a paired *t*-test is reported, the *t* value, degrees of freedom, and *p* value should always be quoted as follows (this allows your reader to double check your result in published tables of the *t*-distribution);

$$t(\text{df}) = t \text{ value}, p = p \text{ value} \tag{12.4}$$

Of course, as we shall see below, modern statistical software packages provide the resulting *p* value for you so that you should not have to look up critical values of *t* in tables of the *t*-distribution.

## Example 12.1 Paired data

Consider the experiment where the heart rate of a group of eight young adult males at rest was recorded immediately before and 15 min following drinking a cup of coffee. The Null Hypothesis would be that a single cup of coffee would have no effect on resting heart rate; this is therefore a two-tailed test as no direction of change in heart rate is indicated. The following table (Table 12.1) summarises the data obtained.

$$t = \frac{4.125}{1.6195} = 2.5471 \qquad (12.5)$$

Table 12.1 Effect of coffee on resting heart rate.

|  | Heart rate (bpm) | | | | |
|  | Before | After | Diff. | Diff. – Mean diff. | (Diff. – Mean diff.)$^2$ |
|---|---|---|---|---|---|
| 1 | 64 | 68 | +4 | −0.125 | 0.0156 |
| 2 | 57 | 65 | +8 | 3.875 | 15.0156 |
| 3 | 75 | 73 | −2 | −6.125 | 37.5156 |
| 4 | 62 | 67 | +5 | 0.875 | 0.7656 |
| 5 | 87 | 86 | −1 | −5.125 | 26.2656 |
| 6 | 55 | 67 | +12 | 7.875 | 62.0156 |
| 7 | 58 | 63 | +5 | 0.875 | 0.7656 |
| 8 | 68 | 70 | +2 | −2.125 | 4.5156 |

From this data we may calculate

- Mean difference in heart rate = **4.125 bpm** (mean of the values in column 4).
- Sum of squared differences of each difference value from the mean difference in heart rate = **146.875 bpm$^2$** (sum of the values in column 6).
- From this latter value, we can further calculate the variance of the differences (by dividing by $n - 1$, the degrees of freedom) = **20.9821 bpm$^2$**,
- the square root of which equals the standard deviation = **4.5806 bpm**.
- If we now divide this value by the square root of the number of subjects, then we calculate the standard error of the differences = **1.6195 bpm**.

We can substitute these values into the earlier equation to determine the paired value of *t*,

The estimate of *t* is therefore 2.5471 with 7 degrees of freedom. If we now refer to the critical values of *t* (see Appendix C) with 7 degrees of freedom, then $p < 0.05$ when $t_{crit} > 2.365$, $p < 0.01$ when $t_{crit} > 3.499$, and $p < 0.001$ when $t_{crit} > 5.408$. From these values, we can see that the probability that coffee had no effect on resting heart rate lay between $p = 0.05$ and $p = 0.01$. We may therefore reject the Null Hypothesis since $p < 0.05$ and conclude that there was a significant change in heart rate. This result may be summarised as follows:

$$t(7) = 2.5471, p < 0.05 \qquad (12.6)$$

The mean resting heart rate is 65.75 bpm, while that following drinking coffee is 69.875 bpm. We may therefore conclude that one cup of coffee significantly elevated resting heart rate in the eight young adult males.

# Example output from statistical software

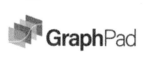 

A

| Paired t test Descriptive statistics | HR Before | HR After | HR After - HR Before |
|---|---|---|---|
| 1 Number of values | 8 | 8 | 8 |
| 2 | | | |
| 3 Minimum | 55.00 | 63.00 | -2.000 |
| 4 25% Percentile | 57.25 | 65.50 | -0.2500 |
| 5 Median | 63.00 | 67.50 | 4.500 |
| 6 75% Percentile | 73.25 | 72.25 | 7.250 |
| 7 Maximum | 87.00 | 86.00 | 12.00 |
| 8 | | | |
| 9 Mean | 65.75 | 69.88 | 4.125 |
| 10 Std. Deviation | 10.77 | 7.180 | 4.581 |
| 11 Std. Error of Mean | 3.807 | 2.539 | 1.619 |
| 12 | | | |
| 13 Lower 95% CI | 56.75 | 63.87 | 0.2955 |
| 14 Upper 95% CI | 74.75 | 75.88 | 7.954 |

| Paired t test | | |
|---|---|---|
| 3 Column Z | | HR After |
| 4 vs. | | vs. |
| 5 Column Y | | HR Before |
| 6 | | |
| 7 **Paired t test** | | |
| 8 P value | | 0.0383 |
| 9 P value summary | | * |
| 10 Significantly different (P < 0.05)? | | Yes |
| 11 One- or two-tailed P value? | | Two-tailed |
| 12 t, df | | t=2.547, df=7 |
| 13 Number of pairs | | 8 |
| 14 | | |
| 15 **How big is the difference?** | | |
| 16 Mean of differences (Z - Y) | | 4.125 |
| 17 SD of differences | | 4.581 |
| 18 SEM of differences | | 1.619 |
| 19 95% confidence interval | | 0.2955 to 7.954 |
| 20 R squared (partial eta squared) | | 0.4810 |

Summary statistical analysis from GraphPad Prism, v8. Panel A shows the summary descriptive statistics together with the paired $t$-test analysis of the heart rate data from Table 12.1.

*Source*: GraphPad Software.

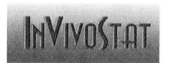

A

View Analysis Log   Export to Html   Export Images     Re-analyse

## InVivoStat Summary Statistics
### Variable selection

Response Heart Rate is analysed in this module, with results categorised by factor Before/After.

### Summary statistics for Heart Rate categorised by Before/After

| Categorisation Factor levels | Mean | N | Std dev | Std error | Lower 95% CI | Upper 95% CI | Min | Max | Median | Lower quartile | Upper quartile |
|---|---|---|---|---|---|---|---|---|---|---|---|
| 1 | 65.7500 | 8 | 10.7670 | 3.8067 | 56.7486 | 74.7514 | 55.0000 | 87.0000 | 63.0000 | 57.5000 | 71.5000 |
| 2 | 69.8750 | 8 | 7.1801 | 2.5385 | 63.8723 | 75.8777 | 63.0000 | 86.0000 | 67.5000 | 66.0000 | 71.5000 |

### Extended paired t-test result

| Effect | Num. df | Den. df | F-value | p-value |
|---|---|---|---|---|
| Before/After | 1 | 7 | 6.49 | 0.0383 |

Comment: The test in this table is a likelihood ratio test.

Conclusion: At the 5% level there is a statistically significant overall difference between the levels of Before/After.

Summary statistical analysis from InVivoStat, v4.0.2. Panel A shows the summary descriptive statistics together with the paired $t$-test analysis of the heart rate data from Table 12.1.

*Source*: InVivoStat.

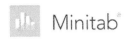

**A**

## Descriptive statistics

| Sample | N | Mean | St Dev | SE mean |
|--------|---|------|--------|---------|
| HR before | 8 | 65.75 | 10.77 | 3.81 |
| HR after | 8 | 69.88 | 7.18 | 2.54 |

## Test

Null hypothesis     $H_0$: μ_difference = 0
Alternative hypothesis     $H_1$: μ_difference ≠ 0

| *T*-Value | *P*-Value |
|-----------|-----------|
| −2.55 | 0.038 |

## Estimation for paired difference

| Mean | St Dev | SE mean | 95% CI for μ_difference |
|------|--------|---------|-------------------------|
| −4.13 | 4.58 | 1.62 | (−7.95, −0.30) |

*μ_difference: population mean of (HR Before - HR After)*

Summary statistical analysis from MiniTab, v19. Panel A shows the summary descriptive statistics together with the paired *t*-test analysis of the heart rate data from Table 12.1.

*Source*: Minitab, LLC.

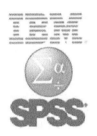

**A**

→ **T-Test**

**Paired Samples Statistics**

| | | Mean | N | Std. Deviation | Std. Error Mean |
|---|---|------|---|----------------|-----------------|
| Pair 1 | HR_Before | 65.7500 | 8 | 10.76701 | 3.80671 |
| | HR_After | 69.875 | 8 | 7.1801 | 2.5385 |

**Paired Samples Correlations**

| | | N | Correlation | Sig. |
|---|---|---|-------------|------|
| Pair 1 | HR_Before & HR_After | 8 | .948 | .000 |

**Paired Samples Test**

| | | Paired Differences | | | | | | | |
|---|---|---|---|---|---|---|---|---|---|
| | | | | | 95% Confidence Interval of the Difference | | | | |
| | | Mean | Std. Deviation | Std. Error Mean | Lower | Upper | t | df | Sig. (2-tailed) |
| Pair 1 | HR_Before - HR_After | -4.12500 | 4.58063 | 1.61950 | -7.95450 | -.29550 | -2.547 | 7 | .038 |

Summary statistical analysis from SPSS, v27. Panel A shows the summary descriptive statistics together with the paired *t*-test analysis of the heart rate data from Table 12.1.

*Source*: IBM Corporation.

# 13 Comparing two sets of data – independent non-parametric data

In the previous chapters, I described how the *t*-test may be used to examine two sets of data (either from independent groups, Chapter 11, or paired, Chapter 12) as long as a number of assumptions were met. Sometimes, however, it's clear that one or more of these assumptions cannot be met, and so a solution to this issue is to employ **non-parametric tests**, also known as **assumption-free**, or **distribution-free tests**. The term distribution-free tests only really mean that the tests do not assume a *normal* distribution. In this chapter and the next, we'll look at a limited number of non-parametric tests that are, essentially, the equivalent of the independent and paired *t*-tests in that they are used to examine two sets of independent or paired data only.

These tests are sometimes referred to as **distribution-free** since the first stage of the analysis involves **ranking** the individual observations in order of magnitude and assigning a rank value to each of the observations. The rank values are then used in the subsequent analysis rather than the values of the original observations.

## The Wilcoxon Rank Sum test and Mann-Whitney *U*-test

### Example 13.1 Independent data

Table 13.1 summarises the number of rears expressed by male rats during a 30 minutes session in an Open Field (this is a common term that refers to a large enclosed area in which activities such as locomotion and rearing behaviour may be quantified), the columns of data are colour coded according to the treatment. There are 15 animals in each group whose rearing behaviour we will compare under the Null Hypothesis that there is no difference in the distribution of the rearing values between the groups; consequently, there should be little or no difference in the respective **median** values.

The data from both groups are then arranged in order of magnitude, with the lowest values first (five rears in the group treated with Drug A) and then increasing in magnitude order all the way through to the highest value (23 rears in the control group), see Table 13.2. The colour coding immediately gives the impression that most of the rearing values of animals treated with Drug A are clustered towards the top of the table and are therefore generally of lower magnitude than the rearing values expressed by the control-treated animals, which are generally clustered towards

**Table 13.1** Effect of Drug A on rodent rearing behaviour.

| Subject | Rears | |
| | Control | Drug A |
| --- | --- | --- |
| 1 | 8 | 6 |
| 2 | 23 | 9 |
| 3 | 14 | 7 |
| 4 | 13 | 8 |
| 5 | 9 | 12 |
| 6 | 11 | 5 |
| 7 | 19 | 10 |
| 8 | 20 | 9 |
| 9 | 19 | 11 |
| 10 | 21 | 8 |
| 11 | 12 | 13 |
| 12 | 11 | 6 |
| 13 | 19 | 7 |
| 14 | 21 | 11 |
| 15 | 20 | 10 |
| **Median** | 19 | 9 |
| **Minimum** | 8 | 5 |
| **Maximum** | 23 | 13 |
| **Range** | 15 | 8 |

Values indicate the number of rears expressed by male rats in a 30-minutes session in an Open Field.

the bottom of the table. Notice also that there are numerous occasions when different subjects, regardless of treatment group, express the same number of rears during the test session. For example, there are two subjects that expressed seven rears and are given the ranks 4 and 5, three subjects that expressed nine rears (with ranks 9, 10 and 11), and four subjects that expressed 11 rears (with ranks 14, 15, 16 and 17). Because these groups of individual subjects expressed the same number of rears as other subjects, we assign a rank equal to the average potential rank for those scores. Thus, the two subjects with seven rears were both assigned the rank of 4.5, the three subjects with nine rears were each assigned a rank of 10, and the four subjects with 11 rears were all assigned a rank of 15.5. These assigned rank values are known as **tied ranks**, and I have indicated the groups of tied ranks in Table 13.2.

Table 13.2 Ranking the rearing behaviour scores.

| Rearing score | Rank | Assigned rank | Treatment |
|---|---|---|---|
| 5 | 1 | 1 | Drug A |
| 6 | 2 | 2.5 | Drug A |
| 6 | 3 | 2.5 | Drug A |
| 7 | 4 | 4.5 | Drug A |
| 7 | 5 | 4.5 | Drug A |
| 8 | 6 | 7 | Control |
| 8 | 7 | 7 | Drug A |
| 8 | 8 | 7 | Drug A |
| 9 | 9 | 10 | Control |
| 9 | 10 | 10 | Drug A |
| 9 | 11 | 10 | Drug A |
| 10 | 12 | 12.5 | Drug A |
| 10 | 13 | 12.5 | Drug A |
| 11 | 14 | 15.5 | Control |
| 11 | 15 | 15.5 | Control |
| 11 | 16 | 15.5 | Drug A |
| 11 | 17 | 15.5 | Drug A |
| 12 | 18 | 18.5 | Control |
| 12 | 19 | 18.5 | Drug A |
| 13 | 20 | 20.5 | Control |
| 13 | 21 | 20.5 | Drug A |
| 14 | 22 | 22 | Control |
| 19 | 23 | 24 | Control |
| 19 | 24 | 24 | Control |
| 19 | 25 | 24 | Control |
| 20 | 26 | 26.5 | Control |
| 20 | 27 | 26.5 | Control |
| 21 | 28 | 28.5 | Control |
| 21 | 29 | 28.5 | Control |
| 23 | 30 | 30 | Control |

There are some important aspects about ranking data in this way.

- Ranking reduces the impact of outliers (values that are greatly smaller or larger than the general distribution of the data would suggest).
- Any information about the magnitude of the differences between scores is lost.
- This loss of information means that non-parametric tests are generally less powerful than their equivalent parametric tests.

The point about outliers is especially important. Consider the first value in Table 13.2; here the observation of five rears was assigned a rank value of 1. In fact, for a single observation any number of rears from 0 to 5 would be assigned a rank of 1. Furthermore, the highest value of rears in Table 13.2, i.e. 23 (which was assigned a rank of 30), could have any value between 22 rears and infinity – it would still be assigned the rank of 30. Notice also that if indeed we change these rearing scores, then neither of these changes would result in any modification of the ranks assigned to any of the other rearing values in the table. Finally, look at the value of 14 rears which was assigned a rank of 22. This observation could have any value between 14 and 18 rears – it would still be assigned the rank value of 22! So, there is a lot of flexibility in the observed values of our data that would have absolutely no effect on the final assigned rank values. Indeed, if the spread of the values in the table were greatly increased, then even more flexibility in the individual rearing values would have little effect on the final ranks assigned to each.

When it comes to choosing a non-parametric test to compare two independent sets of data, then there are just two choices:

1 The Wilcoxon Rank-Sum test
2 The Mann–Whitney $U$-test,

and we shall use the rearing data described earlier to show how each of these tests works.

## The Wilcoxon Rank-Sum test

The first step in the Wilcoxon Rank-Sum test is to rank the data in order of magnitude, taking account of tied ranks, if necessary, as described earlier (see Table 13.2). Once the data have been ranked, then we add up all the assigned rank values for each group. Thus,

$$\text{Control group sum of ranks} = 321$$
$$\text{Drug A group sum of ranks} = 144$$

Our test statistic, denoted by $W_S$, is the lower sum of ranks, thus,

$$W_S = 144$$

If the **Wilcoxon test statistic**, together with the **mean** and the **standard error** of this test statistic are known, then it is a simple process to calculate a **z-score** and associated **p-value** for the data set.

Mean of the Wilcoxon test statistic, denoted by $\overline{W_S}$

$$\overline{W_S} = \frac{n_1(n_1 + n_2 + 1)}{2} \tag{13.1}$$

where $n_1$ and $n_2$ are the sample sizes for the Control and Drug A groups, respectively. Since both groups have 15 observations in each, then,

$$\overline{W_S} = \frac{15(15 + 15 + 1)}{2} = 232.5 \tag{13.2}$$

Standard error of the Wilcoxon test statistic, denoted by $SE_{\overline{W_s}}$

$$SE_{\overline{W_s}} = \sqrt{\frac{n_1 n_2(n_1 + n_2 + 1)}{12}}$$
$$SE_{\overline{W_s}} = \sqrt{\frac{(15 \times 15)(15 + 15 + 1)}{12}} \tag{13.3}$$

So, the result of the M

$$SE_{\overline{W_s}} = \sqrt{\frac{225 \times 31}{12}}$$
$$SE_{\overline{W_s}} = \sqrt{581.25} = 24.1091 \tag{13.4}$$

We can now calculate the $z$-score by

$$z = \frac{x - \bar{x}}{s} = \frac{W_s - \overline{W_s}}{SE_{\overline{W_s}}} = \frac{144 - 232.5}{24.109} = -3.6708 \tag{13.5}$$

For a description on how to interpret $z$-scores see Chapter 7 and Appendix B. Once we know the $z$-score, then Table 7.1 allows us to identify the associated $p$-value. In summary, a $z$-score greater than 1.96 or smaller than $-1.96$ is significant at $p < 0.05$. If the $z$-score is greater than 2.58 or less than $-2.58$ then $p < 0.01$, while if the $z$-score is greater than 3.29 or less than $-3.29$, then $p < 0.001$. The $z$-score for our rearing data of $-3.67$ is clearly less than $-3.29$ and so we may conclude that the probability of the Null Hypothesis being true is less than 1/1000, i.e. $p < 0.001$. We may therefore reject the Null Hypothesis, accept the Alternate Hypothesis, and conclude that the distributions of our two data sets are different such that the relative median scores (see Table 13.1, above) are significantly different; thus, animals treated with Drug A exhibited significantly lower levels of rearing behaviour compared to the control group ($p < 0.001$).

## The Mann–Whitney $U$-test

The Mann–Whitney $U$-test (MWUT) is essentially the same as the Wilcoxon rank-sum test, but uses a slightly different test statistic, $U$. Thus,

$$U = n_1 n_2 + \frac{n_1(n_1 + 1)}{2} - R_1 \tag{13.6}$$

where $n_1$ and $n_2$ are the sample sizes for groups 1 and 2, respectively, and $R_1$ is the sum of ranks for group 1. It doesn't matter which data set we assign to group 1 or group 2 as long as the values we put into the equation are assigned correctly. So, we shall calculate $U$ for both groups and compare the results. Since we have equal group sizes, the first part of the calculation is identical; thus,

$$U = (15 \times 15) + \frac{15(15 + 1)}{2} - R_1$$

$$U = 225 + \frac{240}{2} - R_1 \tag{13.7}$$

$$U = 345 - R_1$$

Then for the control group data:

$$U = 345 - 321 = 24 \tag{13.8}$$

While for the Drug A group data:

$$U = 345 - 144 = 201 \tag{13.9}$$

So, we have generated a pair of $U$ values depending on which set of data we used to determine $U$, but how do these values allow us to determine whether we may accept or reject the Null Hypothesis?

Appendix D contains a number of tables listing the critical values of the Mann–Whitney $U$ at $p = 0.05$ and 0.01 for both one- and two-tailed tests (for one-tailed see Tables D.1 and D.2, for two-tailed see Tables D.3 and D.4). The Null Hypothesis for this experiment was that Drug A had no effect on rearing behaviour compared to control subjects so we need to refer to the two-tailed critical value tables of the Mann–Whitney $U$ to determine the probability that the Null Hypothesis is true.

Table D.3 where $n_1$ and $n_2$ both equal 15 provides two values for $U$, i.e. 64 and 161. If the calculated values of $U$ are either lower than the smallest value or higher than the largest value, then we may conclude that $p < 0.05$. Likewise, Table D.4 also provides two values for $U$ where $n_1$ and $n_2 = 15$, i.e. 51 and 174, so if the calculated values of $U$ lie outside this range, then $p < 0.01$.

For our set of data, the calculated value of $U$ for the control group is 24, which is lower than the smaller critical value provided in Table D.4 for $p < 0.01$. Similarly, the calculated value of $U$ for the Drug A group is 201, which is higher than the larger critical value provided in Table D.4 for $p < 0.01$. So, it doesn't matter which group we choose to examine, in both cases the probability that the Null Hypothesis is true is less than 1/100 (i.e. $p < 0.01$).

As with the result of the Wilcoxon rank-sum test, the results calculated here for the MWUT allow us to reject the Null Hypothesis, accept the Alternate Hypothesis, and conclude that the distributions of our two data sets are different such that the relative median scores (see Table 13.1, above) are significantly different; thus, animals treated with Drug A exhibited significantly lower levels of rearing behaviour compared to the control group ($p < 0.01$).

Notice also that,

**a** it doesn't matter which group we choose to analyse (either the control group or our Drug A group),
**b** the probability that the Null Hypothesis is true is revealed by comparison of the calculated value of $U$ to the critical values of $U$ provided in the Mann–Whitney $U$ tables,
**c** the results of the Wilcoxon rank-sum test and the MWUT agree (phew!).

# Example output from statistical software

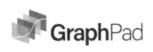 

A

| Mann-Whitney test Descriptive statistics | Rear C | Rear Drg |
|---|---|---|
| 1 Number of values | 15 | 15 |
| 2 | | |
| 3 Minimum | 8.000 | 5.000 |
| 4 25% Percentile | 11.00 | 7.000 |
| 5 Median | 19.00 | 9.000 |
| 6 75% Percentile | 20.00 | 11.00 |
| 7 Maximum | 23.00 | 13.00 |
| 8 | | |
| 9 Mean | 16.00 | 8.800 |
| 10 Std. Deviation | 5.000 | 2.366 |
| 11 Std. Error of Mean | 1.291 | 0.6110 |
| 12 | | |
| 13 Lower 95% CI | 13.23 | 7.490 |
| 14 Upper 95% CI | 18.77 | 10.11 |
| 15 | | |
| 16 Mean ranks | 21.40 | 9.600 |

| Mann-Whitney test Tabular results | |
|---|---|
| 1 Table Analyzed | Complete data set for stats analysis |
| 2 | |
| 3 Column AC | Rear Drg |
| 4 vs. | vs. |
| 5 Column AB | Rear C |
| 6 | |
| 7 **Mann Whitney test** | |
| 8 P value | <0.0001 |
| 9 Exact or approximate P value? | Exact |
| 10 P value summary | **** |
| 11 Significantly different (P < 0.05)? | Yes |
| 12 One- or two-tailed P value? | Two-tailed |
| 13 Sum of ranks in column AB,AC | 321 , 144 |
| 14 Mann-Whitney U | 24 |
| 15 | |

Summary statistical analysis from GraphPad Prism, v8. Panel A shows the summary descriptive statistics together with the Mann–Whitney U-test analysis of the rearing data from Table 13.1.

Source: GraphPad Software.

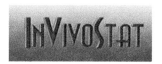

## A

View Analysis Log | Export to Html | Export Images

## InVivoStat Non-parametric Analysis

### Response

The Rearing response is currently being analysed by the Non-parametric Analysis module, with Rear factor fitted as the treatment factor.

### Summary data

| Group | Min | Lower quartile | Median | Upper quartile | Max |
|-------|-------|----------------|--------|----------------|--------|
| 1 | 8.000 | 11.500 | 19.000 | 20.000 | 23.000 |
| 2 | 5.000 | 7.000 | 9.000 | 10.500 | 13.000 |

### Mann-Whitney test

You have selected a factor with only two levels, hence a Mann-Whitney test, also know as a Wilcoxon rank sum test, has been used to analyse the data rather than a Kruskal-Wallis test.

| | Test statistic | p-value | p-value type |
|-------------|----------------|---------|--------------|
| Test result | 201.00 | 0.0003 | Asymptotic |

As there are ties in some of the responses, and/or the number of responses is greater than 50, the asymptotic test result has been calculated.

Summary statistical analysis from InVivoStsat, v4.0.2. Panel A shows the summary descriptive statistics together with the Mann–Whitney $U$-test analysis of the rearing data from Table 13.1.

*Source*: InVivoStat.

 Minitab

| Descriptive statistics | | | Test | | |
|---|---|---|---|---|---|
| **Sample** | **N** | **Median** | Null hypothesis | $H_0$: $\eta_1 - \eta_2 = 0$ | |
| Rear C | 15 | 19 | | | |
| Rear Drg | 15 | 9 | Alternative hypothesis | $H_1$: $\eta_1 - \eta_2 \neq 0$ | |
| | | | **Method** | **W-value** | **P-value** |
| | | | Not adjusted for ties | 321.00 | 0.000 |
| | | | Adjusted for ties | 321.00 | 0.000 |

Summary statistical analysis from MiniTab, v19. Panel A shows the summary descriptive statistics together with the Mann–Whitney $U$-test analysis of the rearing data from Table 13.1.

*Source*: Minitab, LLC.

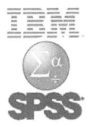

A

→ **NPar Tests**

**Descriptive Statistics**

| | N | Mean | Std. Deviation | Minimum | Maximum | 25th | Percentiles 50th (Median) | 75th |
|---|---|---|---|---|---|---|---|---|
| Rear_C_D | 30 | 12.4000 | 5.30842 | 5.00 | 23.00 | 8.0000 | 11.0000 | 19.0000 |
| Rear_factor | 30 | 1.5000 | .50855 | 1.00 | 2.00 | 1.0000 | 1.5000 | 2.0000 |

**Mann-Whitney Test**

**Ranks**

| | Rear_factor | N | Mean Rank | Sum of Ranks |
|---|---|---|---|---|
| Rear_C_D | 1.00 | 15 | 21.40 | 321.00 |
| | 2.00 | 15 | 9.60 | 144.00 |
| | Total | 30 | | |

**Test Statistics[a]**

| | Rear_C_D |
|---|---|
| Mann-Whitney U | 24.000 |
| Wilcoxon W | 144.000 |
| Z | -3.683 |
| Asymp. Sig. (2-tailed) | .000 |
| Exact Sig. [2*(1-tailed Sig.)] | .000[b] |

a. Grouping Variable: Rear_factor

b. Not corrected for ties.

Summary statistical analysis from SPSS, v27. Panel A shows the summary descriptive statistics together with the Mann–Whitney *U*-test analysis of the rearing data from Table 13.1.

*Source*: IBM Corporation.

# 14 Comparing two sets of data – paired non-parametric data

The previous chapter examined two non-parametric tests that could be used to compare two sets of independent data (i.e. generated by two sets of subjects) whose underlying distribution was non-normal; these tests were therefore the non-parametric equivalent of the independent (Student's) *t*-test. In this chapter, we shall examine a similar situation for data whose distribution is non-normal but where the two sets of observations are generated from the same subject group, i.e. the data is paired, and we are interested in the change in the values rather than the absolute values of each observation. This test is therefore the non-parametric version of the paired *t*-test and is called the **Wilcoxon Signed-Rank test** (*not* to be confused with the Wilcoxon rank-sum test in the previous chapter).

## The Wilcoxon Signed-Rank test

Like the paired *t*-test, the Wilcoxon Signed-Rank test is based upon the *differences* between pairs of observations taken from the same experimental subject.

### Example 14.1 Paired data

Consider the following experiment. Twelve male Hooded Lister rats were trained once daily for 5 consecutive days to find a submerged platform in a Morris-water maze experiment (this is a test of spatial cognitive performance). One week later, the rats were tested once more to see if they remembered the position of the submerged platform. The resulting time values are summarised in Table 14.1 and the data analysed by the Wilcoxon Signed-Rank test. The performances of the test subjects at the end of training and one week later are best described by the median and inter-quartile range values.

Thus,

- Training phase: 66 (50.25, 100.0) seconds
- Testing day: 145.5 (126.5, 169.25) seconds

Once the *differences* between the values have been determined, then they are ranked in order of magnitude (just like the first stage of the Wilcoxon Rank-Sum test or MW*U*T) ignoring whether the difference is positive or negative. Ranking is achieved in exactly the same way as before, including how tied ranks are dealt with. If the difference in scores is zero, then the data is excluded from the ranking process. The sign of the difference is then assigned to the rank value. The total sums of positive ($T_+$) and negative ($T_-$) ranks are then calculated (see Table 14.1). Thus;

- Sum of positive ranks; $T_+ = 72$
- Sum of negative ranks; $T_- = 6$

In the Wilcoxon Signed-Rank test, the test statistics is the sum of the positive ranks, $T_+$. However, as with the Wilcoxon rank sum

**Table 14.1** Performance of male rats in the Morris water maze.

| | Time to find platform (s) | | | | | Positive ranks | Negative ranks |
|---|---|---|---|---|---|---|---|
| | Training | Test | Diff. | Sign | Rank | | |
| 1 | 48 | 120 | 72 | + | 8 | 8 | |
| 2 | 56 | 95 | 39 | + | 3 | 3 | |
| 3 | 139 | 176 | 37 | + | 2 | 2 | |
| 4 | 44 | 210 | 166 | + | 12 | 12 | |
| 5 | 76 | 128 | 52 | + | 5 | 6 | |
| 6 | 115 | 135 | 20 | + | 1 | 1 | |
| 7 | 62 | 154 | 92 | + | 9 | 9 | |
| 8 | 39 | 167 | 128 | + | 10 | 10 | |
| 9 | 208 | 156 | −52 | − | 6 | | 6 |
| 10 | 51 | 210 | 159 | + | 11 | 11 | |
| 11 | 95 | 137 | 42 | + | 4 | 4 | |
| 12 | 70 | 122 | 52 | + | 7 | 6 | |
| | | | | | Total | 72 | 6 |

test (Chapter 13), the significance of the test statistic is determined by calculating the *z*-score which uses the mean (denoted here by $\overline{T}$) and the standard error (denoted here by $SE_{\overline{T}}$), which (if you remember) are both functions of the sample size, *n*. Thus,

$$\overline{T} = \frac{n(n+1)}{4} \tag{14.1}$$

$$SE_{\overline{T}} = \sqrt{\frac{n(n+1)(2n+1)}{24}} \tag{14.2}$$

In this experiment, the number of subjects, *n*, equals 12. However, notice that this reflects the number of participants so if any subject is excluded in the analysis (because the difference in the scores is zero), then the value of *n* must be adjusted accordingly.

Therefore,

$$\overline{T} = \frac{12(12+1)}{4} = 39 \tag{14.3}$$

$$SE_{\overline{T}} = \sqrt{\frac{12(12+1)(2 \times 12 + 1)}{24}} = 12.7474 \tag{14.4}$$

We can now calculate the *z*-score by

$$z = \frac{x - \overline{x}}{s} = \frac{T_+ - \overline{T}}{SE_{\overline{T}}} = \frac{72 - 39}{12.7475} = 2.5887 \tag{14.5}$$

As discussed in the previous chapter, if the *z*-score is greater than 1.96, then $p < 0.05$, if $z > 2.58$, then $p < 0.01$, and if $z > 3.29$, then $p < 0.001$ (note that a resulting negative sign is ignored, it is the absolute value of *z* irrespective of sign that is important). Our calculated *z*-score for the performance of the rats in the

Morris water maze of +2.5887 is clearly greater than 2.58 (! phew), and so we may conclude that the probability of the Null Hypothesis being true (i.e. that there is no difference between the training and test scores for the group of rats) is less than 1/100 (i.e. $p < 0.01$). We may therefore reject the Null Hypothesis and accept the Alternate Hypothesis and conclude that the distributions of our data are different such the relative median scores are significantly different; thus animals performed significantly worse (they failed to remember) on the test day (median score = 145.5 s) than they did at the end of the training phase one week earlier (median score = 66 s).

# Example output from statistical software

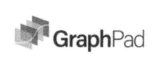 

A

| Wilcoxon test Descriptive statistics | Training | Test | Test - Training |
|---|---|---|---|
| 1 Number of values | 12 | 12 | 12 |
| 2 | | | |
| 3 Minimum | 39.00 | 95.00 | -52.00 |
| 4 25% Percentile | 48.75 | 123.5 | 37.50 |
| 5 Median | 66.00 | 145.5 | 52.00 |
| 6 75% Percentile | 110.0 | 173.8 | 119.0 |
| 7 Maximum | 208.0 | 210.0 | 166.0 |
| 8 | | | |
| 9 Mean | 83.58 | 150.8 | 67.25 |
| 10 Std. Deviation | 49.56 | 35.41 | 61.62 |
| 11 Std. Error of Mean | 14.31 | 10.22 | 17.79 |
| 12 | | | |
| 13 Lower 95% CI | 52.09 | 128.3 | 28.10 |
| 14 Upper 95% CI | 115.1 | 173.3 | 106.4 |

| Wilcoxon test Tabular results | |
|---|---|
| 1 Table Analyzed | Complete data set for stats analysis |
| 2 | |
| 3 Column AF | Test |
| 4 vs. | vs. |
| 5 Column AE | Training |
| 6 | |
| 7 **Wilcoxon matched-pairs signed rank test** | |
| 8 P value | 0.0068 |
| 9 Exact or approximate P value? | Exact |
| 10 P value summary | ** |
| 11 Significantly different (P < 0.05)? | Yes |
| 12 One- or two-tailed P value? | Two-tailed |
| 13 Sum of positive, negative ranks | 72.00 , -6.000 |
| 14 Sum of signed ranks (W) | 66.00 |
| 15 Number of pairs | 12 |
| 16 Number of ties (ignored) | 0 |
| 17 | |
| 18 **Median of differences** | |
| 19 Median | 52.00 |
| 20 96.14% confidence interval | 37.00 to 128.0 |

Summary statistical analysis from GraphPad Prism, v8. Panel A shows the summary descriptive statistics together with the Wilcoxon Signed-Rank test analysis of the Morris water maze data from Table 14.1.

*Source*: GraphPad Software.

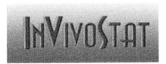

A

View Analysis Log | Export to Html | Export Images | Re-analyse

## InVivoStat Non-parametric Analysis

### Response

The Training response is currently being analysed by the Non-parametric Analysis module, with Test factor fitted as the treatment factor and Subject test fitted as the blocking factor.

### Summary data

| Group | Min | Lower quartile | Median | Upper quartile | Max |
|-------|-----|----------------|--------|----------------|-----|
| 1 | 39.000 | 49.500 | 66.000 | 105.000 | 208.000 |
| 2 | 95.000 | 125.000 | 145.500 | 171.500 | 210.000 |

### All pairwise comparisons - Wilcoxon Signed Rank test

| Comparison Number | Gp 1 | vs. | Gp 2 | p-value | p-value type |
|-------------------|------|-----|------|---------|--------------|
| 1 | 1 | vs. | 2 | 0.0095 | Asymptotic |

As there are ties in some of the response differences, and/or some of the groups have more than 20 responses, the asymptotic test result has been calculated in these cases.

Summary statistical analysis from InVivoStat, v4.0.2. Panel A shows the summary descriptive statistics together with the Wilcoxon Signed-Rank test analysis of the Morris water maze data from Table 14.1.

*Source*: InVivoStat.

 Minitab

| Descriptive statistics | | | | Test | | | | |
|---|---|---|---|---|---|---|---|---|
| **Sample** | **N** | **Median** | | Null hypothesis | | $H_0$: $\eta = 0$ | | |
| Training | 12 | 74.25 | | Alternative hypothesis | | $H_1$: $\eta \neq 0$ | | |
| Test | 12 | 148.50 | | | | | | |

| Sample | N for test | Wilcoxon statistic | P-Value |
|--------|-----------|--------------------|---------|
| Training | 12 | 78.00 | 0.003 |
| Test | 12 | 78.00 | 0.003 |

Summary statistical analysis from MiniTab, v19. Panel A shows the summary descriptive statistics together with the Wilcoxon Signed-Rank test analysis of the Morris water maze data from Table 14.1.

*Source*: Minitab, LLC.

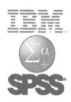

Summary statistical analysis from SPSS, v27. Panel A shows the summary descriptive statistics together with the Wilcoxon Signed-Rank test analysis of the Morris water maze data from Table 14.1.

*Source*: IBM Corporation.

A

→ **NPar Tests**

**Descriptive Statistics**

| | N | Mean | Std. Deviation | Minimum | Maximum | Percentiles 25th | 50th (Median) | 75th |
|---|---|---|---|---|---|---|---|---|
| Training | 12 | 83.5833 | 49.56072 | 39.00 | 208.00 | 48.7500 | 66.0000 | 110.0000 |
| Test | 12 | 150.8333 | 35.41400 | 95.00 | 210.00 | 123.5000 | 145.5000 | 173.7500 |

**Wilcoxon Signed Ranks Test**

**Ranks**

| | | N | Mean Rank | Sum of Ranks |
|---|---|---|---|---|
| Test - Training | Negative Ranks | 1[a] | 6.00 | 6.00 |
| | Positive Ranks | 11[b] | 6.55 | 72.00 |
| | Ties | 0[c] | | |
| | Total | 12 | | |

a. Test < Training
b. Test > Training
c. Test = Training

**Test Statistics[a]**

| | Test - Training |
|---|---|
| Z | -2.593[b] |
| Asymp. Sig. (2-tailed) | .010 |

a. Wilcoxon Signed Ranks Test
b. Based on negative ranks

# Write Your Own Notes

# (15) Parametric one-way analysis of variance

## Introduction

In Chapter 10, I discussed the effect on the Type 1 error rate when multiple pairwise comparisons are performed when there are more than two groups of data generated by our experiment (see sub-section *Comparing several groups of data* and Table 10.2). In these situations, we employ an **Analysis of Variance (ANOVA)** model which examines the whole data set to determine the probability that all the sample data sets come from the same population or whether one or more data sets are likely to come from a different population. The simplest ANOVA model is where there is one Between-Group Factor (see discussion on **Between Group Factors** in the sub-section *Comparing several groups of data*) that generates the number of independent data sets produced by the experiment; this simplest of models is known as a One-way ANOVA.

I shall describe the One-way ANOVA model in detail, since if you can understand how and why this model works, and what it tells us about the sampled data sets, then the reasons why some experimental designs require more complicated ANOVA models that include numerous Between- and/or Within-Group Factors also becomes so much easier to understand.

## One-Way Analysis of Variance

The one-way ANOVA is a method of examining how the *total variance* within a set of data (irrespective of group) is compartmentalised into the variance *between* the different groups in the experiment, referred to as the *Between-Group variance* (and reflects how different the grouped data sets are from each other), and the variance *within* each set of the different groups, referred to as the *Within-Group variance* (and reflects the spread of the data within each group). In its simplest terms, the one-way ANOVA examines the ratio of the Between-Group variance to the Within-Group variance. The ratio of these variances is known as the **F-ratio** (named after Sir Ronald A. Fisher, 1925–1991, who designed this type of analysis), and it is the value of the F-ratio, coupled with its associated probability that the Null Hypothesis is true, that allows us to determine whether our experimental intervention has produced a real change in the magnitude of our data that is unlikely to be produced by chance alone.

Conceptually, there are two ways by which we could try to understand how the ANOVA works, either by considering ANOVA as a special case of a linear model using regression analysis (see Chapter 20) or by simply considering the methods by which separate variance measurements are calculated which in turn are used to calculate the F-ratio. Actually, these are two sides of the same coin. I generally favour the latter of these since conceptually, for simple ANOVA models at least, appreciation of how the Between-Group variance and the Within-Group variance are generated, and what the resulting ratio between these values means in terms of variation in our experimental data is easier to understand.

## Source of variance; Total, Between-Group, and Within-Group

I stated above that the F-ratio generated by the ANOVA is simply the ratio between the Between-Group variance and the Within-Group variance – but let us take a step back to consider these values in terms of the Null Hypothesis.

## Example 15.1

Under the Null Hypothesis, we assume that all the observations produced by our experiment, irrespective of any experimental intervention, come from the same sampled population. So, consider the following experiment which examined the sensitivity of three different strains of rat to the same dose of a hypnotic drug. In each case, the sleeping time (defined as the time during which the righting reflex of each rat was lost) was determined (see Table 15.1).

**Table 15.1** Sleeping time for each strain of rat: original observations.

|        | Strain 1 | Strain 2 | Strain 3 |
|--------|----------|----------|----------|
| 1      | 13       | 20       | 14       |
| 2      | 17       | 17       | 21       |
| 3      | 19       | 23       | 16       |
| 4      | 15       | 26       | 19       |
| 5      | 16       | 19       | 13       |
| Mean   | 16.0     | 21.0     | 16.6     |
| St Dev | 2.24     | 3.54     | 3.36     |

One of the assumptions of examining data using parametric analysis is that the data follow a Normal distribution. Consequently, we assume that the distribution of each independent data set also follow a normal distribution (see Figure 15.1) and may be defined by each groups' mean and standard deviation (see Chapter 4).

If the Null Hypothesis is true, then the mean and spread of the data values for each group should be similar (sampling itself will produce some small differences in the values but nothing too large that should unduly concern us). Consequently, if all the observations do indeed come from the same population, then we can assume that all the observation grouped together should also follow a Normal distribution. So, we can group all the values together (irrespective of group) and calculate the overall mean for all the observations. We'll call this value the Grand Mean, $\overline{X}_{\text{Grand}}$. Thus,

$$\overline{X}_{\text{Grand}} = \frac{\sum x}{N_{\text{total}}} \qquad (15.1)$$

*Experimental Design and Statistical Analysis for Pharmacology and the Biomedical Sciences*, First Edition. Paul J. Mitchell.

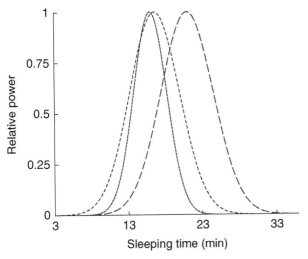

**Figure 15.1  Normal distribution curves of sleeping time data.** Calculated normal distribution curves for the effect of a dose of hypnotic drug on sleeping time in three different strains of rat (see Table 15.1 for original individual sleeping times). *X*-axis indicates sleeping times (min). *Y*-axis indicates relative power distribution. Strain 1 (*N*(16.0, 2.24), dotted curve); Strain 2 (*N*(21.0, 3.54), large dashed curve); and Strain 3 (*N*(16.6, 3.36), small dashed curve).

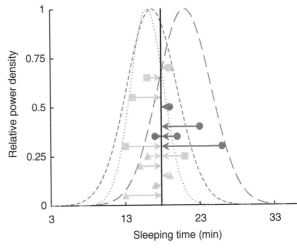

**Figure 15.2  Sleeping time data – individual differences from the Grand Mean.** Figure shows individual data points of sleeping time data colour-coded according to rat strain (see Table 15.1 for original individual sleeping times). *X*-axis indicates sleeping times (min). *Y*-axis indicates relative power distribution of associated normal distribution curves (for details, see Figure 15.1). Strain 1 data, orange solid triangles; Strain 2 data, red solid circles; and Strain 3 data, blue solid squares. Coloured arrows indicate differences from the Grand Mean (solid black line).

We saw back in Chapter 5 that we can calculate the variance of a set of data by first calculating the difference of each observation from the mean, squaring that difference and adding all the squared differences together to produce the Sum of Squares (SSQ) – see Table 5.4. We then simply divide the SSQ value by the appropriate degrees of freedom to produce the variance.

*Total variance*

So, let us apply this procedure to our sleeping time data to calculate the **total variance** for the data irrespective of strain of rat. First, we'll calculate the Grand Mean, thus;

$$\overline{X}_{Grand} = \frac{268}{15} = 17.8667 \tag{15.2}$$

We'll then calculate the difference for each observation in the whole data set from the Grand Mean. This is shown graphically in Figure 15.2. Each difference from the Grand Mean is then squared and these valued added together to produce the Total Sum of Squares (denoted by $SSQ_{total}$). If we do this for the three sets of data arising from our experiment, then the total variance (denoted by $s^2_{total}$) in all our data is simply the total SSQ for all the observations divided by the degrees of freedom (i.e. total number of observations – 1).

Thus,

$$SSQ_{total} = \sum \left( \overline{X}_{Grand} - x \right)^2 \tag{15.3}$$

$$s^2_{total} = \frac{SSQ_{total}}{N_{total} - 1} \tag{15.4}$$

The squared differences of each individual observation from the Grand Mean of the data are summarised in Table 15.2 from which we can calculate the total SSQ, the total variance, and the total standard deviation for the complete data.

**Table 15.2** Sleeping time for each strain of rat: calculation of total SSQ.

| Group | No. | $x$ | $\overline{X}_{Grand} - x$ | $\left( \overline{X}_{Grand} - x \right)^2$ |
|---|---|---|---|---|
| Strain 1 | 1 | 13 | 4.8667 | 23.6844 |
| | 2 | 17 | 0.8667 | 0.7511 |
| | 3 | 19 | −1.1333 | 1.2844 |
| | 4 | 15 | 2.8667 | 8.2178 |
| | 5 | 16 | 1.8667 | 3.4844 |
| Strain 2 | 1 | 20 | −2.1333 | 4.5511 |
| | 2 | 17 | 0.8667 | 0.7511 |
| | 3 | 23 | −5.1333 | 26.3511 |
| | 4 | 26 | −8.1333 | 66.1511 |
| | 5 | 19 | −1.1333 | 1.2844 |
| Strain 3 | 1 | 14 | 3.8667 | 14.9511 |
| | 2 | 21 | −3.1333 | 9.8178 |
| | 3 | 16 | 1.8667 | 3.4844 |
| | 4 | 19 | −1.1333 | 1.2844 |
| | 5 | 13 | 4.8667 | 23.6844 |
| **Total Sum of Squares (SSQ)** | | | | **189.7333** |

Thus,

$$SSQ_{total} = 189.7333 \tag{15.5}$$

$$s^2_{total} = \frac{189.7333}{14} = 13.5524 \tag{15.6}$$

$$\text{Standard deviation}_{Total} = \sqrt{s^2_{total}} = \sqrt{13.5} = 3.6814 \tag{15.7}$$

The Grand Mean (17.87 min) and associated total standard deviation (3.68 min) for all the observations allows us to plot an overarching Normal distribution curve that encompasses all the individual observations in comparison to the normal distribution curves calculated from the data for each strain used in the experiment (see Figure 15.3).

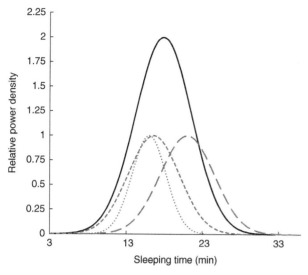

**Figure 15.3** **Normal distribution curves of sleeping time data.** Figure shows the relative power density values for the overarching normal distribution curve ($N$(17.87, 3.68), solid curve) including all observations irrespective of strain group. X-axis indicates sleeping times (min). Y-axis indicates relative power distribution. Strain 1 ($N$(16.0, 2.24), dotted curve); Strain 2 ($N$(21.0, 3.54), large dashed curve); and Strain 3 ($N$(16.6, 3.36), small dashed curve). The relative power density values for the overarching normal distribution have been doubled for clarity.

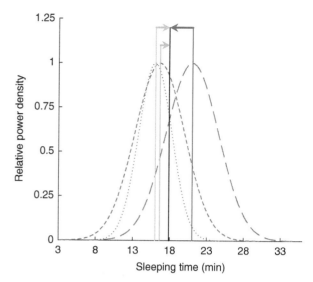

**Figure 15.4** **Normal distribution curves of sleeping time data – calculation of Between-Group variance.** Calculated differences between the Grand Mean and the individual group means for each strain of rat treated with a dose of hypnotic drug. X-axis indicates sleeping times (min). Y-axis indicates relative power distribution. Strain 1, solid orange line indicates mean sleeping time, 16.0 min; Strain 2, solid red line indicates mean sleeping time, 21.0 min; and Strain 3, solid blue line indicates mean sleeping time, 16.6 min. Grand Mean indicated by solid black line = 17.8667 min. Coloured arrows indicate the difference of each group mean to the Grand Mean.

The total variance for the complete data set may be summarised as follows (Table 15.3),

**Table 15.3** Summary of total variance data.

| Source | SSQ | df | Variance |
|--------|-----|-----|----------|
| Total | 189.7333 | 14 | 13.5524 |

### Between-Group variance

As the name suggests, the Between-Group variance reflects the differences in the observation *between* the different groups in the experiment. To calculate the Between-Group variance, we first calculate the difference between each individual group mean and the Grand Mean (see Figure 15.4).

Each difference value is then squared before the contribution of each group to the Between-Group SSQ value is calculated by multiplying the squared difference value by the number of subjects in the appropriate group.

Thus,

$$\text{Strain 1}: \quad \text{SSQ}_{\text{Between 1}} = \left( \left( \overline{X}_{\text{Grand}} - \overline{x}_1 \right)^2 \right) \cdot n_1 \qquad (15.8)$$

$$\text{Strain 2}: \quad \text{SSQ}_{\text{Between 2}} = \left( \left( \overline{X}_{\text{Grand}} - \overline{x}_2 \right)^2 \right) \cdot n_2 \qquad (15.9)$$

$$\text{Strain 3}: \quad \text{SSQ}_{\text{Between 3}} = \left( \left( \overline{X}_{\text{Grand}} - \overline{x}_3 \right)^2 \right) \cdot n_3 \qquad (15.10)$$

The Between-Group SSQ is then calculated by simply adding together the individual Between-Group SSQ contributions from each group in the experiment (see Table 15.4).

**Table 15.4** Calculation of Between-Group Sum of Squares.

| Group | Mean ($\overline{x}$) | Difference from Grand Mean $\overline{X}_{\text{Grand}} - \overline{x}$ | Difference from Grand Mean squared $\left( \overline{X}_{\text{Grand}} - \overline{x} \right)^2$ | (Difference from Grand Mean squared) $\times n$ |
|-------|------|------|------|------|
| Strain 1 | 16.0 | 1.8667 | 3.4844 | 17.4222 |
| Strain 2 | 21.0 | −3.1333 | 9.8178 | 49.0889 |
| Strain 3 | 16.6 | 1.2667 | 1.6044 | 8.0222 |
| | | **Between-Group SSQ** | | **74.5333** |

Once the Between-Group SSQ has been calculated, then it is just a simple matter of dividing this value by the Between-Group degrees of freedom to calculate the Between-Group variance. The Between-Group degrees of freedom is simply the total number of groups in the experiment – 1.

Thus,

$$\text{SSQ}_{\text{Between}} = 74.5333 \qquad (15.11)$$

$$\text{df}_{\text{Between}} = 3 - 1 = 2 \qquad (15.12)$$

$$s^2_{\text{Between}} = \frac{\text{SSQ}_{\text{Between}}}{\text{df}_{\text{Between}}} = \frac{74.5333}{2} = 37.2667 \qquad (15.13)$$

The Between-Group variance data may then be summarised with the total variance data; see Table 15.5

**Table 15.5** Summary of Between-Group and total variance data.

| Source | SSQ | df | Variance |
|--------|-----|-----|----------|
| Between | 74.5333 | 2 | 37.2667 |
| Total | 189.7333 | 14 | 13.5524 |

## Within-Group variance

The final source of variance in our set of data is that within each group of data in our experiment. Here, the variance within each group is determined by first calculating the difference between each observation and its individual group mean. These differences are then squared and then added together to produce each groups' sum of squares.

Thus,

$$\text{Strain } 1: \quad \text{SSQ}_{\text{Within 1}} = \sum (\bar{x}_1 - x)^2 \quad (15.14)$$

$$\text{Strain } 2: \quad \text{SSQ}_{\text{Within 2}} = \sum (\bar{x}_2 - x)^2 \quad (15.15)$$

$$\text{Strain } 3: \quad \text{SSQ}_{\text{Within 3}} = \sum (\bar{x}_3 - x)^2 \quad (15.16)$$

These calculations are summarised graphically in Figure 15.5. The Within-Group SSQ is then calculated by simply adding together the individual Within-Group SSQ contributions from each group in the experiment; Table 15.6 summarises these calculations.

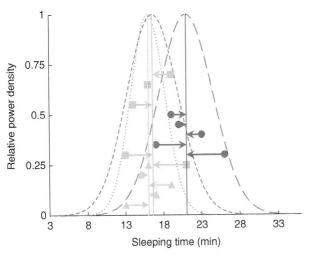

**Figure 15.5  Normal distribution curves of sleeping time data – calculation of Within-Group variance.** Calculated differences between each group mean and the individual observations for each strain of rat treated with a dose of hypnotic drug. X-axis indicates sleeping times (min). Y-axis indicates relative power distribution. Strain 1, solid orange line indicates mean sleeping time (16 min), while solid orange triangles indicate individual observations; Strain 2, solid red line indicates mean sleeping time (21.0 min) while solid red circles indicate individual observations; and Strain 3, solid blue line indicates mean sleeping time (16.6 min) while solid blue squares indicate individual observations. Coloured arrows indicate difference of each individual observation to the appropriate group mean.

Once the Within-Group SSQ has been calculated, then it is just a simple matter of dividing this value by the Within-Group degrees of freedom to calculate the Within-Group variance. The Within-Group degree of freedom is simply the total number of observations in the experiment – the number of groups.

Thus,

$$\text{SSQ}_{\text{Within}} = 115.2 \quad (15.17)$$

$$\text{df}_{\text{Between}} = 15 - 3 = 12 \quad (15.18)$$

$$s^2_{\text{Within}} = \frac{\text{SSQ}_{\text{Within}}}{\text{df}_{\text{Within}}} = \frac{115.2}{12} = 9.6 \quad (15.19)$$

**Table 15.6** Sleeping time for each strain of rat: calculation of within SSQ.

| Group | No. | $x$ | $\bar{x}_{\text{group}}$ | $\bar{x}_{\text{group}} - x$ | $(\bar{x}_{\text{group}} - x)^2$ | $\text{SSQ}_{\text{group}}$ |
|---|---|---|---|---|---|---|
| Strain 1 | 1 | 13 | | 3 | 9 | |
| | 2 | 17 | | −1 | 1 | |
| | 3 | 19 | 16 | −3 | 9 | 20 |
| | 4 | 15 | | 1 | 1 | |
| | 5 | 16 | | 0 | 0 | |
| Strain 2 | 1 | 20 | | 1 | 1 | |
| | 2 | 17 | | 4 | 16 | |
| | 3 | 23 | 21 | −2 | 4 | 50 |
| | 4 | 26 | | −5 | 25 | |
| | 5 | 19 | | 2 | 4 | |
| Strain 3 | 1 | 14 | | 2.6 | 6.76 | |
| | 2 | 21 | | −4.4 | 19.36 | |
| | 3 | 16 | 16.6 | 0.6 | 0.36 | 45.2 |
| | 4 | 19 | | −2.4 | 5.76 | |
| | 5 | 13 | | 3.6 | 12.96 | |
| **Within-Group SSQ** | | | | | **115.2** | |

The Within-Group variance data may then be summarised along with the total and Between-Group variance data; see Table 15.7.

**Table 15.7** Summary of Between-Group, Within-Group, and total variance data.

| Source | SSQ | df | Variance |
|---|---|---|---|
| Between | 74.5333 | 2 | 37.2667 |
| Within | 115.2000 | 12 | 9.6 |
| Total | 189.7333 | 14 | |

This table, known as the one-way ANOVA table (see Table 15.8), now allows the F-ratio of the Between- and Within-Group variance to be calculated which, with the appropriate degrees of freedom, allows the probability that the Null Hypothesis is true to be determined.

**Table 15.8** One-way ANOVA table.

| Source | SSQ | df | Variance | F-ratio | p |
|---|---|---|---|---|---|
| Between | 74.5333 | 2 | 37.2667 | 3.8819 | >0.05 |
| Within | 115.2000 | 12 | 9.6 | | |
| Total | 189.7333 | 14 | | | |

The F-ratio for our experiment examining the effect of a dose of hypnotic drug on the sleeping time of three different strains of rat is equal to 3.8819 with 2 and 12 degrees of freedom. If we now refer to the table of critical values of F with 2 and 12 degrees of freedom (see Appendix E), then $F_{\text{crit}} = 3.89$ for $p = 0.05$, $F_{\text{crit}} = 6.93$ for $p = 0.01$, and $F_{\text{crit}} = 12.97$ for $p = 0.001$. So, the calculated F-ratio from analysis of our experimental data **does not** exceed the critical value of F for $p = 0.05$. Consequently, the probability that the three sets of sleeping time data come from the same population is **greater** than

0.05. We must therefore accept the Null Hypothesis and conclude that there is no difference between the three groups of data.

Generally, it is not appropriate to reproduce the whole ANOVA table in a laboratory report or scientific paper. Instead, the accepted format is that we report the $F$-ratio together with both degrees of freedom for the Between- and Within-Group variances in parenthesis and the resulting $p$-value, as follows,

$$F(2, 20) = 3.8819, p > 0.05 \qquad (15.20)$$

where the first number in parenthesis is the Between-Group degrees of freedom and the second number is the Within-Group degrees of freedom.

Reporting the ANOVA result in this way allows your reader to check that you have arrived at the correct $p$-value. The probability that the Null Hypothesis is true is very important. Indeed, we are only allowed to examine for pairwise differences between the groups of data if the ANOVA result indicates that there are significant differences between two or more of the groups, i.e. if $p < 0.05$ then we may reject the Null Hypothesis. However, in the example used here, $p > 0.05$ and so we must **stop** our inferential analysis at this stage since there is no justification in trawling for differences between these groups when our ANOVA result indicates there is no significant variation between the three groups of data. Thus, we would conclude there is no evidence of any strain differences in the sensitivity to the dose of hypnotic drug used in the experiment.

## Relationship between the *F*-ratio and probability

We saw earlier when discussing the results of the $t$-test that as the value of $t$ increases, so the probability that the Null Hypothesis is true decreases. Such an inverse relationship also exists for the $F$-ratio and the associated $p$-value. Of course, the $F$-ratio in turn is dependent on the relative values of the Between- and Within-Group variance values. Thus, as the $F$-ratio increases so the associated $p$-value decreases, while if the $F$-ratio decreases then the probability of the Null Hypothesis being true increases.

Consider the following pie chart which summarises the proportional values of the Between-Group and Within-Group variance values for our example experiment examining the effect of the hypnotic drug on sleeping time in three strains of rat (see Figure 15.6). The resulting $F$-ratio, with 2 and 12 degrees of freedom, equals 3.8819, $p > 0.05$, as described above.

Let us imagine hypothetically that in the second group of data, the spread of the values within each strain group were maintained so that the Within-Group variance was the same (i.e. 9.6 min$^2$), but the mean values of each group were much closer together so that the Between-Group variance was reduced from 37.2667 to 18.0 min$^2$. The resulting pie chart of the relationship between the two sets of variance values would be as summarised in Figure 15.7. Clearly proportionately the Within-Group variance is now much greater, so there is a reduction in the $F$-ratio and a consequent increase in the value of $p$, thus, $F(2.12) = 1.875, p > 0.10$; the critical value of the $F$-ratio with 2 and 12 degrees of freedom for $p = 0.10$ is 2.8068. A similar effect on the $F$-ratio would occur if the Between-Group variance remained at 37.2667 min$^2$, but the spread of the values within each set of data increased, thereby increasing the Within-Group variance (hypothetically to 19.8756 min$^2$). The resulting $F$-ratio (i.e. 37.2667/19.8756) would still equal 1.875, and so there would be no change in either the pie chart or the associated $p$-value.

Figure 15.7 **Comparison of Between-Group and Within-Group variance values.** Between-Group variance indicated by blue sector and Within-Group variance indicated by orange sector. Identical $F$-ratios occur regardless of whether the Between-Group and Within-Group variance are 18.0 and 9.6 min$^2$, respectively, or 37.2667 and 19.8756 min$^2$, respectively. F(2,12) = 1.875, p > 0.1.

So a reduction in the value of the $F$-ratio may result from either smaller differences between the respective mean values of the sets of data in our experiment (which will reduce the Between-Group variance) and/or greater spread of the individual values within each group (thereby increasing the Within-Group variance).

In contrast, the opposite changes in the Between-Group and Within-Group variances will markedly increase the resultant $F$-ratio. Table 15.9 summarises the critical values of $F$ with 2 and 12 degrees of freedom for $p = 0.05$, $p = 0.01$, and $p = 0.001$ together with example of Between-Group and Within-Group variance values calculated from the sleeping time data (Table 15.1).

Figure 15.6 **Comparison of Between-Group and Within-Group variance values.** Data taken for Table 15.7. Between-Group variance (37.2667 min$^2$) indicated by blue sector, and Within-Group variance (9.6 min$^2$) indicated by orange sector. F(2,12) = 3.8819, p > 0.05.

Table 15.9 Comparison of Between-Group and Within-Group variance values.

| | $p = 0.05$ | $p = 0.01$ | $p = 0.001$ |
|---|---|---|---|
| $F_{crit}(2,12)$ ratio | 3.89 | 6.93 | 12.97 |
| Between Group | 37.2667 | 37.2667 | 37.2667 |
| Within Group | 9.58 | 5.38 | 2.87 |
| Between Group | 37.344 | 66.528 | 124.512 |
| Within Group | 9.60 | 9.60 | 9.60 |

Summary of Between-Group and Within-Group variance values for critical values of $F$ with 2 and 12 degrees of freedom for $p = 0.05$, $p = 0.01$, and $p = 0.001$.

Table 15.9 indicates the required Within-Group variance values for different p values if the Between-Group variance remains at 37.2667 min² (rows 2 and 3 in table body) or the required Between-Group variance values if the Within-Group variance remains at 9.60 min² (rows 3 and 4). Table 15.9 shows that if the Between-Group variance remains constant, (at 37.2667 min²) then progressive reductions in the Within-Group variance, which would occur if the spread of data within each group of data became less and less as the data became more tightly packed, results in greater values for the $F$-ratio which, in turn, results in lower probability values for the Null Hypothesis being true. Similarly, if the Within-Group variance remained constant (at 9.60 min²) but the Between-Group variance became progressively larger, which would occur if the mean values of the individuals groups of data became increasingly different from the grand mean as the relative distributions of the different groups became progressively further and further apart, then the resultant $F$-ratio would also become progressively larger, again resulting in lower probability values for the Null Hypothesis being true. These progressive increases in the $F$-ratio (together with percentage values for the Between-Group and Within-Group variances) can be seen in the summary pie charts shown in Figure 15.8.

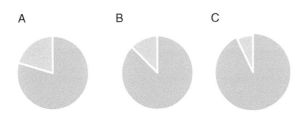

A          B          C

Figure 15.8 **Comparison of Between-Group and Within-Group variance values.** Between-Group variance indicated by blue sector, and Within-Group variance indicated by orange sector. Increasing $F_{crit}$-ratios occur as proportion of Between-Group variance increases in relation to the Within-Group variance. Panel A: $F_{crit}(2,12) = 3.89$, $p = 0.05$, Between = 79.6%, and Within = 20.4%. Panel B: $F_{crit}(2,12) = 6.93$, $p = 0.01$, Between = 87.4%, and Within = 12.6%. Panel C: $F_{crit}(2,12) = 12.97$, $p = 0.001$, Between = 92.84%, and Within = 7.16%. Data from Table 15.9.

In summary, therefore, the resulting $F$-ratio following ANOVA is not dependent on the values of the Between-Group or Within-Group variance alone, but on the *relationship* between the two. Increased $F$-ratio value may be achieved by either increasing the degree of separation between the groups in the experiment (i.e. to increase the Between-Group variance) or by reducing the spread of the individual values within each group (i.e. to decrease the Within-Group variance). Of course, the number of subjects in the experiment also has profound effects on the values of both the Between-Group and Within-Group variances and also on the Within-Group degrees of freedom, and so increasing the number of subjects in your experiment may allow you to resolve your experimental conclusions when perhaps the initial results of your studies are somewhat equivocal (see also discussion on statistical power in Chapter 10).

## So, what do we do next?

The Null Hypothesis for the one-way ANOVA is that the Between-Group Factor of our experimental intervention (i.e. the single factor that creates the independence of our experimental groups) has no effect on the experimental parameter we are measuring, i.e. all the data values, irrespective of group, come from the same population. If the result of the one-way ANOVA analysis, however, indicates that the probability that this statement is true is less than 5% (i.e. $p < 0.05$), then we may reject the Null Hypothesis and accept that the alternate hypothesis is likely to be true. Consequently, we may therefore conclude that there is sufficient variation between the groups to indicate that at least one of the groups is different from at least one of the others. So, while the ANOVA analysis provides a general overview as to whether our experimental intervention had an effect on the experimental output, it fails to identify exactly where that difference lies; i.e. it fails to identify which groups differ from each other. The one-way ANOVA analysis may therefore be considered as the **first** stage of our inferential analysis, and whether we move on to stage two is dependent on the resulting probability that the Null Hypothesis is true. If $p \geq 0.05$, then we accept the Null Hypothesis and we stop our analysis as there is *no evidence* of any difference between our experimental groups. If, however (and only if!), $p < 0.05$, then we move to the **second** stage of the analysis to determine which groups are likely to be different from each other by using **multiple pairwise comparisons**.

## Multiple pairwise comparisons; *post hoc* and *a priori* analysis

Let us assume that the result of our one-way ANOVA allows us to reject the Null Hypothesis and instead accept the alternate hypothesis that there is sufficient variation between our experimental groups to suggest that there may be differences between some of the groups of data. The problem now is how do we identify which groups are likely to be different from each other?

Well, we could use the independent 'Student's' $t$-test, but this raises the problem of increasing the Type 1 error rate (see sub-section **Comparing several groups of data** and Tables 10.2 and 10.3) and so this strategy should not be used unless you are willing to apply a correction factor to all of the resulting $p$-values (e.g. Bonferroni correction). The more common approach is to subject the data to *post hoc* (Latin; made or happening only after an event). **Post hoc** procedures are statistical tests that consist of multiple pairwise comparisons that compare some or all of the different combinations of the independent groups on our experiment, but they do so in ways which, in most cases, control the familywise error rate by ensuring that the overall Type 1 error rate (the $\alpha$ value, remember? If not see Chapter 10) remains at 0.05. So, this family of statistical procedures has a built-in Bonferroni-type correction factor applied to the resulting $p$-value for each comparison performed.

But how do we know which *post hoc* test to use? Consider the two following experiments.

## Example 15.2 Experiment 1: All Means comparisons

Eighteen young age- and weight-matched mice were randomly allocated to one of three groups and their weights recorded. Each group was fed a different diet for a month and then the mice were reweighed. The weight increase for each subject is given in the table below.

Table 15.10 shows that in all cases the Kolmogorov–Smirnov and Shapiro–Wilk tests for normality (i.e. $D$ or $W$ scores, respectively; see Chapter 6) show that all three sets of data approximate to a normal distribution (i.e. $p > 0.05$ in all cases). Furthermore, the Fisher–Pearson coefficient values of skewness indicate that none of the data sets show significant positive or negative skew (all $z$-scores $< 1.96$, $p > 0.05$ in all cases). Finally, the Levene's test indicates homogeneity of variance across all three sets of data $[F(2,15) = 1.078, p = 0.365]$. Consequently, we may conclude that the sets of weight gain data each approximate to a normal distribution with homogeneity of variance and so further analysis by parametric one-way ANOVA is justified.

## Example 15.3 Experiment 2: Control group comparisons

The systolic blood pressure of four groups of conscious male rats (six rats per group), measured by the tail-cuff method, were recorded prior to and 30 minutes following oral treatment with either 0.1% methyl cellulose ($^w/_v$ in water, dose volume 2.5 ml/kg) or 20 mg/kg (dose volume 2.5 ml/kg) of three new experimental drugs (Drug A, Drug B, or Drug C). The changes in systolic blood pressure are summarised in Table 15.11.

As seen with the data from Experiment 1, Table 15.11 indicates that in all cases the Kolmogorov–Smirnov and Shapio–Wilk tests for normality (i.e. $D$ or $W$ scores, respectively; see Chapter 6) show that all three sets of data approximate to a normal distribution (i.e. $p > 0.05$ in all cases). Furthermore, the Fisher–Pearson coefficient values of skewness indicate that none of the data sets show significant positive or negative skew (all $z$-scores $< 1.96$, $p > 0.05$ in all cases). Finally, the Levene's test indicates homogeneity of variance

**Table 15.10** Effect of diet on weight gain in mice.

| Subject | Diet 1 | Diet 2 | Diet 3 |
|---|---|---|---|
| 1 | 2.0 | 2.2 | 3.6 |
| 2 | 2.5 | 2.5 | 5.2 |
| 3 | 1.9 | 3.3 | 3.1 |
| 4 | 0.2 | 2.8 | 5.1 |
| 5 | 3.5 | 2.5 | 4.1 |
| 6 | 2.2 | 2.9 | 3.7 |
| Mean | 2.050 | 2.700 | 4.133 |
| St Dev | 1.075 | 0.385 | 0.850 |
| SEM | 0.439 | 0.157 | 0.347 |
| Kolmogorov–Smirnov | $D(6) = 0.278, p = 0.163$ | $D(6) = 0.198, p = 0.200$ | $D(6) = 0.206, p = 0.200$ |
| Shapiro–Wilk | $W(6) = 0.922, p = 0.522$ | $W(6) = 0.967, p = 0.873$ | $W(6) = 0.903, p = 0.394$ |
| Fisher–Pearson skewness | $-0.771 \pm 0.845, z = 0.912$ $p > 0.05$ | $0.443 \pm 0.845, z = 0.524$ $p > 0.05$ | $0.381 \pm 0.845, z = 0.451$ $p > 0.05$ |
| Levene's test | | $F(2,15) = 1.078, p = 0.365$ | |

Descriptive analysis of the effect of diet on weight gain in mice. Table shows individual weight gain ($g$) together with summary statistics and data distribution analysis for all three sets of data.

**Table 15.11** Effect of drug treatment on systolic blood pressure.

| Subject | 1% Methyl cellulose | Drug A | Drug B | Drug C |
|---|---|---|---|---|
| 1 | 3 | −1 | 12 | 3 |
| 2 | −2 | −8 | 3 | 1 |
| 3 | −1 | 1 | 6 | 2 |
| 4 | 5 | −5 | 9 | 0 |
| 5 | 0 | −6 | 7 | 5 |
| 6 | 1 | 2 | 8 | 2 |
| Mean | 1.000 | −2.833 | 7.500 | 2.167 |
| St dev | 2.608 | 4.070 | 3.017 | 1.722 |
| SEM | 1.065 | 1.662 | 1.232 | 0.703 |
| Kolmogorov–Smirnov | $D(6) = 0.167$ $p = 0.200$ | $D(6) = 0.203$ $p = 0.200$ | $D(6) = 0.143$ $p = 0.200$ | $D(6) = 0.205$ $p = 0.200$ |
| Shapiro–Wilk | $W(6) = 0.960$ $p = 0.817$ | $W(6) = 0.924$ $p = 0.533$ | $W(6) = 0.992$ $p = 0.993$ | $W(6) = 0.961$ $p = 0.830$ |
| Fisher–Pearson skewness | $0.609 \pm 0.845$ $z = 0.039$ $p > 0.05$ | $-0.02 \pm 0.85$ $z = 0.024$ $p > 0.05$ | $0.00 \pm 0.845$ $z = 0.000$ $p > 0.05$ | $0.678 \pm 0.845$ $z = 0.802$ $p > 0.05$ |
| Levene's test | | $F(3,20) = 2.525, p = 0.087$ | | |

Descriptive analysis of the effect of drug treatment on changes in systolic blood pressure (mmHg). Table shows individual changes in systolic blood pressure together with summary statistics and data distribution analysis for all four sets of data.

across all four sets of data [$F(3,20) = 2.525$, $p = 0.087$]. Consequently, we may conclude that the sets of changes in systolic blood pressure data each approximate to a normal distribution with homogeneity of variance and so further analysis by parametric one-way ANOVA is justified.

## Data analysis step 1: one-way ANOVA

Analysis of the data arising from Experiment 1 and Experiment 2 by one-way ANOVA may be summarised as follows:

- **Experiment 1:** $F(2,15) = 10.096$, $p = 0.002$
- **Experiment 2:** $F(3,20) = 12.335$, $p < 0.001$

In both cases, the probability that the Null Hypothesis is true is less than 0.05. Consequently, the Null Hypothesis (that there is no difference between the groups of data in each experiment) may be rejected for both experiments. This means that there is sufficient evidence in each experiment to indicate that at least one group is different from one other group. But as we have already seen, the one-way ANOVA alone does not indicate which groups in our experiment differ and so we must resort to one of the *post hoc* procedures to identify groups of data that differ from each other.

There are a number of issues we need to consider when choosing the best *post hoc* test to use for our experimental data.

- Do I wish to compare all the groups against each other or am I only interested in comparisons to a control group?
- Are the group sizes equal?
- Are the variances of the groups equal?
- Does the test control the Type 1 error rate?
- Does the test control the Type 2 error rate (is the statistical power good)?
- Is the test robust?

The decision about whether to use a multiple All Means pairwise comparison test or multiple pairwise comparisons to a control group is absolutely critical, since the adjustment of the *p*-value for each individual comparison in order to control the overall Type 1 error rate is dependent on the total number of comparisons being made (see Table 10.3). The total number of comparisons made by standard *post hoc* procedures is dependent on whether we wish to compare all groups against each other or just compare a number of test groups to a control group (see Table 10.2). The following table (see Table 15.12) summarises the resulting effect on the adjusted *p*-value of individual comparisons after applying the Bonferroni correction to control the Type 1 error rate according to the type of *post hoc* procedure we wish to use. In all cases, the All Means procedures require a greater number of comparisons for a given number of groups in the experiment and consequently there is a greater adjustment of the *p*-value for an individual comparison in order to maintain the overall familywise Type 1 error rate.

In the experiments described above, Experiment 1 does not have an obvious control group and therefore the appropriate type of *post hoc* procedure should be a multiple All Means pairwise comparison test. In contrast, Experiment 2 clearly contains a control group and so the appropriate type of *post hoc* procedure should be multiple pairwise comparisons to a control group. In addition, we have already seen that there is a trade-off between the Type 1 error rate and statistical power (see Chapter 10). Table 15.13 summarises the most-commonly used *post hoc* procedures together with comments for general guidance regarding their use. *Post hoc* procedures that are very conservative and rigidly control the Type 1 error rate will consequently have low power resulting in meaningful differences being rejected. Getting the correct balance is important.

For multiple All Means pairwise comparisons, both the Fisher's least significant difference (LSD) and Studentised Newman-Keuls (SNK) fail to control the Type 1 error rate. In contrast, the Bonferroni (All Means) and Tukey tests control the Type 1 error rate but lack statistical power; generally, the Bonferroni has more power when the number of groups is small, while same is true for the Tukey test with a large number of groups. The Duncan and Scheffé procedures are less powerful than the Tukey test. If the group sizes are the same, then the REGWQ is a suitable alternative to the Bonferroni (All Means) or Tukey tests, while the Hochberg's GT2 and Gabriel's procedures are useful when the group sizes vary (N.B. the Hochberg's GT2 should not be used when the variances differ and the Gabriel's test risk Type 1 errors when the group sizes are very different). The remainder of the listed All Means comparison tests are useful in situations when the variances of the groups differ (of these the Games–Howell procedure is generally the best except when sample sizes are small).

For multiple pairwise comparisons to a control group, then the choice is between the Bonferroni (Control) procedure and the less-conservative Dunnett's test.

As a general guide then for All Means comparisons, I would recommend the REGWQ or Tukey test if the group variances are similar since both exert control over the Type 1 error rate and have good power – the Bonferroni (All Means) procedure is a good alternative as it has very good control over the Type 1 error rate but, consequently, has less statistical power. For Control Means

**Table 15.12** Adjusted *p*-values following Bonferroni correction to maintain the familywise Type 1 error rate at 0.05.

| Number of groups (N) | All Means comparisons | | Comparisons to control group | |
| | Comparisons N(N − 1)/2 | Bonferroni adjusted p | Comparisons N − 1 | Bonferroni adjusted p |
|---|---|---|---|---|
| 3 | 3 | 0.0167 | 2 | 0.025 |
| 4 | 6 | 0.0083 | 3 | 0.0167 |
| 5 | 10 | 0.005 | 4 | 0.0125 |
| 6 | 15 | 0.0033 | 5 | 0.01 |
| 7 | 21 | 0.00238 | 6 | 0.0083 |
| 8 | 28 | 0.00179 | 7 | 0.00714 |
| 9 | 36 | 0.00139 | 8 | 0.00625 |
| 10 | 45 | 0.00111 | 9 | 0.00556 |

Table values indicate the dependency of the total number of comparisons on the number of experimental groups for either All Means pairwise comparisons or pairwise comparisons to a control group.

98

Experimental Design and Statistical Analysis for Pharmacology and the Biomedical Sc...

**Table 15.13** *Post hoc* procedures.

| Test | Comment |
|---|---|
| **All Means comparisons** | |
| Fisher's least significant difference (LSD) | No control over Type 1 error rate, equivalent to multiple *t*-tests. |
| Studentised Newman–Keuls (SNK) | Lacks control over Type 1 error rate. More powerful but less conservative than Tukey. |
| Bonferroni (All Means) | Control Type 1 error, conservative. Better for small number of comparisons |
| Sidak | Based on *t* statistic but with control over Type 1 error rate (tighter than Bonferroni) |
| Tukey | Control Type 1 error, conservative. Better for large number of comparisons |
| Duncan's multiple range test (MRT) | Less power than Tukey. Similar to LSD but more power than SNK |
| Scheffé | Less power than Tukey. Used with unequal sample sizes |
| Ryan, Einot, Gabriel and Welch Q (REGWQ) | Modified SNK with control of Type 1 error rate and good power |
| Hochberg's GT2 | Similar to Tukey and Scheffé but used with unequal group sizes |
| Gabriel's | Similar to Hochberg's GT2 but more powerful |
| Tamhane's T2 | Unequal variances, conservative |
| Dunnett's T3 | Unequal variances, conservative |
| Games–Howell | Useful with unequal variances and group sizes |
| Dunnett's C | Unequal variances, conservative |
| **Control group comparisons** | |
| Bonferroni (Control) | Control Type 1 error, conservative. |
| Dunnett | Less conservative than Bonferroni |

comparisons, then there is little to choose between the Bonferroni (Control Means) and Dunnett's procedures, although the Dunnett's test is probably the test of choice where a large number of groups are involved.

## Data analysis step 2: *Post hoc* analysis

Given the above discussion, *post hoc* analysis of the data arising from Experiment 1 and Experiment 2 may be summarised as follows:

### Experiment 1:

Results of the multiple All Means pairwise comparisons are summarised in Table 15.14 (*post hoc* analysis following one-way ANOVA by Bonferroni (All Means) – results of Tukey test provided for comparison).

**Table 15.14** *Post hoc* analysis of Experiment 1 data.

| | Comparator groups | | Bonferroni (All Means) | Tukey test |
|---|---|---|---|---|
| 1 | Diet 1 | Diet 2 | 0.572 | 0.381 |
| 2 | Diet 1 | Diet 3 | 0.002 | 0.001 |
| 3 | Diet 2 | Diet 3 | 0.026 | 0.022 |

Table values indicate probability for Null Hypothesis is true according to *post hoc* test.

All Means *post hoc* analysis by either Bonferroni (All Means) test or Tukey test revealed that mice fed Diet 3 showed a significant difference in weight gain compared to that of mice fed Diet 1 ($p < 0.01$) or Diet 2 ($p < 0.05$), but there was no significant difference between the weight changes for mice fed Diet 1 compared to those fed Diet 2. I stated above that the Bonferroni (All Means) procedure is a good alternative to the Tukey test as it has very good control over the Type 1 error rate and is good for small group numbers but, consequently, has less statistical power. This is borne out by

the results in Table 15.14, where the adjusted *p*-values following Bonferroni correction are slightly greater than the corresponding *p*-values produced by the Tukey test. This means that for small group numbers, at least, we are slightly less likely to make a Type 1 error with the Bonferroni (All Means) test than with the Tukey test. Overall, however, the general conclusions to our experiment are the same (that Diet 3 induced a significantly different weight gain compared to mice fed Diets 1 or 2). It is important to note, however, that the results of the *post hoc* analysis alone do not indicate whether mice fed Diet 3 showed increased or decreased weight gain compared to that produced by the other diets used in the experiment. To identify the relative magnitude of the change in weight, we need to refer back to the results of the Descriptive Statistics (see Table 15.10). These results may be summarised in Figure 15.9. The results indicate that mice fed Diet 3 showed significantly increased weight gain compared to mice fed Diets 1 and 2.

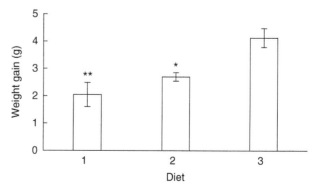

**Figure 15.9** **Effect of diet on weight gain in mice.** Three groups of weight- and age-matched mice ($n = 6$ per group) were allowed free access to palatable diet. Water was available *ad libitum*. Weights were recorded prior to diet access and after one month. X-axis indicates diet and Y-axis indicates weight gain (*g*) over one month. One-way ANOVA indicates significant variation in weight gain between the diets [$F(2,15) = 10.096$, $p = 0.002$]. *Post hoc* analysis (Bonferroni [All Means]); *$p < 0.05$, **$p < 0.01$ compared to Diet 3.

## Experiment 2:

Results of the multiple pairwise comparisons to a control group are summarised in Table 15.15 (*post hoc* analysis following one-way ANOVA by Dunnett's test for multiple comparisons).

Table 15.15 *Post hoc* analysis of Experiment 2 data.

| | Comparator groups | | Dunnett's test |
|---|---|---|---|
| 1 | Control | Drug A | 0.093 |
| 2 | Control | Drug B | 0.003 |
| 3 | Control | Drug C | 0.837 |

Table values indicate probability for Null Hypothesis is true according to *post hoc* Dunnett's test.

*Post hoc* analysis by Dunnett's test for multiple comparisons to a control group revealed that only Drug B induced a significant change in systolic blood pressure compared to the change observed in the control group ($p < 0.01$). In contrast, neither Drug A nor Drug C induced a significant change in systolic blood pressure compared to Control ($p > 0.05$ in both cases). As we saw with the results from Experiment 1, the results of the Dunnett's test similarly do not indicate whether Drug B induced a significant increase or decrease in systolic blood pressure. To identify the direction of change in systolic blood pressure induced by Drug B, we need to look at the results of the Descriptive Statistics (see Table 15.11). These results may be summarised in Figure 15.10. The results indicate that Drug B induced a significant increase in systolic blood pressure.

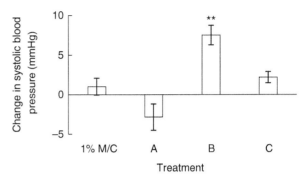

Figure 15.10 **Effect of drug treatment on systolic blood pressure in rats.** Four groups of rats ($n = 6$ per group) were treated orally with 1% methyl cellulose (1% M/C, 2.5 ml/kg) or Drugs A, B, or C, 20 mg/kg. *X*-axis indicates treatment and *Y*-axis indicates mean change in systolic blood pressure. One-way ANOVA indicates significant variation in systolic blood pressure [$F(3,20) = 12.335$, $p < 0.001$]. *Post hoc* analysis (Dunnett's test); **$p < 0.01$ compared to Control (1% M/C).

# Example output from statistical software

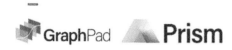

**A**

**B**

**C**

Summary statistical analysis from GraphPad Prism, v8. Panel A shows the results of the one-way ANOVA of the sleeping time data from Table 15.1. Panel B shows the results of the one-way ANOVA of the weight gain data from Table 15.10 together with the results of *post hoc* Bonferroni and Tukey (All Means) multiple comparison tests. Panel C summarises the results of the one-way ANOVA of the systolic blood pressure data from Table 15.11 together with the results of *post hoc* Dunnett's (Control) multiple comparison test.

*Source*: GraphPad Software.

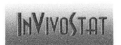

## A

View Analysis Log   Export to Html   Export Images

### InVivoStat Summary Statistics

#### Variable selection

Response Strain response is analysed in this module, with results categorised by factor Strain factor.

#### Summary statistics for Strain response categorised by Strain factor

| Categorisation Factor levels | Mean | N | Variance | Std dev | Lower 95% CI | Upper 95% CI |
|---|---|---|---|---|---|---|
| 1 | 16.0000 | 5 | 5.0000 | 2.2361 | 13.2236 | 18.7764 |
| 2 | 21.0000 | 5 | 12.5000 | 3.5355 | 16.6101 | 25.3899 |
| 3 | 16.6000 | 5 | 11.3000 | 3.3615 | 12.4261 | 20.7739 |

#### Analysis of variance (ANOVA) table

| Effect | Sums of squares | Degrees of freedom | Mean square | F-value | p-value |
|---|---|---|---|---|---|
| Strain factor | 74.533 | 2 | 37.267 | 3.88 | 0.0501 |
| Residual | 115.200 | 12 | 9.600 | | |

Comment: ANOVA table calculated using a Type III model fit, see Armitage et al. (2001).

Conclusion: There is no statistically significant overall difference between the levels of the treatment factor.

## B

View Analysis Log   Export to Html   Export Images

### InVivoStat Summary Statistics

#### Variable selection

Response Diet response is analysed in this module, with results categorised by factor Diet factor.

#### Summary statistics for Diet response categorised by Diet factor

| Categorisation Factor levels | Mean | N | Std dev | Lower 95% CI | Upper 95% CI |
|---|---|---|---|---|---|
| 1 | 2.0500 | 6 | 1.0747 | 0.9222 | 3.1778 |
| 2 | 2.7000 | 6 | 0.3847 | 2.2963 | 3.1037 |
| 3 | 4.1333 | 6 | 0.8501 | 3.2412 | 5.0255 |

#### All pairwise comparisons using Bonferroni's procedure

| Comparison | Difference | Lower 95% CI | Upper 95% CI | Std error | p-value |
|---|---|---|---|---|---|
| '1' - '2' | -0.650 | -1.661 | 0.361 | 0.474 | 0.5724 |
| '1' - '3' | -2.083 | -3.095 | -1.072 | 0.474 | 0.0016 |
| '2' - '3' | -1.433 | -2.445 | -0.422 | 0.474 | 0.0258 |

Conclusion: The following pairwise tests are statistically significantly different at the 5% level: '1' - '3', '2' - '3'.

#### Analysis of variance (ANOVA) table

| Effect | Sums of squares | Degrees of freedom | Mean square | F-value | p-value |
|---|---|---|---|---|---|
| Diet factor | 13.634 | 2 | 6.817 | 10.10 | 0.0017 |
| Residual | 10.128 | 15 | 0.675 | | |

Comment: ANOVA table calculated using a Type III model fit, see Armitage et al. (2001).

Conclusion: There is a statistically significant overall difference between the levels of Diet factor.

#### All pairwise comparisons using Tukey's procedure

| Comparison | Difference | Lower 95% CI | Upper 95% CI | Std error | p-value |
|---|---|---|---|---|---|
| '1' - '2' | -0.650 | -1.661 | 0.361 | 0.474 | 0.3806 |
| '1' - '3' | -2.083 | -3.095 | -1.072 | 0.474 | 0.0014 |
| '2' - '3' | -1.433 | -2.445 | -0.422 | 0.474 | 0.0221 |

Conclusion: The following pairwise tests are statistically significantly different at the 5% level: '1' - '3', '2' - '3'.

## C

View Analysis Log   Export to Html   Export Images                    Re-analyse

### InVivoStat Summary Statistics

#### Variable selection

Response SBP response is analysed in this module, with results categorised by factor SBP factor.

#### Summary statistics for SBP response categorised by SBP factor

| Categorisation Factor levels | Mean | N | Std dev | Lower 95% CI | Upper 95% CI | Min | Max | Median | Lower quartile | Upper quartile |
|---|---|---|---|---|---|---|---|---|---|---|
| 1 | 1.0000 | 6 | 2.6077 | -1.7366 | 3.7366 | -2.0000 | 5.0000 | 0.5000 | -1.0000 | 3.0000 |
| 2 | -2.8333 | 6 | 4.0702 | -7.1048 | 1.4381 | -8.0000 | 2.0000 | -3.0000 | -6.0000 | 1.0000 |
| 3 | 7.5000 | 6 | 3.0166 | 4.3343 | 10.6657 | 3.0000 | 12.0000 | 7.5000 | 6.0000 | 9.0000 |
| 4 | 2.1667 | 6 | 1.7224 | 0.3591 | 3.9742 | 0.0000 | 5.0000 | 2.0000 | 1.0000 | 3.0000 |

#### All to one comparisons using Dunnett's procedure

| Comparison | Difference | Lower 95% CI | Upper 95% CI | Std error | p-value |
|---|---|---|---|---|---|
| '2' - '1' | -3.833 | -7.418 | -0.249 | 1.718 | 0.0927 |
| '3' - '1' | 6.500 | 2.916 | 10.084 | 1.718 | 0.0034 |
| '4' - '1' | 1.167 | -2.418 | 4.751 | 1.718 | 0.8373 |

#### Analysis of variance (ANOVA) table

| Effect | Sums of squares | Degrees of freedom | Mean square | F-value | p-value |
|---|---|---|---|---|---|
| SBP factor | 327.792 | 3 | 109.264 | 12.33 | < 0.0001 |
| Residual | 177.167 | 20 | 8.858 | | |

Comment: ANOVA table calculated using a Type III model fit, see Armitage et al. (2001).

Conclusion: There is a statistically significant overall difference between the levels of SBP factor.

Summary statistical analysis from InVivoStat, v4.0.2. Panel A shows the summary descriptive statistics together with the results of the one-way ANOVA of the sleeping time data from Table 15.1. Panel B shows the summary descriptive statistics together with the results of the one-way ANOVA of the weight gain data from Table 15.10 and the results of *post hoc* Bonferroni and Tukey (All Means) multiple comparison tests. Panel C summarises the summary descriptive statistics together with the results of the one-way ANOVA of the systolic blood pressure data from Table 15.11 and the results of *post hoc* Dunnett's (Control) multiple comparison test.

*Source*: InVivoStat.

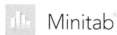 Minitab

## A

### Means

| Factor | N | Mean | St Dev | 95% CI |
|---|---|---|---|---|
| Strain 1 | 5 | 16.00 | 2.24 | (12.98, 19.02) |
| Strain 2 | 5 | 21.00 | 3.54 | (17.98, 24.02) |
| Strain 3 | 5 | 16.60 | 3.36 | (13.58, 19.62) |

*Pooled St Dev = 3.09839*

### Analysis of variance

| Source | DF | Adj SS | Adj MS | F-value | P-value |
|---|---|---|---|---|---|
| Factor | 2 | 74.53 | 37.267 | 3.88 | 0.050 |
| Error | 12 | 115.20 | 9.600 | | |
| Total | 14 | 189.73 | | | |

## B

### Means

| Factor | N | Mean | St Dev | 95% CI |
|---|---|---|---|---|
| Diet 1 | 6 | 2.050 | 1.075 | (1.335, 2.765) |
| Diet 2 | 6 | 2.700 | 0.385 | (1.985, 3.415) |
| Diet 3 | 6 | 4.133 | 0.850 | (3.418, 4.848) |

*Pooled St Dev = 0.821719*

### Analysis of variance

| Source | DF | Adj SS | Adj MS | F-value | P-value |
|---|---|---|---|---|---|
| Factor | 2 | 13.63 | 6.8172 | 10.10 | 0.002 |
| Error | 15 | 10.13 | 0.6752 | | |
| Total | 17 | 23.76 | | | |

### Tukey simultaneous tests for differences of means

| Difference of levels | Difference of means | SE of difference | 95% CI | T-Value | Adjusted P-value |
|---|---|---|---|---|---|
| Diet 2 – Diet 1 | 0.650 | 0.474 | (−0.581, 1.881) | 1.37 | 0.381 |
| Diet 3 – Diet 1 | 2.083 | 0.474 | (0.852, 3.314) | 4.39 | 0.001 |
| Diet 3 – Diet 2 | 1.433 | 0.474 | (0.202, 2.664) | 3.02 | 0.022 |

*Individual confidence level = 97.97%*

## C

### Means

| Factor | N | Mean | St Dev | 95% CI |
|---|---|---|---|---|
| SBP C | 6 | 1.00 | 2.61 | (−1.53, 3.53) |
| SBP DrgA | 6 | −2.83 | 4.07 | (−5.37, −0.30) |
| SBP DrgB | 6 | 7.50 | 3.02 | (4.97, 10.03) |
| SBP DrgC | 6 | 2.167 | 1.722 | (−0.368, 4.701) |

*Pooled St Dev = 2.97630*

### Analysis of variance

| Source | DF | Adj SS | Adj MS | F-value | P-value |
|---|---|---|---|---|---|
| Factor | 3 | 327.8 | 109.264 | 12.33 | 0.000 |
| Error | 20 | 177.2 | 8.858 | | |
| Total | 23 | 505.0 | | | |

### Dunnett simultaneous tests for level mean - control mean

| Difference of levels | Difference of means | SE of difference | 95% CI | T-value | Adjusted P-value |
|---|---|---|---|---|---|
| SBP DrgA – SBP C | −3.83 | 1.72 | (−8.20, 0.53) | −2.23 | 0.093 |
| SBP DrgB – SBP C | 6.50 | 1.72 | (2.13, 10.87) | 3.78 | 0.003 |
| SBP DrgC – SBP C | 1.17 | 1.72 | (−3.20, 5.53) | 0.68 | 0.837 |

*Individual confidence level = 98.05%*

Summary statistical analysis from MiniTab, v19. Panel A shows the summary descriptive statistics together with the results of the one-way ANOVA of the sleeping time data from Table 15.1. Panel B shows the summary descriptive statistics together with the results of the one-way ANOVA of the weight gain data from Table 15.10 and the results of *post hoc* Tukey (All Means) multiple comparison test. Panel C summarises the summary descriptive statistics together with the results of the one-way ANOVA of the systolic blood pressure data from Table 15.11 and the results of *post hoc* Dunnett's (Control) multiple comparison test.

*Source*: Minitab, LLC.

## A

➡ Oneway

**Descriptives**

Strains

| | | N | Mean | Std. Deviation | Std. Error | 95% Confidence Interval for Mean Lower Bound | Upper Bound | Minimum | Maximum | Between-Component Variance |
|---|---|---|---|---|---|---|---|---|---|---|
| 1.00 | | 5 | 16.0000 | 2.23607 | 1.00000 | 13.2236 | 18.7764 | 13.00 | 19.00 | |
| 2.00 | | 5 | 21.0000 | 3.53553 | 1.58114 | 16.6101 | 25.3899 | 17.00 | 26.00 | |
| 3.00 | | 5 | 16.6000 | 3.36155 | 1.50333 | 12.4261 | 20.7739 | 13.00 | 21.00 | |
| Total | | 15 | 17.8667 | 3.68136 | .95052 | 15.8280 | 19.9053 | 13.00 | 26.00 | |
| Model | Fixed Effects | | | 3.09839 | .80000 | 16.1236 | 19.6097 | | | |
| | Random Effects | | | | 1.57621 | 11.0848 | 24.6486 | | | 5.53333 |

**ANOVA**

Strains

| | Sum of Squares | df | Mean Square | F | Sig. |
|---|---|---|---|---|---|
| Between Groups | 74.533 | 2 | 37.267 | 3.882 | .050 |
| Within Groups | 115.200 | 12 | 9.600 | | |
| Total | 189.733 | 14 | | | |

## B

Oneway

**Descriptives**

Diets

| | | N | Mean | Std. Deviation | Std. Error | 95% Confidence Interval for Mean Lower Bound | Upper Bound | Minimum | Maximum | Between-Component Variance |
|---|---|---|---|---|---|---|---|---|---|---|
| 1.00 | | 6 | 2.0500 | 1.07471 | .43875 | .9222 | 3.1778 | .20 | 3.50 | |
| 2.00 | | 6 | 2.7000 | .38471 | .15706 | 2.2963 | 3.1037 | 2.20 | 3.30 | |
| 3.00 | | 6 | 4.1333 | .85010 | .34705 | 3.2412 | 5.0255 | 3.10 | 5.20 | |
| Total | | 18 | 2.9611 | 1.18229 | .27867 | 2.3732 | 3.5491 | .20 | 5.20 | |
| Model | Fixed Effects | | | .82172 | .19368 | 2.5483 | 3.3739 | | | |
| | Random Effects | | | | .61541 | .3132 | 5.6090 | | | 1.02367 |

**ANOVA**

Diets

| | Sum of Squares | df | Mean Square | F | Sig. |
|---|---|---|---|---|---|
| Between Groups | 13.634 | 2 | 6.817 | 10.096 | .002 |
| Within Groups | 10.128 | 15 | .675 | | |
| Total | 23.763 | 17 | | | |

**Post Hoc Tests**

**Multiple Comparisons**

Dependent Variable: Diets

| | (I) Diet_factor | (J) Diet_factor | Mean Difference (I-J) | Std. Error | Sig. | 95% Confidence Interval Lower Bound | Upper Bound |
|---|---|---|---|---|---|---|---|
| Tukey HSD | 1.00 | 2.00 | -.65000 | .47442 | .381 | -1.8823 | .5823 |
| | | 3.00 | -2.08333* | .47442 | .001 | -3.3156 | -.8510 |
| | 2.00 | 1.00 | .65000 | .47442 | .381 | -.5823 | 1.8823 |
| | | 3.00 | -1.43333* | .47442 | .022 | -2.6656 | -.2010 |
| | 3.00 | 1.00 | 2.08333* | .47442 | .001 | .8510 | 3.3156 |
| | | 2.00 | 1.43333* | .47442 | .022 | .2010 | 2.6656 |
| Bonferroni | 1.00 | 2.00 | -.65000 | .47442 | .572 | -1.9280 | .6280 |
| | | 3.00 | -2.08333* | .47442 | .002 | -3.3613 | -.8054 |
| | 2.00 | 1.00 | .65000 | .47442 | .572 | -.6280 | 1.9280 |
| | | 3.00 | -1.43333* | .47442 | .026 | -2.7113 | -.1554 |
| | 3.00 | 1.00 | 2.08333* | .47442 | .002 | .8054 | 3.3613 |
| | | 2.00 | 1.43333* | .47442 | .026 | .1554 | 2.7113 |

*. The mean difference is significant at the 0.05 level.

## C

➡ Oneway

**Descriptives**

SBPs

| | | N | Mean | Std. Deviation | Std. Error | 95% Confidence Interval for Mean Lower Bound | Upper Bound | Minimum | Maximum | Between-Component Variance |
|---|---|---|---|---|---|---|---|---|---|---|
| 1.00 | | 6 | 1.0000 | 2.60768 | 1.06458 | -1.7366 | 3.7366 | -2.00 | 5.00 | |
| 2.00 | | 6 | -2.8333 | 4.07022 | 1.66166 | -7.1048 | 1.4381 | -8.00 | 2.00 | |
| 3.00 | | 6 | 7.5000 | 3.01662 | 1.23153 | 4.3343 | 10.6657 | 3.00 | 12.00 | |
| 4.00 | | 6 | 2.1667 | 1.72240 | .70317 | .3591 | 3.9742 | .00 | 5.00 | |
| Total | | 24 | 1.9583 | 4.68559 | .95644 | -.0202 | 3.9369 | -8.00 | 12.00 | |
| Model | Fixed Effects | | | 2.97630 | .60753 | .6910 | 3.2256 | | | |
| | Random Effects | | | | 2.13370 | -4.8320 | 8.7487 | | | 16.73426 |

**ANOVA**

SBPs

| | Sum of Squares | df | Mean Square | F | Sig. |
|---|---|---|---|---|---|
| Between Groups | 327.792 | 3 | 109.264 | 12.335 | .000 |
| Within Groups | 177.167 | 20 | 8.858 | | |
| Total | 504.958 | 23 | | | |

**Post Hoc Tests**

**Multiple Comparisons**

Dependent Variable: SBPs
Dunnett t (2-sided)[a]

| (I) SBP_factors | (J) SBP_factors | Mean Difference (I-J) | Std. Error | Sig. | 95% Confidence Interval Lower Bound | Upper Bound |
|---|---|---|---|---|---|---|
| 2.00 | 1.00 | -3.83333 | 1.71836 | .093 | -8.1986 | .5320 |
| 3.00 | 1.00 | 6.50000* | 1.71836 | .003 | 2.1347 | 10.8653 |
| 4.00 | 1.00 | 1.16667 | 1.71836 | .837 | -3.1986 | 5.5320 |

*. The mean difference is significant at the 0.05 level.

a. Dunnett t-tests treat one group as a control, and compare all other groups against it.

Summary statistical analysis from SPSS, v27. Panel A shows the summary descriptive statistics together with the results of the one-way ANOVA of the sleeping time data from Table 15.1. Panel B shows the summary descriptive statistics together with the results of the one-way ANOVA of the weight gain data from Table 15.10 and the results of *post hoc* Bonferroni and Tukey (All Means) multiple comparison tests. Panel C summarises the summary descriptive statistics together with the results of the one-way ANOVA of the systolic blood pressure data from Table 15.11 and the results of *post hoc* Dunnett's (Control) multiple comparison test.

*Source*: IBM Corporation.

# 16 Repeated measure analysis of variance

## Introduction

In Chapter 10, I described how data sets may be differentiated either by Between-Group factors (e.g. different treatment groups) or Within-Group Factors (i.e. repeated measurements taken from the same set of subjects), and in Chapters 11 and 12, I described how this gave rise to two different types of *t*-test to compare two groups of parametric data depending on whether our data were obtained from two independent groups of subjects (i.e. independent *t*-test, Chapter 11) or from two measurements obtained from a single group of subjects (i.e. paired *t*-test, Chapter 12). In the same way, we need to employ different models of Analysis of Variance when we analyse more than two groups of data. Chapter 15 described (in depth!) the one-way ANOVA to analyse more than two groups of independent data sets. But what model do we use when we have a single group of subjects but take successive readings from them during the course of the experiment? Clearly, it is appropriate to think of such data sets as **paired** rather than independent. This raises a problem since one assumption of the one-way ANOVA is that the data sets are independent. Consequently, when repeated measurements are obtained in an experiment, then this assumption of independency is violated, and so it would be incorrect to employ a one-way ANOVA model with one Between-Group Factor (if you don't know why this is so then go back and read Chapter 15 again!); instead, we need to use a model that has one Within-Group Factor which reflects the paired nature of the data. If data from a repeated measures design experiment were analysed by a one-way ANOVA, then the result would lack accuracy since the individual scores obtained at each time point within the experiment are likely to be related as they come from the same subjects. So, the ANOVA model to use here is called a **Repeated Measures Analysis of Variance,** and the values used in the analysis are the *differences* between the observed values at different time points during the experiment. To my mind, therefore, Within-Group Factors in an experiment are always a function of time; such experiments may be the time course of drug-induced changes in the behaviour of subjects induced by psychotropic drugs, the sequential changes in blood pressure or heart rate observed over time following treatment with drugs that act on the cardiovascular system, and even the sequential estimates of the number of cells in a cell culture incubated in a particular medium (e.g. population dynamics of a mammalian cell line).

## Repeated measures ANOVA

We have already seen that a repeated measures design of experiment violates the assumption of independency that underpins a one-way ANOVA. In addition, because the scores at different time points in the experiment come from the same subjects and that we are interested in the difference between these scores, then we must assume that there is a relationship between these scores which is constant throughout the experiment. If this is being true, then the variance in the observed differences from the first to the second time point would be similar to the variance in the differences from the second to the third time point, and so on right through successive time points until the penultimate and last set of observations. If

this is the case, then the same argument would apply to alternate time points (i.e. time 1 to time 3, time 2 to time 4, etc.). This is akin to the assumption of homogeneity of variance that underpins a one-way ANOVA, and for repeated measures design of experiments is known as **sphericity** (sometimes referred to as *circularity*) and denoted by the symbol $\varepsilon$ by statisticians. So, to put it more simply, sphericity is the equality of variances of the *differences* between sets of observations taken at different time points throughout the experiment. Thus, if we were to take each pair of time points and calculate the differences for each pair of observations, then these differences would have near equal variances in order to preserve the assumption of sphericity. It is important to note that sphericity is not an issue for the paired *t*-test since there are only one set of differences in the analysis; for sphericity to be an issue, there must be at least three sets of repeated measurements in the data set.

## Assessing sphericity

Assume, we run an experiment where the heart rates of a single group of subjects are measured at the beginning of the experiment ($T_0$) and then again after 30 ($T_{30}$) and 60 ($T_{60}$) minutes. The assumption of sphericity may be summarised as follows:

$$\text{variance}_{(T_0 - T_{30})} \approx \text{variance}_{(T_0 - T_{60})} \approx \text{variance}_{(T_{30} - T_{60})} \quad (16.1)$$

The sphericity of the data may be assessed by using **Mauchly's test** which tests the hypothesis that the variances of the differences between the various time points of the experiment are equal. The Null Hypothesis of Mauchly's test is that there are no differences between the variances of the differences between the sets of data obtained in the experiment, i.e. that the variances of the differences are almost equal. In contrast, the assumption of sphericity is not met if the probability of Mauchly's test statistic is <0.05; here we would reject the Null Hypothesis of equality of the variances of the differences between the sets of data and conclude that the assumption of sphericity has been violated. If this happens, then there are implications for the Type 1 error rate associated not only with the ANOVA model (so the risk of concluding that there are differences between our observations at different time points is erroneously increased, i.e. the ANOVA model has less power), but also for any *post hoc* pairwise comparisons.

The amount of sphericity in a set of data may be estimated and this value may then be used to adjust the degrees of freedom for any *F*-ratio resulting from the ANOVA model to compensate if the assumption of sphericity is violated. If the complete data set is spherical, then the estimate of sphericity equals 1, but progressively less than 1 as the level of violation increases. It is then simply a matter of multiplying the degrees of freedom by the amount of sphericity. The logic behind this approach is that if there is no violation of sphericity then the degrees of freedom (and hence the *p*-value for a given F-ratio) do not change. However, smaller degrees of freedom (which obviously follow when each original value is multiplied by a sphericity estimate less than 1) result in a larger *p*-value for a given *F*-ratio, thereby making the *F*-ratio more conservative which in turn exerts a level of control over the Type 1 error rate (see above).

*Experimental Design and Statistical Analysis for Pharmacology and the Biomedical Sciences*, First Edition. Paul J. Mitchell.

There are two estimates of sphericity that are used to adjust the degrees of freedom: the **Greenhouse–Geisser** and **Huynh–Feldt** estimates.

- *Greenhouse–Geisser estimate*

This estimate of sphericity has a range of values from 1 down to $1/(k-1)$, where $k$ is the number of repeated measure time points in the experiment. The lower value is known as the *lower-bound estimate* of sphericity.

- *Huynh–Feldt estimate*

The Huynh–Feldt estimate of sphericity is generally used when the Greenhouse–Geisser estimate is greater than 0.75 where the resulting correction of the probability associated with the $F$-ratio would be too conservative.

As a general rule, the Greenhouse–Geisser estimate is the preferred value of sphericity used to adjust the degrees of freedom whenever a repeated measures ANOVA is used except where the Greenhouse–Geisser estimate is greater than 0.75 whereupon the Huynh–Feldt estimate should be used.

Conceptually the Repeated Measures ANOVA is very similar to the one-way ANOVA discussed in Chapter 15 (*indeed the Repeated Measures ANOVA is often referred to as a Repeated Measures one-way ANOVA or one-way Repeated Measures ANOVA; I personally avoid this terminology as there is no clear distinction between these two names which subsequently only leads to confusion, especially for those of us – myself included – trying to get to grips with the vagaries of statistical analysis*). If you remember (if not go back to Chapter 15, do not pass Go, do not collect £200, etc.) in a one-way ANOVA, the sum of squares and variance are compartmentalised into the Between-Group and Within-Group compartments, which when added together gives the Total Sum of Squares and variance in the data set (see Table 15.7). The same general approach is taken in the Repeated Measures ANOVA.

In the repeated measures ANOVA, the total sum of squares, and hence the total variance, is calculated in exactly the same way as for the one-way ANOVA. So, the first stage of the analysis is to calculate the Grand Mean and the total variance of the data.

### Grand mean and sum of squares

$$\overline{X}_{\text{Grand}} = \frac{11\,646}{48} = 242.625 \tag{16.2}$$

We then calculate the difference for each observation in the whole data set from the Grand Mean. Each difference from the Grand Mean is then squared and these valued added together to produce the Total Sum of Squares (denoted by $SSQ_T$), thus,

$$SSQ_T = \sum \left(\overline{X}_{\text{Grand}} - x\right)^2 = 1\,893\,497.25 \tag{16.3}$$

### Grand variance

If we do this for all the locomotor activity scores arising from our experiment, then the total variance (denoted by $s^2_{\text{Total}}$) is simply the total SSQ for all the observations divided by the degrees of freedom (i.e. total number of observations – 1), thus,

$$s^2_{\text{Total}} = \frac{SSQ_T}{N_{\text{total}} - 1} = \frac{1\,893\,497.25}{47} = 40\,287.17553 \tag{16.4}$$

In the one-way ANOVA described in Chapter 15, we saw that the variance may be compartmentalised into the variance *between* the different groups and *within* each group (see Chapter 15). In a Repeated Measures ANOVA, the total variability is compartmentalised into the between-subject variability and the variance component for the individual differences for each subject throughout the course of the experiment; this is referred to as the within-subject (sometimes called within-participant) variance.

## Example 16.1 Repeated measures data

Consider the following experiment. The locomotor activity of a single group of eight adult male Wistar rats was monitored in an activity monitor. Each rat was placed into the monitor and its activity recorded in 5 minutes time bins for 30 minutes. Notice that there is no treatment involved in this experiment as we are simply interested in how the animals' activity changes over time. The resulting activity measurements are shown in Table 16.1. The Null Hypothesis for the Repeated Measures ANOVA would state that there is no variation in the observed data throughout the duration of the experiment.

**Table 16.1** Locomotor activity of male Wistar rats.

| | 0–5 | 5–10 | 10–15 | 15–20 | 20–25 | 25–30 | Mean |
|---|---|---|---|---|---|---|---|
| 1 | 583 | 347 | 200 | 120 | 75 | 72 | 232.83 |
| 2 | 654 | 475 | 325 | 140 | 82 | 60 | 289.33 |
| 3 | 555 | 333 | 203 | 65 | 126 | 78 | 226.67 |
| 4 | 590 | 354 | 110 | 232 | 29 | 57 | 228.67 |
| 5 | 727 | 462 | 210 | 129 | 78 | 128 | 289.00 |
| 6 | 479 | 250 | 115 | 76 | 148 | 55 | 187.17 |
| 7 | 614 | 370 | 229 | 143 | 56 | 20 | 238.67 |
| 8 | 622 | 357 | 300 | 60 | 32 | 121 | 248.67 |
| Mean | 603.0 | 368.5 | 211.5 | 120.6 | 78.3 | 73.9 | |

The columns 0–5 to 25–30 are grouped under the heading **Time (min)**.

Table values indicate locomotor activity counts for each animal ($n = 8$) according to each five-min time bin. Mean values indicate the arithmetic mean for each subject (far right column) and each time bin (bottom row).

### Within-subject sum of squares and variance

In the one-way ANOVA, we had different subjects for each Between-Group factor in the experiment. In the Repeated Measures ANOVA, however, we are interested in the variation of the scores for each subject *across* the different conditions (e.g. time points) of the experiment. Consequently, the within-subject sum of squares (denoted by $SSQ_W$) is determined by first calculating the mean and sum of squares value for each subject throughout the experiment and then adding all these values together. So, if you refer to Table 16.1, this means we need to calculate the mean and sum of squares values for each *row* of data (corresponding to each individual subject; see far right column in Table 16.1 for the calculated mean values) rather than calculating the mean and sum of squares values for each *column* of data as we would if each group of data were obtained from independent groups of subjects at each time point of the experiment. From these values, we can calculate the within-subject variance for each subject by dividing the sum of squares value by the appropriate degrees of freedom for each subject (i.e. number of observations for each subject minus 1). The resulting data for each subject are summarised in Table 16.2.

Table 16.2 Within-subject mean, sum of squares, and variance.

| Subject | Mean | Sum of Squares | Variance |
|---------|--------|----------------|-----------|
| 1 | 232.83 | 200 238.83 | 40 047.77 |
| 2 | 289.33 | 286 607.33 | 57 321.47 |
| 3 | 226.67 | 178 041.33 | 35 608.27 |
| 4 | 228.67 | 229 699.33 | 45 939.87 |
| 5 | 289.00 | 324 056.00 | 64 811.20 |
| 6 | 187.17 | 125 682.83 | 25 136.57 |
| 7 | 238.67 | 248 551.33 | 49 710.27 |
| 8 | 248.67 | 252 587.33 | 50 517.47 |
| Within-subject $SSQ_W$ | | 1 845 464.33 | |

If we now calculate the sum of all the individual sum of squares values, then we obtain the total within-subject sum of squares, thus,

$$SSQ_W = 1\ 845\ 464.33 \qquad (16.5)$$

The within-subject degrees of freedom are calculated by adding all the individual degrees of freedom together for each subject. For the current data set, this is equal to the number of repeated measurements per subject minus 1 multiplied by the number of subjects, i.e.,

$$df_w = N(n_s - 1) = 8(6-1) = 8 \times 5 = 40 \qquad (16.6)$$

where $N$ = number of subjects and $n_s$ = the number of repeated observations per subject.

The within-subject variance may then be summarised as follows (Table 16.3).

Table 16.3 Summary of within-subject variance data.

| Source | $SSQ_W$ | df | Variance |
|--------|---------|------|----------|
| Total | 1 845 464.33 | 40 | 46 136.61 |

So, at this stage, we know that the total amount of variation in the data set, i.e. the total sum of squares, is 1 893 497.25, while 1 845 464.33 of that is due to the change in the scores of each individual throughout the course of the experiment. The next stage of the analysis is to determine how much of the change in the individual scores is due to experimental manipulation (in this experiment this is the effect of time) or just random variation.

### The model sum of squares and variance

In the independent one-way ANOVA, we determined how much variation was due to the Between-Group factor by comparing the mean for each group to the Grand Mean of the whole set of data (see *Between-Group* variance in Chapter 15). In the Repeated Measures ANOVA, we do exactly the same thing where we compare the mean of the data obtained at each stage of the experiment (i.e. the various stages for the Within-Group Factor) to the Grand Mean of all the observations (see above). The resulting **model sum of squares (denoted by $SSQ_M$) and variance** reflect the differences in the observations taken at each stage of the experiment.

So, the first step is to determine the mean value for each stage of the experiment (see bottom row in Table 16.1) following which the difference between the mean value for each stage of the experiment and the Grand Mean is calculated (Grand Mean = 242.625; see equation 16.2). Each difference is then squared before the contribution of each stage of the experiment to the model sum of squares value is calculated by multiplying the squared difference value by the number of subjects in the appropriate sample. The model sum of squares, $SSQ_M$, is then calculated by adding together the contributions from each stage of the experiment (see Table 16.4). Once the $SSQ_M$ has been calculated, then it is just a simple matter of dividing this value by the model degrees of freedom to calculate the model variance. The model degrees of freedom ($df_M$) is simply the number of repeated measures in the experiment – one. If you look back at Chapter 15, you will see this is *exactly* the same procedure as that used to determine the Between-Group SSQ for the independent one-way ANOVA.

Thus,

$$SSQ_M = 1\ 736\ 354.83 \qquad (16.7)$$

$$df_M = 6 - 1 = 5 \qquad (16.8)$$

$$s_M^2 = \frac{SSQ_M}{df_M} = \frac{1\ 736\ 354.83}{5} = 347\ 270.966 \qquad (16.9)$$

Table 16.4 Calculation of Between-Sample variance.

| | Time (min) | | | | | |
|---|---|---|---|---|---|---|
| | 0–5 | 5–10 | 10–15 | 15–20 | 20–25 | 25–30 |
| Mean ($\bar{x}$) | 603.0 | 368.5 | 211.5 | 120.6 | 78.3 | 73.9 |
| Difference from Grand Mean $\bar{X}_{Grand} - \bar{x}$ | 360.375 | 125.875 | −31.125 | −122.025 | −164.325 | −168.253 |
| Difference from Grand Mean squared $(\bar{X}_{Grand} - \bar{x})^2$ | 129 870.141 | 15 844.516 | 968.766 | 14 890.101 | 27 002.706 | 28 468.126 |
| (Difference from Grand Mean squared) × N | 1 038 961.13 | 126 756.13 | 7750.13 | 119 120.81 | 216 021.65 | 227 745.01 |

Table values indicate locomotor activity counts calculated from raw values provided in Table 16.1. Grand Mean value = 242.625 activity units
Model $SSQ_M$ = 1 736 354.83

The model sum of squares and variance data may then be summarised with the total within-subject variance data; see Table 16.5.

Table 16.5 Summary of model and within-subject variance data.

| Source | SSQ | df | Variance |
|---|---|---|---|
| Model | 1 736 354.83 | 5 | 347 270.966 |
| Within subject | 1 845 464.33 | 40 | 46 136.61 |

So, at this stage, we know that the total amount of variation in the data set, i.e. the total sum of squares, is 1 893 497.25, while 1 845 464.33 of that is due to the change in the scores of each individual throughout the course of the experiment. Furthermore, the change in the individual scores due to the experimental manipulation is able to account for 1 736 354.83 of this variation. Any remaining variation is consequently due to factors outside of our experimental control and is known as the residual sum of squares.

### Residual sum of squares and variance

We have already calculated the within-subject and model sum of squares, $SSQ_W$ and $SSQ_M$, respectively, and the easiest way to calculate the remaining residual sum of squares (denoted by $SSQ_R$) is to subtract the model sum of squares from the within-subject sum of squares, thus,

$$SSQ_R = SSQ_W - SSQ_M$$
$$= 1\ 845\ 464.33 - 1\ 736\ 354.83 \qquad (16.10)$$
$$= 109\ 109.5$$

Similarly, we can calculate the residual degrees of freedom ($df_R$) in the same way:

$$df_R = df_W - df_M = 40 - 5 = 35 \qquad (16.11)$$

The residual data may then be summarised along with the appropriate model and within-subject data, see Table 16.6.

Table 16.6 Summary of model, residual, and within-subject variance data.

| Source | SSQ | df | Variance |
|---|---|---|---|
| Model | 1 736 354.83 | 5 | 347 270.966 |
| Residual | 109 109.50 | 35 | 3 117.414 |
| Within subject | 1 845 464.33 | 40 | |

This table now allows the $F$-ratio of the model and residual variance values to be calculated which, with the appropriate degrees of freedom, allows the probability of the Null Hypothesis is true to be determined (see Table 16.7).

Table 16.7 Repeated measures ANOVA.

| Source | SSQ | df | Variance | F-ratio | p |
|---|---|---|---|---|---|
| Model | 1 736 354.83 | 5 | 347 270.966 | 111.397 | <0.001 |
| Residual | 109 109.50 | 35 | 3 117.414 | | |
| Within subject | 1 845 464.33 | 40 | | | |

As with the independent one-way ANOVA, the value of the $F$-ratio may be compared to the critical values of $F$ according to the degrees of freedom for the model and residual values. The critical values of the $F$ distribution are provided in Appendix E, indeed Table E.3 indicates that the critical value for $F$ with 5 and 35 degrees of freedom where $p = 0.001$ is approximately 5.30. The calculated $F$-ratio from the experiment described here is 111.397 which far exceeds the critical value 5.30 and so you might assume that this result provides sufficient statistical support to reject the Null Hypothesis and conclude that there is significant variation across the duration of the experiment suggesting that locomotor activity changes over time. The resulting F-ratio and associated $p$-value provided in Table 16.7 should not be taken at face value, however, since at this stage we have not examined the possible issue of sphericity. Indeed, the values reported in Table 16.7 only apply where sphericity is assumed. To complete the Repeated Measures ANOVA, we therefore need to run Mauchly's test to assess the sphericity of the data. I shall return to this issue in a moment (see below).

I mentioned at the beginning of this chapter that the total variability of a Repeated Measures ANOVA is partitioned into the between- and within-subject variances. The between-subject variance is not required to calculate the F-ratio, but it is important to look at this value since it represents the differences between individual subjects in our experiment. We have already calculated the total and within-subject sum of squares values ($SSQ_T$ and $SSQ_W$, respectively) so it is easy to calculate the between-subject SSQ (denoted by $SSQ_B$).

Thus,

$$SSQ_B = SSQ_T - SSQ_W$$
$$= 1\ 893\ 497.25 - 1\ 845\ 464.33 \qquad (16.12)$$
$$= 48\ 032.92$$

In the experiment described here, the between-subject SSQ suggests that less than 3% of the total variability in the differences in locomotor activity across the course of the experiment may be explained by individual differences between the subjects alone.

## Mauchly's test

Applying Mauchly's test to the experimental data reveals Mauchly's $W = 0.031$ with $\chi^2(14) = 17.76$, $p = 0.265$ (see screenshots from SPSS v27 at the end of this chapter). Since the probability is greater than the critical value of 0.05, we may assume that the assumption of sphericity has not been violated and consequently we may accept the result of the repeated measures ANOVA without any modification of the degrees of freedom by either the Greenhouse–Geiser or Huynh–Feldt estimates. Interestingly, for the Greenhouse–Geiser estimate for these data $\hat{\varepsilon} = 0.559$, while for the Huynh–Feldt estimate $\hat{\varepsilon} = 0.967$. For the Greenhouse–Geiser estimate, the range of possible values lies between 1 (where the data are perfectly spherical) down to the lower-bound value (see description of Greenhouse–Geiser estimate above). For the set of data described here, the lower-bound value of the Greenhouse–Geiser estimate = $1/(6 - 1) = 0.2$. Consequently, the Greenhouse–Geiser estimate of sphericity lies approximately mid-way between its possible range of values, while that for the Huynh–Feldt lies very close to 1. Taken together, these results indicate that for this data set at least sphericity has not been violated.

Consequently, the result of the Repeated Measures ANOVA may be summarised as follows: $F(5,35) = 111.397$, $p < 0.001$. Remember, when you report the results of a Repeated Measures ANOVA, then you _must_ support your ANOVA summary with the results of the Mauchly's test. In those situations where

Mauchly's test suggests that the assumption of sphericity has been violated, then you *must* correct your degrees of freedom by applying the Greenhouse–Geiser or Huynh–Feldt estimate; in both cases you simply multiply the original degrees of freedom by the appropriate $\hat{\varepsilon}$ value and then test the $F$-ratio against the adjusted degrees of freedom.

## Post hoc tests

The result of the Repeated Measures ANOVA for the experimental data used here strongly suggests that the probability of the Null Hypothesis (which states that there is no variation in locomotor activity of the experimental subjects across the course of the experiment) is very low. Consequently, we may reject the Null Hypothesis and conclude that there is very strong evidence of variability between the locomotor activity at different time points during the experiment. As we saw earlier with the independent one-way ANOVA, such an analysis does not tell us which groups are significantly different from each other; to determine which groups differ significantly we need to examine the data using *post hoc* tests. Again, the same question arises as to whether we wish to compare each group against all the others, or whether we are only interested in a limited number of comparisons due to the presence of a group of data that could legitimately be labelled a control group.

As already stated at the beginning of this chapter, we need to consider the data sets in a repeated measures experimental design as paired rather than independent. This, coupled with the sphericity-related issues described above, indicates that the standard *post hoc* tests for independent experimental designs (as listed in Table 15.13) should **not** be used for multiple comparison analysis of repeated measures (i.e. paired) data sets.

## All Means comparisons

Recommended All Means multiple comparisons *post hoc* tests are primarily the Tukey test, which may be used when sphericity is not violated (see Mauchly's test above), or preferably the Games–Howell procedure (which uses a pooled error term) if sphericity cannot be assumed. Some software programmes allow the Fisher's LSD *post hoc* test, but this test does not adjust the reported $p$-value and therefore has no control over the Type 1 error rate and so is not recommended. An alternative procedure is to examine the **Confidence Intervals** of the differences using the Tukey test with either Bonferroni or Sidak correction. These *post hoc* multiple comparisons are performed across the three levels of the within-subject factor. Tables 16.8 and 16.9 summarise the $p$-values for each comparison of the confidence intervals of the differences with Bonferroni and Sidak correction, respectively, which provide control over the Type 1 error rate and essentially provide the same information, although the Sidak test is slightly less conservative.

**Table 16.8** Bonferroni-corrected *post hoc* analysis.

| Time bin (min) | Time bin (min) | | | | |
|---|---|---|---|---|---|
| | 5–10 | 10–15 | 15–20 | 20–25 | 25–30 |
| 0–5 | $p < 0.001$ | $p < 0.001$ | $p < 0.001$ | $p < 0.001$ | $p < 0.001$ |
| 5–10 | | 0.003 | 0.001 | 0.001 | $p < 0.001$ |
| 10–15 | | | 0.732 | 0.089 | 0.019 |
| 15–20 | | | | 1.000 | 1.000 |
| 20–25 | | | | | 1.000 |

Table values indicate probability values for each pairwise comparison, as indicated. Data analysed using SPSS, v27.

**Table 16.9** Sidak-corrected *post hoc* analysis.

| Time bin (min) | Time bin (min) | | | | |
|---|---|---|---|---|---|
| | 5–10 | 10–15 | 15–20 | 20–25 | 25–30 |
| 0–5 | $p < 0.001$ | $p < 0.001$ | $p < 0.001$ | $p < 0.001$ | $p < 0.001$ |
| 5–10 | | 0.003 | 0.001 | 0.001 | $p < 0.001$ |
| 10–15 | | | 0.528 | 0.085 | 0.019 |
| 15–20 | | | | 0.969 | 0.874 |
| 20–25 | | | | | 1.000 |

Table values indicate probability values for each pairwise comparison, as indicated. Data analysed using SPSS, v27.

## Control group comparisons

It may be possible in some experimental designs to identify a potential control group within the resulting groups of data. In this particular experiment, there seems to be a decline in the magnitude of locomotor activity expressed by the group of rats during the experiment which appears to stabilise after about 25 minutes. The initial elevated levels of locomotion are often referred to as exploratory locomotor activity where the subjects explore their new environment. In contrast, the latter, stable, level of locomotion is usually referred to as the baseline locomotor activity. One possible aim of this experiment would be to determine whether the elevated level of locomotion during the exploratory phase is significantly different from the baseline. It makes sense therefore to set either the first or the last epoch as the control level. By doing this, we also limit the number of possible pairwise comparisons of the data, which therefore has a less detrimental effect on the adjusted $p$-value (see Table 10.2). One possible strategy to compare these groups of data would be to perform multiple comparisons using the paired $t$-test with Bonferroni correction to control the Type 1 error rate. Table 16.10 summarises the results of multiple comparisons using the paired $t$-test applied to the locomotor activity where the final time bin (25–30 minutes) has been set as the control group.

**Table 16.10** Multiple paired $t$-tests with Bonferroni correction.

| Control (min) | Test (min) | $T$ | df | $p$ | Corrected $p$ |
|---|---|---|---|---|---|
| 25–30 | 0–5 | 23.578 | 7 | <0.001 | <0.01 |
| 25–30 | 5–10 | 11.882 | 7 | <0.001 | <0.01 |
| 25–30 | 10–15 | 5.178 | 7 | 0.001 | <0.01 |
| 25–30 | 15–20 | 1.721 | 7 | 0.129 | >0.05 |
| 25–30 | 20–25 | 0.212 | 7 | 0.838 | >0.05 |

Table values summarise the results of repeated paired $t$-tests of locomotor activity data with the original probability ($p$) and the adjusted probability (Corrected $p$) after applying the Bonferroni correction.

The results of this experiment are summarised in Figure 16.1 and indicate that the group of eight male Wistar rats expressed elevated levels of locomotor activity during the first 15 minutes of the recording period that progressively returned to baseline levels by 20–25 following introduction of each subject to the activity monitor.

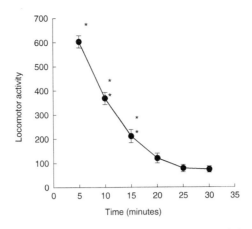

**Figure 16.1** Effect of time on locomotor activity expressed by male Wistar rats. Locomotor activity was recorded every 5 minutes for a total of 30 minutes. $N = 8$ subjects. Repeated measures ANOVA revealed significant variation in locomotion throughout the period of recording [$F(5,35) = 111.397$, $p < 0.001$. Mauchly's test, $p = 0.265$]. $**p < 0.01$ (paired $t$-test with Bonferroni correction) compared to time period 25–30 minutes.

# Example output from statistical software

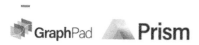

**A**

Summary statistical analysis from GraphPad Prism, v8. Panel A shows the summary of the descriptive statistics of the rodent locomotor activity data from Table 16.1, together with the results of the Repeated Measures ANOVA (compared to Table 16.7), the results of the *post hoc* Bonferroni and Sidak (All Means) multiple comparison tests (compared to Tables 16.8 and 16.9, respectively) and the Bonferroni multiple comparison test where the final 25–30 minutes time period was assigned as the baseline control group (see Table 16.10 for comparison to multiple paired *t*-tests with Bonferroni correction).

*Source*: GraphPad Software.

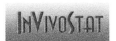

*Analysis of a single Within Group factor not available at the time of writing.*

Minitab®

A

### Statistics

| Variable | Mean | SE mean | St Dev |
|---|---|---|---|
| 0–5 | 603.0 | 25.6 | 72.4 |
| 5–10 | 368.5 | 25.4 | 71.9 |
| 10–15 | 211.5 | 27.0 | 76.4 |
| 15–20 | 120.6 | 19.9 | 56.2 |
| 20–25 | 78.3 | 14.8 | 41.8 |
| 25–30 | 73.9 | 12.6 | 35.7 |

### Analysis of variance

| Source | DF | Adj SS | Adj MS | F-value | P-value |
|---|---|---|---|---|---|
| Time | 5 | 1736505 | 347301 | 111.56 | 0.000 |
| Subject | 7 | 48033 | 6862 | 2.20 | 0.058 |
| Error | 35 | 108959 | 3113 | | |
| Total | 47 | 1893497 | | | |

### Estimation for paired difference

| | | | 95% CI for |
|---|---|---|---|
| Mean | St Dev | SE mean | μ_difference |
| −529.1 | 63.5 | 22.4 | (−582.2,−476.1) |

μ_difference: population mean of (25-30-0-5)

### Test

Null hypothesis $H_0$: μ_difference = 0
Alternative $H_1$: μ_difference ≠ 0
hypothesis

| T-value | P-value |
|---|---|
| −23.58 | 0.000 |

### Estimation for paired difference

| | | | 95% CI for |
|---|---|---|---|
| Mean | St Dev | SE mean | μ_difference |
| −294.6 | 70.1 | 24.8 | (−353.3,−236.0) |

μ_difference: population mean of (25-30 - 5-10)

### Test

Null hypothesis $H_0$: μ_difference = 0
Alternative $H_1$: μ_difference ≠ 0
hypothesis

| T-value | P-value |
|---|---|
| −11.88 | 0.000 |

### Estimation for paired difference

| | | | 95% CI for |
|---|---|---|---|
| Mean | St Dev | SE mean | μ_difference |
| −137.6 | 75.2 | 26.6 | (−200.5,−74.8) |

μ_difference: population mean of (25-30 -10-15)

### Test

Null hypothesis $H_0$: μ_difference = 0
Alternative $H_1$: μ_difference ≠ 0
hypothesis

| T-value | P-value |
|---|---|
| −5.18 | 0.001 |

### Estimation for paired difference

| | | | 95% CI for |
|---|---|---|---|
| Mean | St Dev | SE mean | μ_difference |
| −46.8 | 76.8 | 27.2 | (−111.0, 17.5) |

μ_difference: population mean of (25-30-15-20)

### Test

Null hypothesis $H_0$: μ_difference = 0
Alternative $H_1$: μ_difference ≠ 0
hypothesis

| T-value | P-value |
|---|---|
| −1.72 | 0.129 |

### Estimation for paired difference

| | | | 95% CI for |
|---|---|---|---|
| Mean | St Dev | SE mean | μ_difference |
| −4.4 | 58.3 | 20.6 | (−53.1, 44.4) |

μ_difference: population mean of (25-30-20-25)

### Test

Null hypothesis $H_0$: μ_difference = 0
Alternative $H_1$: μ_difference ≠ 0
hypothesis

| T-value | P-value |
|---|---|
| −0.21 | 0.838 |

*Analysis of a single Within Group factor not available at the time of writing.*

*Source*: InVivoStat.

Summary statistical analysis from MiniTab, v19. Panel A shows the summary of the descriptive statistics of the rodent locomotor activity data from Table 16.1, together with the results of the Repeated Measures ANOVA (compared to Table 16.7).

The remaining section lists the results of multiple paired *t*-tests (where the final 25–30 minutes time period was assigned as the baseline control group) prior to application of the Bonferroni correction (see Table 16.10 for Bonferroni corrected probability values following multiple paired *t*-tests).

*Source*: Minitab, LLC.

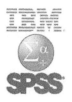

A

**Descriptive Statistics**

| | Mean | Std. Deviation | N |
|---|---|---|---|
| Time_0_5 | 603.0000 | 72.41547 | 8 |
| Time_5_10 | 368.5000 | 71.90669 | 8 |
| Time10_15 | 211.5000 | 76.38437 | 8 |
| Time15_20 | 120.6250 | 56.20355 | 8 |
| Time20_25 | 78.2500 | 41.79798 | 8 |
| Time25_30 | 73.8750 | 35.67087 | 8 |

**Mauchly's Test of Sphericity[a]**

Measure: Time2

| | | | | | | Epsilon[b] | | |
|---|---|---|---|---|---|---|---|---|
| Within Subjects Effect | Mauchly's W | Approx. Chi-Square | df | Sig. | Greenhouse-Geisser | Huynh-Feldt | Lower-bound |
| Timefactor | .031 | 17.760 | 14 | .265 | .559 | .967 | .200 |

Tests the null hypothesis that the error covariance matrix of the orthonormalized transformed dependent variables is proportional to an identity matrix.

a. Design: Intercept
Within Subjects Design: Timefactor

b. May be used to adjust the degrees of freedom for the averaged tests of significance. Corrected tests are displayed in the Tests of Within-Subjects Effects table.

**Tests of Within-Subjects Effects**

Measure: Time2

| Source | | Type III Sum of Squares | df | Mean Square | F | Sig. |
|---|---|---|---|---|---|---|
| Timefactor | Sphericity Assumed | 1736505.000 | 5 | 347301.000 | 111.560 | .000 |
| | Greenhouse-Geisser | 1736505.000 | 2.793 | 621703.797 | 111.560 | .000 |
| | Huynh-Feldt | 1736505.000 | 4.836 | 359065.905 | 111.560 | .000 |
| | Lower-bound | 1736505.000 | 1.000 | 1736505.000 | 111.560 | .000 |
| Error(Timefactor) | Sphericity Assumed | 108959.333 | 35 | 3113.124 | | |
| | Greenhouse-Geisser | 108959.333 | 19.552 | 5572.805 | | |
| | Huynh-Feldt | 108959.333 | 33.853 | 3218.582 | | |
| | Lower-bound | 108959.333 | 7.000 | 15565.619 | | |

**Paired Samples Test**

Paired Differences

| | | Mean | Std. Deviation | Std. Error Mean | 95% Confidence Interval of the Difference Lower | Upper | t | df | Sig. (2-tailed) |
|---|---|---|---|---|---|---|---|---|---|
| Pair 1 | Time25_30 - Time_0_5 | -529.12500 | 63.47426 | 22.44154 | -582.19081 | -476.05919 | -23.578 | 7 | .000 |

**Paired Samples Test**

Paired Differences

| | | Mean | Std. Deviation | Std. Error Mean | 95% Confidence Interval of the Difference Lower | Upper | t | df | Sig. (2-tailed) |
|---|---|---|---|---|---|---|---|---|---|
| Pair 1 | Time25_30 - Time_5_10 | -294.62500 | 70.13240 | 24.79555 | -353.25715 | -235.99285 | -11.882 | 7 | .000 |

**Paired Samples Test**

Paired Differences

| | | Mean | Std. Deviation | Std. Error Mean | 95% Confidence Interval of the Difference Lower | Upper | t | df | Sig. (2-tailed) |
|---|---|---|---|---|---|---|---|---|---|
| Pair 1 | Time25_30 - Time10_15 | -137.62500 | 75.17967 | 26.58003 | -200.47677 | -74.77323 | -5.178 | 7 | .001 |

**Paired Samples Test**

Paired Differences

| | | Mean | Std. Deviation | Std. Error Mean | 95% Confidence Interval of the Difference Lower | Upper | t | df | Sig. (2-tailed) |
|---|---|---|---|---|---|---|---|---|---|
| Pair 1 | Time25_30 - Time15_20 | -46.75000 | 76.81657 | 27.15876 | -110.97026 | 17.47026 | -1.721 | 7 | .129 |

**Paired Samples Test**

Paired Differences

| | | Mean | Std. Deviation | Std. Error Mean | 95% Confidence Interval of the Difference Lower | Upper | t | df | Sig. (2-tailed) |
|---|---|---|---|---|---|---|---|---|---|
| Pair 1 | Time25_30 - Time20_25 | -4.37500 | 58.30202 | 20.61288 | -53.11670 | 44.36670 | -.212 | 7 | .838 |

Summary statistical analysis from SPSS, v27. Panel A shows the summary of the descriptive statistics of the rodent locomotor activity data from Table 16.1, together with the results of Mauchly's test for sphericity and the Repeated Measures ANOVA (compared to Table 16.7). The final section details the results of multiple paired *t*-tests (where the final 25–30 minutes time period was assigned as the baseline control group) prior to application of the Bonferroni correction (see Table 16.10 for Bonferroni corrected probability values following multiple paired *t*-tests).

*Source*: IBM Corporation.

# Write Your Own Notes

# 17 Complex Analysis of Variance Models

The previous two chapters examined how different ANOVA models are required to examine data sets that arise from two very different types of experiment.

• In Chapter 15, three different strains of rat (with five rats per strain) were treated with the same dose of a hypnotic drug and the resulting sleeping time of each individual animal recorded. This experiment, therefore, composed of three independent groups of experimental subjects, where the factor that differentiated each group was the *strain* of rat, and the data were initially analysed by a one-way ANOVA. In statistical parlance, the factor that differentiated the groups is known as a **Between-Group Factor**.

• In Chapter 16, in contrast, a single group of rats was used to determine how rodent exploratory activity changes over time. This experiment, therefore, did not have a Between-Group Factor to differentiate each set of data but simply relied on obtaining a series of successive measurements from the same subjects, and the data were initially analysed by a Repeated Measures ANOVA. In statistical terms, the factor that differentiated the data sets was the *time* at which each measurement of locomotor activity was obtained and is known as a **Within-Group Factor**.

In both these cases, each ANOVA test provided a *single F* value with associated degrees of freedom and *p* value for the Between-Group Factor or Within-Group Factor, respectively, and this is known as the **Main Factor**. As previously described, if the *p* value is less than 0.05, then the Null Hypothesis may be rejected, and appropriate multiple comparisons *post hoc* analysis employed to identify which groups of data are different from which others.

In this chapter, I will describe how more complex experimental designs, involving one or more Between-Group Factors coupled with or without a Within-Group Factor, require a more complicated ANOVA model to analyse the resulting data. As previously described, significant differences between groups of data are only revealed following pairwise comparisons subsequent to the initial ANOVA test (i.e. *post hoc* analysis). However, the more complex the ANOVA model employed, the greater the number of outputs from that analysis. These outputs consist of the Main effects of the Between-Group and Within-Group Factors and **all possible** interactions between two or more of these factors. Whether the *p* value associated with each Main factor or interaction is less than 0.05 directly determines the number and type of multiple pairwise comparisons that may be legitimately performed. Interestingly (and surprisingly!), there is a definite logic to identifying which pairwise comparisons are justified by each ANOVA result. I have purposely divided this chapter into two distinct parts in order to guide you through the complexity of identifying which ANOVA model to use, and which multiple pairwise comparisons are subsequently permissible.

In part A, I shall describe different ANOVA models that include one or more Between-Group Factors with or without one Within-Group Factor. Once you see how the experimental design and the associated Between-Group and/or Within-Group Factors determine which ANOVA model is appropriate, then you will be able to identify the correct ANOVA model for your own experiments.

In part B, I shall describe the guidelines for determining which pairwise comparisons are appropriate for each ANOVA models described in Part A. At the end of this section, you should understand the simple rules that will allow you to identify which multiple pairwise comparisons are permissible according to the results of the ANOVA model used.

## Part A: choice of suitable Analysis of Variance models.

*Every* experiment we perform in pharmacology, or related biomedical area, will comprise of one or more Between-Group Factor(s) and/or Within-Group Factor(s). Where an experimental design includes one or more Between-Group Factors *and* a Within-Group Factor (i.e. the design includes a Repeated Measures component), then this is known as a **mixed design**. It is absolutely vital that we identify each Between-Group Factor and Within-Group Factor in our experiments since this ensures that not only may we design a perfectly balanced experiment, but that we also identify which ANOVA model to use to analyse the resulting data.

There are two principle questions to ask here

1 How many Between-Group Factors are there in the data?
2 Is there a Within-Group Factor in the data?

### Between-Group Factors

These reflect the number of variables (different factors) in the experiment that differentiate one group from another such that there are different subjects in each group according to each factor. Table 17.1 provides some typical examples of Between-Group Factors used in experimental pharmacology. In all cases, there is only a single measured output obtained at the end of the experiment. If there is only a single Between-Group Factor that differentiates the groups in the experiment, then a one-way ANOVA is required to analyse the data (see Chapter 15). However, if there is more than one Between-Group Factor involved, then a more complex ANOVA model is required.

For example, consider the following experimental designs:

• the effect of pre-treatment with a receptor antagonist on the response to a receptor agonist,
• the effect of chronic treatment on the response to a receptor agonist.

Both of these experimental designs contain two Between-Group Factors and consequently require a two-way ANOVA to analyse the data sets. Adding an additional Between-Group Factor into the experimental design (e.g. gender) will consequently require initial analysis by a three-way ANOVA.

*Experimental Design and Statistical Analysis for Pharmacology and the Biomedical Sciences*, First Edition. Paul J. Mitchell.

**Table 17.1** Examples of Between-Group Factors

| Between-Group Factor | Comment |
|---|---|
| Acute treatment | Reflects a single treatment, e.g. receptor agonists. Such experiments may include where each group of subjects is administered a different drug or where the different groups are given the different doses of the same drug. The factor here is the act of a single treatment, not what that treatment is comprised of. |
| Chronic treatment | Reflects a treatment given repeatedly over days/weeks/months, etc. As in the above example, the factor here is the act of the repeated treatment, not what that treatment is comprised of. |
| Pre-treatment | Where a pre-treatment is administered before a subsequent treatment. Examples include<br>• a single drug treatment followed by a second single drug treatment (antagonist/agonist interaction),<br>• a period of repeated drug treatment followed by a single drug treatment,<br>• a period of repeated drug treatment followed by a second period of repeated drug treatment. |
| Differences in cell media | Experiments where cells were incubated in different media |
| Gender | Experiments where the effect of gender is examined |
| Diet | Experiments where subjects were fed different diets. |

## Within-Group Factors

The Within-Group Factor reflects the situation where repeated measurements are taken from the same group regardless of whether the experimental design includes one or more Between-Group Factors or not. This invariably involves a *Time* variable in the experiment. Such an experiment may simply involve a single group examined repeatedly on more than two occasions (these data should be analysed by a Repeated Measures ANOVA, sometimes referred to as a one-way Repeated Measures ANOVA, as described in Chapter 16). If an experiment involves a number of different treatment groups (one Between-Group Factor) examined over a series of time points, then such data should be analysed by a **one-way ANOVA with Repeated Measures** to take account of the Between-Group Factor. More complicated ANOVA models will be required with the addition of further Between-Group Factors.

## Using spreadsheets in experimental design

Way back in Chapter 1 I argued that important decisions about statistical analysis are integral to the experimental design process. Consequently, identifying the appropriate strategy (and hence which descriptive statistics and inferential tests to use) to analyse your experimental data should occur *before* you run your experiment. An important component of my experimental design process is to develop a spreadsheet as an overview to enable me to design well-balanced experiments and to identify the most appropriate inferential tests to analyse the resulting data.

The following spreadsheets (Excel is useful here!) may provide an easier way to visualise the different models of ANOVA required by different experimental designs. In each case, the Between-Group Factors are presented as different columns with the single measured output provided in the final column (where there will be one cell for each measurement obtained from the

subjects in each group), while the Within-Group Factors run across a number of columns reflecting the number of different time points involved.

For brevity, I have omitted specific data sets from the experimental examples described in this chapter to limit any discussion to the experimental design and consequent decisions on the statistical analysis required. However, I have included two further experimental examples (for two-way ANOVA (see Example 17.2) and one-way ANOVA with Repeated Measures [see Example 17.5], respectively) in the screen shot section at the end of this chapter so that the reader may appreciate the differences in how the results of statistical analysis are provided by the different software programmes. *It is absolutely vital that care should be taken here since each statistical analysis programme requires data to be provided in a specific structure/format, consequently you must ensure that the experimental data is in the correct spreadsheet format according to the requirements of the software programme you intend to use.*

## Example 17.1 One Between-Group Factor only

In a single Between-Group Factor experimental design, there is just one factor that differentiates the different groups in the experiment. The general plan of the experimental group structure is provided in Table 17.2; here the first column summarises the different treatments administered to the different groups of subjects. The second column will contain a separate row for each subject in each group (in Table 17.2 I've condensed the individual subject rows into one cell row only for brevity), while the final column will eventually contain the experimental output (i.e. observation) for each subject.

**Table 17.2** One Between-Group Factor = one-way ANOVA.

| Between Factor 1 (e.g. treatment) | Subject numbers | Measured output (observations) |
|---|---|---|
| Drug/dose 1 | N per group | |
| Drug/dose 2 | N per group | |
| Drug/dose 3 | N per group | |
| Drug/dose 4 | N per group | |

Summary spreadsheet plan of a typical experimental design where treatment is the one Between-Group Factor.

Further examples of a single Between-Group Factor experimental design include the following.

• Different diets on weight gain (Between-Group Factor = diet).
• Different media on cell growth (Between-Group Factor = growth media).
• Different doses of same drug compared to control (Between-Group Factor = single treatment).
• Different drugs compared to control (Between-Group Factor = single treatment).

Another example of a single Between-Group Factor design is the sleeping time data used to describe the one-way ANOVA in Chapter 15; Table 17.3 shows how the sleeping time data would be input into such a summary spreadsheet. In this and the following spreadsheet plans, the row colours simply enable identification of independent groups indicating the different drugs or doses of drug used. In the final table, the number of rows per group will be equal to the number of subjects in each group.

**Table 17.3** One Between-Group Factor = one-way ANOVA.

| Between Factor 1 (e.g. strain) | Subject numbers | Measured output (sleeping time, min) |
|---|---|---|
| Strain 1 | 1 | 13 |
| | 2 | 17 |
| | 3 | 19 |
| | 4 | 15 |
| | 5 | 16 |
| Strain 2 | 1 | 20 |
| | 2 | 17 |
| | 3 | 23 |
| | 4 | 26 |
| | 5 | 19 |
| Strain 3 | 1 | 14 |
| | 2 | 21 |
| | 3 | 16 |
| | 4 | 19 |
| | 5 | 13 |

Values in the final column indicate sleeping time (min) for each subject following treatment with a standard dose of hypnotic drug. Data taken from Table 15.1.

## Example 17.2 Two Between-Group Factors only

As the title indicates, in a two Between-Group Factor experimental design there are two factors which give rise to the experimental groups.

Consider the following experiment where we are interested in whether male and female subjects show a difference in sensitivity to the effect of four different treatments. The resulting experimental plan may be summarised as shown in Table 17.4.

**Table 17.4** Two Between-Group Factor = two-way ANOVA.

| Between Factor 2 (gender) | Between Factor 1 (treatment) | Subject numbers | Measured output (observations) |
|---|---|---|---|
| Female | Drug/dose 1 | N per group | |
| | Drug/dose 2 | N per group | |
| | Drug/dose 3 | N per group | |
| | Drug/dose 4 | N per group | |
| Male | Drug/dose 1 | N per group | |
| | Drug/dose 2 | N per group | |
| | Drug/dose 3 | N per group | |
| | Drug/dose 4 | N per group | |

In this experimental design there are two important points to note:

**1** In order to maintain the balance of the experimental design, all the four different treatments administered to female subjects must also be administered to the corresponding male subjects.
**2** None of the eight resulting groups of subjects are truly independent from each other. Thus, both the total female and male data sets contain all four treatments, and consequently, the total observations for each treatment contains both male and female subjects.

Consider another typical experimental design. Here we are interested in the pharmacodynamic interaction between a drug that has antagonist activity at a specific receptor and a second drug that possess agonist (i.e. stimulating) activity at the same receptor. The resulting experimental plan may be summarised as shown in Table 17.5.

**Table 17.5** Two Between-Group Factor = two-way ANOVA.

| Between Factor 2 (pre-treatment) | Between Factor 1 (acute treatment) | Subject numbers | Measured output |
|---|---|---|---|
| Control | Control | N per group | |
| | Agonist drug | N per group | |
| Antagonist drug | Control | N per group | |
| | Agonist drug | N per group | |

Again, the experimental design is perfectly balanced in that the control treatment for the agonist drug and the agonist treatment itself are both administered to those subjects that were previously treated with either the antagonist drug or the appropriate control for that drug. Furthermore, the resulting four treatment combinations are not independent from each other since the experimental subjects treated with either the pre-treatment control or antagonist drug *both* received either the control treatment for the agonist drug or the agonist drug itself. Similarly, the experimental subjects treated with either the control treatment for the agonist drug or the agonist drug itself *both* received either the pre-treatment control or antagonist drug.

In both the latter two examples summarised in Tables 17.4 and 17.5, the appropriate ANOVA model to analyse such data is the two-way ANOVA, where the 'two-' indicates the two- Between-Group Factors. As the complexity of the ANOVA model used to analyse different sets of experimental data increases, so the output of the analysis also increases. The reason for this is that not only are the **main** effects of each Between-Group Factor analysed, but so are the various **interactions** between the different Between-Group Factors.

So, the output following analysis by a two-way ANOVA will comprise:

- Main effect of Between-Group Factor 1
- Main effect of Between-Group Factor 2
- Interaction between both Between-Group Factors 1 and 2,

and in all three cases the output will include the $F$-ratio, the degrees of freedom, and the resulting $p$ value. When reporting such results, then all three of these results **must** be quoted regardless of whether the resulting $p$ value in each case is greater or smaller than the family error rate (i.e. $p = 0.05$).

## Example 17.3 Three Between-Group Factors only

Imagine the experimental scenario where we wanted to determine whether the pharmacodynamic interaction between the receptor agonist and antagonist described above differed between male and female subjects. This would require an additional Between-Group Factor in the design of our experiment, resulting in a three Between-Group Factor design as summarised in Table 17.6.

**Table 17.6** Three Between-Group Factor = three-way ANOVA.

| Between Factor 3 (gender) | Between Factor 2 (pre-treatment) | Between Factor 1 (acute treatment) | Subject numbers | Measured output |
| --- | --- | --- | --- | --- |
| Female | Control | Control | N per group | |
| | | Agonist drug | N per group | |
| | Antagonist drug | Control | N per group | |
| | | Agonist drug | N per group | |
| Male | Control | Control | N per group | |
| | | Agonist drug | N per group | |
| | Antagonist drug | Control | N per group | |
| | | Agonist drug | N per group | |

Once again, the summary spreadsheet plan demonstrates that not only is the experimental design perfectly balanced, but also none of the eight different combinations of gender plus pre-treatment-plus acute treatment are entirely independent from each other.

The appropriate ANOVA model to analyse such data is a three-way ANOVA as indicated by the three Between-Group Factors. In this case, the resulting output will include not only the main effects of the Between-Group Factors but also all possible interactions between these factors. Thus, the output following analysis by a three-way ANOVA will comprise:

- Main effect of Between-Group Factor 1
- Main effect of Between-Group Factor 2
- Main effect of Between-Group Factor 3
- Interaction between both Between-Group Factors 1 and 2,
- Interaction between both Between-Group Factors 1 and 3,
- Interaction between both Between-Group Factors 2 and 3,
- Interaction between all Between-Group Factors 1, 2, and 3

In Chapter 15, I discussed a number of *post hoc* procedures that are commonly used to perform multiple pairwise comparisons following a one-way ANOVA (see Table 15.13). These *post hoc* tests either compare each group against all the others in the data set (i.e. All Means *post hoc* tests), or only compare each test group against a control group (i.e. control group *post hoc* tests). In both cases, every group is compared to one or more of the other groups in the data set. As previously described, this approach is perfectly justified in the situation where there is just one Between-Group Factor. However, where the experimental design includes two or three Between-Group Factors then such an approach is **only** justified when there is a significant interaction between **all** the factors in the experiment, i.e. between the Between-Group Factors 1 and 2 following a two-way ANOVA and between the Between-Group Factors 1, 2 and 3 following a three-way ANOVA. If either of these full interactions fail to show significant variation between the groups (i.e. if $p > 0.05$ for the full interaction), then the number of permissible pairwise comparisons is limited. I shall describe which pairwise comparisons are justified later in this chapter.

## Example 17.4 Zero Between-Group Factor plus one Within-Group Factor

Table 17.7 summarises a typical spreadsheet from an experiment where there is only one group of subjects from which a measurement is recorded at six sequential time points. Such an experimental design only has one Within-Group Factor but no Between-Group Factors. The appropriate ANOVA model to analyse such data is the Repeated Measures ANOVA as previously described in Chapter 16 (see Table 16.1).

**Table 17.7** Zero Between-Group Factor plus one Within-Group Factor = Repeated Measures ANOVA.

| Subject | Measured output (observations) | | | | | |
| --- | --- | --- | --- | --- | --- | --- |
| | Time 1 | Time 2 | Time 3 | Time 4 | Time 5 | Time 6 |
| 1 | | | | | | |
| 2 | | | | | | |
| 3 | | | | | | |
| 4 | | | | | | |
| 5 | | | | | | |
| 6 | | | | | | |

Examples of experimental designs where there is one Within-Group Factor include the following:

- Measurement of locomotor activity exhibited by untreated subjects (zero Between-Group Factor) over six time points (Within-Group Factor).
- Measurement of cell population growth in separate cell cultures in identical conditions (zero Between-Group Factor) over six time points (Within-Group Factor).

As mentioned previously (see Chapter 16), the Repeated Measures ANOVA is essentially a one-way ANOVA but over time (which is why it is sometimes referred to as a one-way Repeated Measures ANOVA). The main problem with a Repeated Measures ANOVA (or any ANOVA model containing a Repeated Measures factor), however, is that the experimental design contains a whole series of paired data sets rather than independent data sets required by the conditions for a simple one-way ANOVA. This introduces a phenomenon known as sphericity. If the assumptions of sphericity are violated (as determined by *Mauchly's* test), then the ANOVA values are corrected using either the Greenhouse–Geisser or the Huynh–Feldt estimates of sphericity to correct the degrees of freedom values (see the discussion in Chapter 16). The resulting corrected *p* value indicates whether there is significant variation in the data across time or not (i.e. the Null Hypothesis is that there is no variation in the data across the various time points of the experiment).

## Example 17.5 One Between-Group Factor plus one Within-Group Factor

Table 17.2 summarises the experimental spreadsheet for an experimental design with one Between-Group Factor. If we now add a single Within-Group Factor into our experimental design, then we produce an experimental design as summarised in Table 17.8. In this experiment, we have four different drug or doses (comprising the one Between-Group Factor) the effects of which are measured at six sequential time points (indicated by T1–T6).

The correct ANOVA model to analyse these data is a one-way ANOVA with Repeated Measures and is our first example of a **mixed-design ANOVA model**.

**Table 17.8** One Between-Group Factor plus one Within-Group Factor = one-way ANOVA with Repeated Measures.

| Between Factor 1 (e.g. treatment) | Subject numbers | Measured output (observations) | | | | | |
|---|---|---|---|---|---|---|---|
| | | T1 | T2 | T3 | T4 | T5 | T6 |
| Drug/dose 1 | N per group | | | | | | |
| Drug/dose 2 | N per group | | | | | | |
| Drug/dose 3 | N per group | | | | | | |
| Drug/dose 4 | N per group | | | | | | |

In this example, the resulting output will include not only the main effects of the Between-Group and Within-Group Factors but also the interaction between these factors. Thus, the output following analysis by a one-way ANOVA with Repeated Measures will comprise:

- Main effect of Between-Group Factor 1 (i.e. treatment)
- Main effect of Within-Group Factor 1 (i.e. time)
- Interaction between both Between-Group Factor 1 and Within-Group Factor 1; i.e. treatment * time.

## Example 17.6 Two Between-Group Factors plus one Within-Group Factor

Table 17.5 summarises the experimental spreadsheet for an experimental design with two Between-Group Factors. If we now add a single Within-Group Factor into our experimental design, then we produce an experiment as summarised in Table 17.9. In this experimental design, we are interested how the pharmacodynamic interaction between an agonist and antagonist for a specific receptor (comprising the two Between-Group Factors) changes over time (by taking measurements at six sequential time points indicated by T1–T6). The correct ANOVA model to analyse these data is a two-way ANOVA with Repeated Measures and is a second example of a mixed-design ANOVA model.

**Table 17.9** Two Between-Group Factors plus one Within-Group Factor = two-way ANOVA with Repeated Measures.

| Between Factor 2 | Between Factor 1 | Subject numbers | Measured output (observations) | | | | | |
|---|---|---|---|---|---|---|---|---|
| | | | T1 | T2 | T3 | T4 | T5 | T6 |
| Control | Control | N per group | | | | | | |
| | Agonist drug | N per group | | | | | | |
| Antagonist drug | Control | N per group | | | | | | |
| | Agonist drug | N per group | | | | | | |

As with the previous examples, the resulting output of the ANOVA model will include not only the main effects of the Between-Group and Within-Group Factors but also all possible interactions between two or more factors. Thus, the output following analysis by a two-way ANOVA with Repeated Measures will comprise:

- Main effect of Between-Group Factor 1 (i.e. acute treatment)
- Main effect of Between-Group Factor 2 (i.e. pre-treatment)
- Main effect of Within-Group Factor 1 (i.e. time)
- Interaction between the Between-Group Factor 1 and the Between-Group Factor 2, i.e. acute treatment * pre-treatment.
- Interaction between the Between-Group Factor 1 and the Within-Group Factor 1, i.e. acute treatment * time.
- Interaction between the Between-Group Factor 2 and the Within-Group Factor 1, i.e. pre-treatment * time.
- Interaction between the Between-Group Factor 1, Between-Group Factor 2 and the Within-Group Factor 1, i.e. acute treatment * pre-treatment * time

## Part B: choice of suitable *post hoc* pairwise comparisons

In Chapters 15 and 16, I discussed a number of *post hoc* procedures that may be employed to perform multiple pairwise comparisons following either a one-way ANOVA or a Repeated Measures ANOVA (see Table 17.10).

**Table 17.10** Summary of suitable *post hoc* procedures.

| Data type | ANOVA model | Required comparisons | Suitable *post hoc* tests |
|---|---|---|---|
| Independent | One-way ANOVA | All Means Control | See Table 15.13 • Dunnett's test, • Bonferroni (control) |
| Paired | Repeated Measures ANOVA | All Means | • Comparison of CI using Tukey test with Bonferroni or Sidak correction, • Multiple paired *t*-test with Bonferroni correction. |
| | | Control | • Multiple paired *t*-test with Bonferroni correction. |

CI indicates confidence intervals.

In all cases, each group is compared to one or more of the other groups in the data set. This approach, to identify significant differences between experimental groups, is perfectly justified in the situation where there is just one Between-Group Factor **or** one Within-Group Factor in the experiment.

However, in experiments that include multiple Between-Group Factors **only** (i.e. two-way and three-way ANOVA models), then the use of the multiple comparison *post hoc* tests listed in Tables 15.13 and 17.10 is **only** justified when the Null Hypothesis according to the highest level interaction (i.e. that which includes **all** the factors in the experiment) may be rejected (i.e. $p < 0.05$). These highest level interactions are indicated at the bottom of the respective list of outputs to be reported for these ANOVA models in Table 17.11 (indicated by [a]). If the highest level interaction fails to show significance, then the number of permissible pairwise comparisons is limited but must be in accordance with significant variation identified by the remaining outputs from the ANOVA model. The problem then arises for the experimenter to identify *which* pairwise comparisons are fully justified according to the other outputs of the ANOVA model.

**Table 17.11** Summary of ANOVA output according to model of ANOVA used.

| ANOVA model | Output to be reported ($F(df) = f\ value$, $p = p\ value$) | | |
|---|---|---|---|
| One-way ANOVA | Main effect: | Between-Group Factor[a] | |
| Two-way ANOVA | Main effects: | Between-Group Factor 1 | |
| | | Between-Group Factor 2 | |
| | Interaction: | Factor 1 × Factor 2[a] | |
| Three-way ANOVA | Main effects: | Between-Group Factor 1 | |
| | | Between-Group Factor 2 | |
| | | Between-Group Factor 3 | |
| | Interaction: | Factor 1 × Factor 2 | |
| | | Factor 1 × Factor 3 | |
| | | Factor 2 × Factor 3 | |
| | | Factor 1 × Factor 2 × Factor 3[a] | |
| Repeated Measures ANOVA | Main effect: | Within-Group Factor, i.e. time[a] | |
| One-way ANOVA with Repeated Measures | Main effects: | Between-Group Factor | |
| | | Within-Group factor, i.e. Time | |
| | Interaction: | Between Factor × Time | |
| Two-way ANOVA with Repeated Measures | Main effects: | Between-Group Factor 1 | |
| | | Between-Group Factor 2 | |
| | | Within-Group Factor, i.e. Time | |
| | Interactions: | Factor 1 × Factor 2 | |
| | | Factor 1 × Time | |
| | | Factor 2 × Time | |
| | | Factor 1 × Factor 2 × Time | |

[a] Indicates the sole Main effect or highest level interaction from the ANOVA output where standard multiple comparison *post hoc* tests should be used (see Chapters 15 and 16 and also Table 17.10). In all other cases, where the data are analysed by a mixed ANOVA model then the number of permissible multiple pairwise comparisons based on Main effects or lower level interactions are limited (see Examples 17.11 and 17.12).

Table 17.11 summarises all the outputs from each of the complex ANOVA models described in the first part of this chapter. Whenever it is necessary to report the results of such complex ANOVA models, then the full ANOVA data, i.e. [$F(df) = f\ value$, $p = p\ value$] (where df = degrees of freedom), for each main effect (i.e. each Between-Group and Within-Group Factor) **and** for each possible interaction between two or more of these main effects *must* be reported. It should be noted that ***it is wholly unacceptable to make bland statements that only highlight those ANOVA results where p < 0.05, or just simply provide the resulting p values without the corresponding ANOVA data as evidence in support of the findings.***

Throughout the discussions on ANOVA techniques in the present chapter, and also in Chapters 15 and 16, I've loosely used the term *post hoc* to refer to the array of multiple pairwise comparisons that are performed following the ANOVA test to identify which groups of data are significantly different from which others. The term *post hoc* comes from the Latin (which is why

the term is italicised) and literally means 'after this'. In statistical analysis, the term *post hoc* refers to those standard tests that occur *following* the ANOVA where all groups are compared to either *one* other group (as in the case of comparisons to a control group) or *all* other groups (as in the case of All Means comparisons). The important point to note here is that the experimenter does not identify which specific pairwise comparisons to perform. There are, however, situations where the experimenter must decide which comparisons he/she identifies as important. Such decisions must be made *before* the ANOVA test and are generally in accordance with *a priori* predictions about the data collected. The term *a priori* (again from the Latin) literally means 'from the earlier'; this infers that we have some prior knowledge about what changes in the data we expect as a direct result of the experimental interventions. Consequently, in complex experimental designs, there will be a number of pairwise comparisons in which we are interested and a range of comparisons that hold no interest whatsoever. Of course, by limiting the number of comparisons, then we reduce the impact of the multiple pairwise comparisons on the Type 1 error rate (see Tables 10.2 and 10.3), so it is always beneficial to reduce the number of pairwise comparisons we perform rather than trawling for as many significant differences between groups as possible.

I've already argued that the standard *post hoc* tests are only appropriate when a one-way ANOVA or a Repeated Measures ANOVA or the highest level interaction from a two-way or three-way ANOVA model suggests that the appropriate Null Hypothesis may be rejected (see Table 17.11). In the case of two-way or three-way ANOVA, the significant highest level interaction allows us to treat all the groups as being independent from each other, and consequently, the use of the standard *post hoc* tests is justified.

This raises the question what strategy do we adopt when only Main effects or low-level interactions resulting from the more complex ANOVA models suggest that there may be significant variation between the different experimental groups? To answer this question, we need to carefully consider all the outputs of the ANOVA model and identify which multiple pairwise comparisons are justified according to the result of each output in turn. This sounds more complicated than it actually is, and the decision-making process should be apparent if we work carefully through the ANOVA models described above in Part A.

The first point to note is that any pairwise comparison is only justified if the ANOVA model suggests that there is significant variation between the groups according to the Main effects and/or any level of interaction between the various Between-Group and Within-Group Factors; in all cases, significant variation is identified where $p < 0.05$.

## Example 17.7 Pairwise comparisons following one-way ANOVA (see Ex 17.1)

If the Main effect of the Between-Group Factor suggests significant variation in the data, then any subsequent *post hoc* analysis depends on whether the experiment contains a clear control group or not (see Chapter 15 and especially Table 15.13 and Table 17.10).

Consider the experiment summarised in Table 17.2 where there are four independent treatment groups. If these four groups are all different drugs, then we may be interested in comparing each group to each of the others, as summarised in Table 17.12. In this situation, the All Means multiple pairwise comparison tests listed in Table 15.13 would be appropriate.

120

Experimental Design and Statistical Analysis for Pharmacology and the Biomedical Sc...

**Table 17.12** All Means pairwise comparisons of independent groups following one-way ANOVA

|  | Drug 1 | Drug 2 | Drug3 | Drug 4 |
|---|---|---|---|---|
| Drug 1 | / | * | * | * |
| Drug 2 |  | / | * | * |
| Drug 3 |  |  | / | * |

\* Indicate permissible All Means multiple pairwise comparisons of independent data sets.

In contrast, if we assume the first treatment group (drug/dose 1) is a control group and the remaining groups are different doses of the same drug, then the only pairwise comparisons we are interested in are summarised in Table 17.13. In this situation, the control group multiple pairwise comparison *post hoc* tests listed at the bottom of Table 15.13 would be appropriate.

**Table 17.13** Control group pairwise comparisons of independent groups following one-way ANOVA.

|  | Drug 1 | Drug 2 | Drug 3 | Drug 4 |
|---|---|---|---|---|
| Drug 1 | / | * | * | * |

\* Indicate permissible Control Group multiple pairwise comparisons of independent data sets.

## Example 17.8 Pairwise comparisons following two-way ANOVA (see Ex 17.2)

Consider the experimental design summarised in Table 17.5 where we are interested in the ability of pre-treatment with an antagonist drug for a specific receptor to block the stimulant activity of an agonist drug (acute treatment) at the same receptor. In this example, there are two Between-Group Factors resulting in four possible combinations of drug or drug vehicle (i.e. respective control treatments). These treatment combinations are as follows:

**1** Control 1 (pre-treatment drug vehicle) plus Control 2 (acute treatment drug vehicle)
**2** Control 1 plus Agonist (acute treatment)
**3** Antagonist pre-treatment plus Control 2
**4** Antagonist pre-treatment plus Agonist

Consequently, there are a maximum of six possible pairwise comparisons that we could perform according to the equation $N(N-1)/2$, where N equals the number of treatment combinations. Where the two-way ANOVA model indicates a significant interaction between both Between-Group Factors (i.e. pre-treatment and acute treatment in this example), then theory allows the different treatment combinations indicated above to be assumed to be independent from each other. For example, Control 1 plus Control 2

may be assumed to be independent from Control 1 plus Agonist *even though both groups received Control 1 treatment*. Consequently, a significant Between-Group Factor interaction (where $p < 0.05$) allows all the data sets to be compared to each other by an All Means *post hoc* test (as summarised in Table 17.14).

However, if the two-way ANOVA reveals **only** the Main effects of Between-Group Factor 1 and/or Between-Group Factor 2, then the justified comparisons are somewhat limited. Where there is only a Main effect of a single Between-Group or Within-Group Factor, then the only **simple** comparisons that are justified are those where the sole Between-Group Factor concerned differs between the two groups being compared, with the variants of all other factors remaining constant.

### Main effect of Between-Group Factor 1 (Acute Treatment)

Where there is significant variation in the acute treatment factor, then the only comparisons allowed are where Control 2 is compared to the Agonist but the Control 1 or Antagonist treatment remains the same in both groups being compared (see Table 17.14). Thus,

- Control 1 + **Control 2** compared to Control 1 + **Agonist**
- Antagonist + **Control 2** v Antagonist + **Agonist**

(here, the treatment that differs between the groups being compared is in bold type for identification purposes only).

### Main effect of Between-Group Factor 2 (Pre-treatment)

Where there is significant variation in the pre-treatment factor, then the only comparisons allowed are where Control 1 is compared to the Antagonist but the Control 2 or Agonist treatment remains the same in both groups being compared (see Table 17.14). Thus,

- **Control 1** + Control 2 compared to **Antagonist** + Control 2
- **Control 1** + Agonist compared to **Antagonist** + Agonist

(again, the treatment that differs between the groups being compared is in bold type).

In addition, it is vitally important to recognise that where only Main effects of the Between Factors are identified, then comparisons where *both* Factors change are *not* justified. In the above experiment, therefore, neither of the following two comparisons may be performed, since both the pre-treatments and the acute treatments differ between the two groups in each comparison!

- Control 1 + Control 2 compared to Antagonist + Agonist
- Control 1 + Agonist v Antagonist + Control 2

In cases where a limited number of pairwise comparisons are justified due to a significant Main effect of one or more Between-Group Factor(s) (see Table 17.14), then multiple pairwise comparisons using either the independent *t*-test or one-way ANOVA between two groups may be performed. However, the resulting *p* value must be adjusted to account for the total number of pairwise comparisons performed using the Bonferroni method to correct for the subsequent changes in the Type 1 error rate (as indicated at the bottom of Table 17.14).

**Table 17.14** Pairwise comparisons following two-way ANOVA.

| Treatment combination A | Treatment combination B | Main effects | | Interaction |
|---|---|---|---|---|
| | | Between Factor 1 | Between Factor 2 | Between Factor 1 × Between Factor 2 |
| Control plus control | Control plus Agonist | * | | * |
| Control plus control | Antagonist plus control | | * | * |
| Control plus control | Antagonist plus Agonist | | | * |
| Control plus Agonist | Antagonist plus control | | | * |
| Control plus Agonist | Antagonist plus Agonist | | * | * |
| Antagonist plus control | Antagonist plus Agonist | * | | * |
| Bonferroni correction (see Table 10.3) | | 0.05/2 = 0.025 0.05/4 = 0.0125 | 0.05/2 = 0.025 | Multiple All Means *post hoc* test |

* Indicate permissible multiple pairwise comparisons of independent data sets. Note: Comparisons 3 and 4 above are only justified if there is a significant interaction between the factors as identified by the two-way ANOVA.

## Example 17.9 Pairwise comparisons following three-way ANOVA (see Ex 17.3)

Consider the experimental design summarised in Table 17.6 where we are interested in whether there is an effect of gender on the ability of pre-treatment with an antagonist drug for a specific receptor to block the stimulant activity of an agonist drug (acute treatment) at the same receptor. Consequently, there are three Between-Group Factors (1 = gender, 2 = pre-treatment with the control [drug vehicle] or antagonist drug and 3 = acute treatment with the control [drug vehicle] and agonist drug) resulting in eight possible combinations of these factors as summarised in Table 17.15. Thus, according to the equation $N(N - 1)/2$, where $N$ equals the number of different factor combinations, there are a maximum of 28 possible pairwise comparisons that we could perform if we wished to compare each group against each of the others. (N.B. if we were to perform all these comparisons by the independent $t$-test *without* applying the Bonferroni correction, then the probability of no Type 1 error would reduce from 0.95 down to 0.238, resulting in a Type 1 error rate increasing from 0.05 to 0.762; see Table 10.2).

**Table 17.15** All possible combinations of 3 Between-Group Factors.

| | Between-Group Factor 1 (Gender) | Between-Group Factor 2 (Pre-treatment) | Between-Group Factor 3 (Acute treatment) |
|---|---|---|---|
| 1 | Female | Control 1 | Control 2 |
| 2 | Female | Control 1 | Agonist |
| 3 | Female | Antagonist | Control 2 |
| 4 | Female | Antagonist | Agonist |
| 5 | Male | Control 1 | Control 2 |
| 6 | Male | Control 1 | Agonist |
| 7 | Male | Antagonist | Control 2 |
| 8 | Male | Antagonist | Agonist |

If the highest order interaction between the three Between-Group Factors (i.e. Gender, Pre-treatment, and Acute treatment)

shows that $p < 0.05$ (i.e. significant variation between all the groups), then the data sets may be assumed to be independent from each other and all the data sets may be compared to each other by an All Means *post hoc* test (as summarised in Table 17.16). However, if the three-way ANOVA reveals only main effects of the Between-Group Factors or lower order interactions between any two of the Between-Group Factors, then the justified comparisons are somewhat limited.

In these cases, then the only *simple* comparisons that are justified are those where only the Between-Group Factor (for Main effects) or the interaction of two Between-Group Factors (for lower order interactions) concerned differs between the two groups being compared. For the sake of brevity, I'm not going to identify all the simple effects in detail as I did above when discussing the two-way ANOVA, but if you followed the logic in the previous section, then the justification for the allowed pairwise comparisons should be apparent by studying Table 17.16 carefully for each of the possible results of the three-way ANOVA. As in the previous example, the resulting $p$ value for each pairwise comparison must be adjusted to account for the total number of comparisons performed using the Bonferroni method to correct for the subsequent changes in the Type 1 error rate.

The general rule of thumb to follow when identifying which *simple* pairwise comparisons are justified following complex models of ANOVA is to ensure that only the Between-Group Factor or Factors for the Main effects or low-order interactions, respectively, differ between the groups being compared. Such groups may be compared by using the independent $t$-test. It is important to note that Bonferroni correction of the resulting $p$ value must be applied, and this must reflect the **total** number of pairwise comparisons being made across the whole data set. Each column in Table 17.16 carries a Bonferroni correction factor of 4 (i.e. each Main effect or low-order interaction identifies four possible pairwise comparisons) so if the three-way ANOVA identifies multiple Main effects or low-order interactions, then the final Bonferroni correction factor will be $4 \times n$, where $n$ = total number of Main effects or low-order interactions identified.

**Table 17.16** Pairwise comparisons following three-way ANOVA.

| Pairwise comparison | Main effects (Between-Group Factors) | | | Low-order interactions | | | High-order interaction |
|---|---|---|---|---|---|---|---|
| | 1 | 2 | 3 | 1 × 2 | 1 × 3 | 2 × 3 | 1 × 2 × 3 |
| 1 v 2 | | | * | | | | * |
| 1 v 3 | | * | | | | | * |
| 1 v 4 | | | | | | * | * |
| 1 v 5 | * | | | | | | * |
| 1 v 6 | | | | | * | | * |
| 1 v 7 | | | | * | | | * |
| 1 v 8 | | | | | | | * |
| 2 v 3 | | | | | | * | * |
| 2 v 4 | | * | | | | | * |
| 2 v 5 | | | | | * | | * |
| 2 v 6 | * | | | | | | * |
| 2 v 7 | | | | | | | * |
| 2 v 8 | | | | * | | | * |
| 3 v 4 | | | * | | | | * |
| 3 v 5 | | | | * | | | * |
| 3 v 6 | | | | | | | * |
| 3 v 7 | * | | | | | | * |
| 3 v 8 | | | | | * | | * |
| 4 v 5 | | | | | | | * |
| 4 v 6 | | | | * | | | * |
| 4 v 7 | | | | | * | | * |
| 4 v 8 | * | | | | | | * |
| 5 v 6 | | | * | | | | * |
| 5 v 7 | | * | | | | | * |
| 5 v 8 | | | | | | * | * |
| 6 v 7 | | | | | | * | * |
| 6 v 8 | | * | | | | | * |
| 7 v 8 | | | * | | | | * |

Summary of justified pairwise comparisons following three-way ANOVA. Group numbers according to the combination of Between-Group Factors in each pairwise comparison are summarised in Table 17.15 to which the reader is directed for explanation.
* Justified comparisons according to Main effects or interactions identified by three-way ANOVA. Between-Group Factor 1 = Gender (Male or Female), Between-Group Factor 2 = Pre-treatment (Control 1 or Antagonist drug), Between-Group Factor 3 = Acute treatment (Control 2 or Agonist drug). Interactions according to Between-Group Factors as indicated. It is important to note that some pairwise comparisons (i.e. 1 v 8, 2 v 7, 3 v 6, and 4 v 5) are **only justified** if the highest order interaction between all three Between-Group Factors is identified by the three-way ANOVA.

## Example 17.10 Pairwise comparisons following Repeated Measures ANOVA (one Within-Group Factor only) (see Ex 17.4)

Consider the experimental design summarised in Table 17.7 where there is only a single group of subjects from which a measurement is recorded at six sequential time points. The resulting ANOVA model is similar to the one-way ANOVA, except that the data sets are paired rather than independent. The output of the Repeated Measures ANOVA is just the Main effect of the Within-Group Factor (Time), and if the analysis suggests significant variation between the data sets then any subsequent *post hoc* analysis depends on whether the experiment contains a clear control group or not (see Chapter 16 and Table 17.10). If we were interested in comparing each time point to each of the others, then the subsequent pairwise comparisons would be performed by comparing the confidence intervals of the *differences* using the Tukey test with either Bonferroni or Sidak correction, as summarised in Table 17.17.

In contrast, if we assume the first time point is the control group and the remaining groups are sequential time points, then the only pairwise comparisons we are interested in are summarised in Table 17.18. In this situation, multiple comparisons using the paired t-test with Bonferroni correction reflecting the five pairwise comparisons would be appropriate.

**Table 17.17** All Means comparisons of sequential time points following Repeated Measures ANOVA.

| | Time 1 | Time 2 | Time 3 | Time 4 | Time 5 | Time 6 |
|---|---|---|---|---|---|---|
| Time 1 | / | * | * | * | * | * |
| Time 2 | | / | * | * | * | * |
| Time 3 | | | / | * | * | * |
| Time 4 | | | | / | * | * |
| Time 5 | | | | | / | * |

* Indicate permissible All Means multiple pairwise comparisons of paired data sets.

**Table 17.18** Control group comparisons of sequential time points following Repeated Measures ANOVA.

| | Time 1 | Time 2 | Time 3 | Time 4 | Time 5 | Time 6 |
|---|---|---|---|---|---|---|
| Time 1 | / | * | * | * | * | * |

* Indicate permissible Control Group multiple pairwise comparisons of paired data sets.

## Mixed ANOVA models

The discussion so far on which multiple pairwise comparison tests are appropriate following ANOVA has been limited to those ANOVA models that have either **only** Between-Group Factors or a Within-Group Factor. The important point to note here is that any subsequent pairwise comparison is based on the independent or paired nature of the data being analysed. Thus, ANOVA techniques with one or more Between-Group Factors require multiple pairwise comparison tests appropriate for **independent** groups, while multiple pairwise comparison tests following significant variation in any Within-Group Factor should reflect the **paired nature** of the data sets concerned; this is especially important in the following examples of **mixed-design** models of ANOVA. Mixed ANOVA models include one or more Between-Group Factors *and* a Within-Group Factor. Just as we saw in the preceding discussion for multiple Between-Group Factors, identification of the justified pairwise comparisons is determined by the results of the ANOVA model. However, the additional issue to consider here, however, is that we also need to use the appropriate pairwise comparison tests according to whether the data sets being compared are independent or paired! The knock-on effect of this, *in my view*, is that the standard *post hoc* tests, as indicated in Tables 15.13 and 17.10, are inappropriate when the experimental design includes **both** Between- and Within-Group Factors!

## Example 17.11 Pairwise comparisons following one-way ANOVA with Repeated Measures (see Ex 17.5)

Consider the experimental design summarised in Table 17.8 where the experimental design includes four different treatment groups from which a measurement is recorded from each subject in each group at six sequential time points. Consequently, there is one Between-Group Factor (treatment) and one Within-Group Factor (time). The output following one-way ANOVA with Repeated Measures will therefore comprise the main effects of these two factors and the interaction between the two factors.

### Main effect of the Between-Group Factor

If the ANOVA model reveals significant variation in the data that is solely dependent on the Between-Group Factor, then the only pairwise comparisons that may be made are those between the different treatment groups at the same time point, i.e. the time at which the treatment groups are compared (the Within-Group factor) **must** remain constant. At any one time point in the experiment, the different treatment groups comprise different subjects and are thus independent from each other.

One may argue that it should be possible to perform either an All Means or Control Group multiple pairwise comparison test for independent groups at a single time point within the experiment and to repeat this approach for all the time points. However, this would be an incorrect approach since the inherent correction of the resulting *p* values to control the Family Error Rate using a standard *post hoc* test at a single time point would not correct for the total number of comparisons made across **all** the time points.

In this experiment (see Table 17.8), there are four treatment groups. Consequently, the standard All Means multiple pairwise comparison tests would perform six pairwise comparisons (as summarised in Table 17.12), whereas the Control Group multiple pairwise comparison test would perform three comparisons (as summarised in Table 17.13) *at each time point* of the experiment. However, since there are 6 time points in the experiment, this would result in a total of either 36 All Means multiple pairwise comparisons (see Table 17.19) or 18 Control Group multiple pairwise comparisons (see Table 17.20) depending on which type of test was used. To use standard *post hoc* tests for independent data sets would therefore risk a Type 1 error since the correction of the *p* values produced by these multiple pairwise comparison tests would greatly underestimate the *total* number of comparisons made by each *post hoc* test. In addition, performing All Means or Control Group multiple pairwise comparisons across *all* the data groups irrespective of treatment or time point would also be incorrect since this approach would perform independent comparisons on paired data groups within each treatment group and thereby also greatly over-compensate the correction of the *p* value (due to the overestimation of the total number of comparisons made), thereby risking a Type 2 error.

**Table 17.19** All Means multiple pairwise comparisons of independent groups following one-way ANOVA with Repeated Measures (Main effect of Between-Group Factor).

| Time point | | Drug 1 | Drug 2 | Drug3 | Drug 4 |
|---|---|---|---|---|---|
| T1 | Drug 1 | / | * | * | * |
| | Drug 2 | | / | * | * |
| | Drug 3 | | | / | * |
| T2 | Drug 1 | / | * | * | * |
| | Drug 2 | | / | * | * |
| | Drug 3 | | | / | * |
| T3 | Drug 1 | / | * | * | * |
| | Drug 2 | | / | * | * |
| | Drug 3 | | | / | * |
| T4 | Drug 1 | / | * | * | * |
| | Drug 2 | | / | * | * |
| | Drug 3 | | | / | * |
| T5 | Drug 1 | | * | * | * |
| | Drug 2 | | / | * | * |
| | Drug 3 | | | / | * |
| T6 | Drug 1 | / | * | * | * |
| | Drug 2 | | / | * | * |
| | Drug 3 | | | / | * |

* Indicate permissible All Means multiple pairwise comparisons of independent groups while keeping the Within-Group Factor (Time) constant.

**Table 17.20** Control Group multiple pairwise comparisons of independent groups following one-way ANOVA with Repeated Measures (Main effect of Between-Group Factor).

| Time Point | | Drug 1 | Drug 2 | Drug3 | Drug 4 |
|---|---|---|---|---|---|
| T1 | Drug 1 | / | * | * | * |
| T2 | Drug 1 | / | * | * | * |
| T3 | Drug 1 | / | * | * | * |
| T4 | Drug 1 | / | * | * | * |
| T5 | Drug 1 | / | * | * | * |
| T6 | Drug 1 | / | * | * | * |

*Indicate permissible Control Group multiple pairwise comparisons of independent groups while keeping the Within-Group Factor (Time) constant.

Consequently, the most appropriate strategy is for the experimenter to make *a priori* decisions about those independent comparisons in which s/he is interested. The experimenter should then perform an *independent t*-test on each comparison of interest and use the Bonferroni correction to control the Family Error Rate for *the total number* of comparisons performed.

### Main effect of the Within-Group Factor

A very similar strategy to that described above should be adopted if the ANOVA model reveals significant variation in the data that is solely dependent on the Within-Group Factor. Here the only pairwise comparisons that may be made are those across the time-course of the experiment for each individual treatment group in turn, i.e. where different time points are compared the treatment group (the Between-Group Factor) **must** remain constant. The various time points throughout the experiment contain the same subjects within a single treatment group and thus such data are paired.

In accordance with the previous discussion, one may argue that it should be possible to perform either a standard All Means or control group *post hoc* multiple pairwise comparison test for paired data groups across the time points for each treatment group in turn. However, this would be an incorrect approach since the inherent correction of the resulting *p* values to control the Family Error Rate for each treatment group for all the paired comparisons across all time points throughout the experiment would not correct for the *total* number of comparisons made for *all* the treatment groups. In this experiment (see Table 17.8), there are 6 time points. Consequently, the standard All Means multiple pairwise comparison tests would perform 15 pairwise comparisons (as summarised in Table 17.17), while the Control Group multiple pairwise comparisons would perform 5 comparisons (as summarised in Table 17.18) *for each treatment group* in the experiment.

However, since there are four treatment groups in the experiment this would result in a total of either 60 All Means multiple pairwise comparisons (see Table 17.21) or 20 Control Group comparisons (see Table 17.22) depending on which type of test was used. So using a standard *post hoc* multiple pairwise comparison test for paired data groups for each treatment group in turn would risk a Type 1 error (see discussion above) since the correction of the *p* values produced by these multiple pairwise comparison tests would greatly underestimate the *total* number of comparisons made by each *post hoc* test. In addition, performing All Means or Control Group multiple pairwise comparisons across

all data groups irrespective of treatment or time point would also be incorrect since this approach would perform paired comparisons on independent data sets at each time point in the experiment and thereby also greatly over compensate the correction of the *p* value (due to the overestimation of the total number of comparisons made), thereby risking a Type 2 error.

**Table 17.21** All Means multiple pairwise comparisons of paired group data following one-way ANOVA with Repeated Measures (Main effect of Within-Group Factor).

| Treatment | | T1 | T2 | T3 | T4 | T5 | T6 |
|---|---|---|---|---|---|---|---|
| Drug 1 | T1 | / | * | * | * | * | * |
| | T2 | | / | * | * | * | * |
| | T3 | | | / | * | * | * |
| | T4 | | | | / | * | * |
| | T5 | | | | | / | * |
| Drug 2 | T1 | / | * | * | * | * | * |
| | T2 | | / | * | * | * | * |
| | T3 | | | / | * | * | * |
| | T4 | | | | / | * | * |
| | T5 | | | | | / | * |
| Drug 3 | T1 | / | * | * | * | * | * |
| | T2 | | / | * | * | * | * |
| | T3 | | | / | * | * | * |
| | T4 | | | | / | * | * |
| | T5 | | | | | / | * |
| Drug 4 | T1 | / | * | * | * | * | * |
| | T2 | | / | * | * | * | * |
| | T3 | | | / | * | * | * |
| | T4 | | | | / | * | * |
| | T5 | | | | | / | * |

*Indicate permissible All Means multiple pairwise comparisons of paired data groups while keeping the Between-Group Factor (Treatment) constant. T1–T6 indicate sequential time points.

**Table 17.22** Control Group multiple pairwise comparisons of paired group data following one-way ANOVA with Repeated Measures (Main effect of Within-Group Factor).

| Treatment | | T1 | T2 | T3 | T4 | T5 | T6 |
|---|---|---|---|---|---|---|---|
| Drug/dose 1 | T1 | / | * | * | * | * | * |
| Drug/dose 2 | T1 | / | * | * | * | * | * |
| Drug/dose 3 | T1 | / | * | * | * | * | * |
| Drug/dose 4 | T1 | / | * | * | * | * | * |

*Indicate permissible Control Group multiple pairwise comparisons of paired data groups while keeping the Between-Group Factor (Treatment) constant. T1–T6 indicate sequential time points, where T1 is the assumed control group.

Consequently, the most appropriate strategy is for the experimenter to make *a priori* decisions about which paired comparisons s/he is interested in. The experimenter should then perform a *paired t*-test to compare those time points of interest within a single treatment group, repeat this strategy for each treatment group in turn, and then use the Bonferroni correction to control the Family Error Rate for *the total number* of comparisons performed.

### Interaction between the Between-Group and Within-Group Factors

If we follow the previous logic for the two- and three-way ANOVA examples described earlier in this chapter but apply that discussion to experimental situations requiring data analysis by a mixed ANOVA model, then any high-level interaction revealed by a one-way ANOVA with Repeated Measures should allow for any group of data to be compared to any other group of data.

However, to employ a standard *post hoc* multiple pairwise All Means or Control Group comparison tests for independent or paired data sets in situations requiring analysis by a mixed ANOVA would be inappropriate since the total number of data sets include **both** independent and paired data. Indeed, the previous discussion with respect to deciding how to identify simple effects in the data following analysis by one-way ANOVA with Repeated Measures reveals that simply applying standard *post hoc* tests for independent or paired data sets across all the data irrespective of either the Between- or Within-Group Factors also risks making both Type 1 and Type 2 errors. The experimenter therefore needs to make *a priori* decisions about which independent and paired comparisons s/he wishes to make. The experimenter should then compare the different groups of data using the independent or paired *t*-test as appropriate and correct the resulting *p* values by applying the Bonferroni correction according to the *total* number of comparisons performed.

## Example 17.12 Pairwise comparisons following two-way ANOVA with Repeated Measures (see Ex 17.6)

The two-way ANOVA with Repeated Measures example described earlier (see Table 17.9) is probably one of the most complicated analysis procedures encountered in experimental pharmacology. As with earlier examples, if the high-order interaction between the both Between-Group Factors and the Within-Group Factor (i.e. Factor 1 * Factor 2 * Time) shows that $p < 0.05$ then all the data sets, regardless of either of the Between-Group Factors or the Within-Group Factor (i.e. across *Time*) may be compared to each other. However, *a priori* decisions are required to identify which comparisons to make and these are then performed with either repeated independent or paired *t*-tests, according to type of data sets involved, and the Bonferroni correction applied according to the **total** number of comparisons performed. As argued in the preceding section, to apply standard *post hoc* multiple pairwise comparison tests to data containing both independent and paired data sets would be an inappropriate strategy and potentially lead to both Type 1 and Type 2 errors.

Furthermore, where only Main effects of the Between or Within-Group Factors are identified by the ANOVA model, or where there are low-order interactions between only 2 of these factors, then the number of pairwise comparisons are severely limited. For the sake of brevity, I'm not going to describe the strategy of identifying which pairwise comparisons are permitted for all possible Main effects and low-order interactions since the arguments provided in the previous section should provide sufficient general guidance. Therefore, I shall just provide a summary of the strategy to adopt in these circumstances.

## Main Effects

### Main Effect of Between-Group Factor 1

Comparison of all groups to each other within Between-Group Factor 1 is allowed as long as the Between-Group Factor 2 and the Within-Group Factor remain constant. All data sets would be independent from each other and so multiple independent *t*-tests with Bonferroni correction should be performed.

### Main effect of Between-Group Factor 2

Comparison of all groups to each other within Between-Group Factor 2 is allowed as long as the Between-Group Factor 1 and the Within-Group Factor remain constant. All data sets would be independent from each other and so multiple independent *t*-tests with Bonferroni correction should be performed.

### Main effect of Within-Group Factor

Comparison of all groups to each other across all time points of the experiment is allowed for each treatment combination in turn; this will ensure that the two Between-Group Factors remain constant. All data sets would contain the same individual subjects and so multiple paired *t*-tests with Bonferroni correction should be performed.

## Low-order interactions

### Between-Group Factor 1 * Between-Group Factor 2

Comparison of all groups to each other within both Between-Group Factor 1 and Between-Group Factor 2 is allowed as long as the Within-Group Factor remains constant. All data sets would be independent from each other and so multiple independent *t*-tests with Bonferroni correction should be performed.

### Between-Group Factor 1 * Within-Group Factor

Comparison of all groups to each other within Between-Group Factor 1 and across all time points of the experiment is allowed as long as the Between-Group Factor 2 remains constant. Pairwise comparisons should be performed by multiple independent and paired *t*-tests, as appropriate according to the nature of the data being compared, with Bonferroni correction.

### Between-Group Factor 2 * Within-Group Factor

Comparison of all groups to each other within Between-Group Factor 2 and across all time points of the experiment is allowed as long as the Between-Group Factor 1 remains constant. Pairwise comparisons should be performed by multiple independent and paired *t*-tests, as appropriate according to the nature of the data being compared, with Bonferroni correction.

## Bonferroni and alternative correction procedures

Throughout this chapter, I have emphasised how multiple pairwise comparisons by either the independent or paired *t*-test may be used with Bonferroni correction whenever it is inappropriate to use the

126

Experimental Design and Statistical Analysis for Pharmacology and the Biomedical S...

standard *post hoc* tests, thereby forcing the experimenter to make *a priori* decisions about which pairwise comparisons to perform. I have argued previously why the Bonferroni correction is important (see Chapter 10, especially Tables 10.2 and 10.3).

The Bonferroni correction is generally calculated by two methods; it doesn't matter which method is used as the final conclusions are identical.

**1** The first method (and easiest to understand) is to multiply the *p* value determined by the pairwise comparison test by the total number of comparisons that are performed (*n*) across all the data. If the modified *p* value is still less than the chosen Family Error Rate (i.e. $\alpha$, usually 0.05), then the Null Hypothesis may be rejected, and the user may conclude that the two groups are different at the 0.05 level.

**2** The second method is to divide the Family Error Rate (i.e. 0.05) by the number of comparisons made (i.e. $0.05/n$). If the *p* value determined by the pairwise comparison test is less than the modified probability level, then the Null Hypothesis may be rejected, and the user may conclude that the two groups are different at the 0.05 level.

Of course, the greater the number of pairwise comparisons required, then the greater the Bonferroni correction procedure has on the adjusted *p* value to decide whether to accept or reject the Null hypothesis. A less conservative approach is provided by the Holme correction procedure.

## Holme correction procedure

The Holme correction procedure is a modified, less conservative approach to the Bonferroni method.

Consider a large experiment where, following a suitable ANOVA analysis, the *a priori* decision has identified 10 pairwise comparisons performed by multiple independent *t*-tests in which we are interested. Table 17.23 summarises the resulting *p* values from each *t*-test listed in order of magnitude (lowest *p* value first). The multistage Holme correction procedure corrects the *p* value by dividing the Family Error Rate ($\alpha$) by the number of pairwise comparisons remaining to be performed (see Table 17.23 second column); thus,

$$\alpha' = \alpha/c \qquad (17.1)$$

where $\alpha$ is the Family Error Rate and *c* is the number of comparisons remaining.

**Table 17.23** Summary of Holme correction procedure.

| Comparison | No of comparisons remaining | $\alpha'$ | Original p value (t-test) | Decision |
|---|---|---|---|---|
| 1 | 10 | 0.005 | $p < 0.001$ | Reject $H_0$ |
| 2 | 9 | 0.00556 | $p < 0.001$ | Reject $H_0$ |
| 3 | 8 | 0.00625 | $p = 0.000412$ | Reject $H_0$ |
| 4 | 7 | 0.00714 | $p = 0.000998$ | Reject $H_0$ |
| 5 | 6 | 0.00833 | $p = 0.00708$ | Reject $H_0$ |
| 6 | 5 | 0.01 | $p = 0.0115$ | Accept $H_0$ |
| 7 | 4 | 0.0125 | $p = 0.0121$ | Non- |
| 8 | 3 | 0.0167 | $p = 0.0164$ | applicable |
| 9 | 2 | 0.025 | $p = 0.0355$ | as $H_0$ |
| 10 | 1 | 0.05 | $p = 0.25$ | accepted |

For the first comparison $0.05/10 = 0.005$ and since the calculated *p* from the *t*-test is less than $\alpha'$, then the Null Hypothesis is rejected. For the second comparison $0.05/9 = 0.00556$. The calculated *p* from the second *t*-test is still less than $\alpha'$ and so the Null Hypothesis is rejected for a second time. This procedure is repeated by dividing 0.05 by the sequentially adjusted denominator until the **first** occasion where the original *p* value exceeds the adjusted $\alpha'$; whereupon the Null Hypothesis is accepted (see comparison 6). At this point, the sequential procedure stops and the Null Hypothesis accepted for all the remaining pairwise comparisons, even if subsequent values of *p* are less than the calculated value of $\alpha'$ (see comparison 7).

## General comments on complex ANOVA models

If you've managed to keep up with the discussions in this chapter, then I admire your tenacity in staying with it (either that or you've been successfully bribed by your statistics lecturer)! It is quite clear from the foregoing pages that complex models of ANOVA raise a number of issues that standard statistical inferential tests struggle to address – in particular the appropriate multiple pairwise comparisons to perform following analysis by mixed ANOVA models. Indeed, many readers at this point must be left wondering '**Why bother?**' and, indeed, that was a question I asked myself repeatedly while writing this chapter!

The actual reason is simply that because we wish to make accurate, justifiable, inferences from our experimental data about the real world then we must have confidence in the results produced by whatever strategy we wish to adopt to analyse our data. By extension, therefore, we need to minimise the possibility of making Type 1 and Type 2 errors, i.e. we do not wish to identify statistical differences between groups where no difference exists (a Type 1 error), nor do we wish to conclude that there is no difference between two sets of data when, in the real world, the difference between two groups is real (a Type 2 error).

And there, in a nutshell, is the sole reason why we need to analyse our experimental data in a statistically robust manner – as I've stated before, it's simply to stop ourselves making a balls-up by drawing ridiculous conclusions from our data!

The discussions on the previous pages show how quickly these complex ANOVA models may produce a plethora of multiple pairwise comparisons. But one question you must always ask yourself is '**Are all these possible pairwise comparisons necessary?**' For example, if a mixed ANOVA model reveals a significant high-order interaction between the Between-Group Factor(s) and the Within-Group Factor, then is it really necessary to compare two different treatments (or treatment combinations) at diverse time points in the experiment? This is a question that only the experimenter may answer, but in most cases, the answer is probably 'No!' Consequently, an understanding of how to make suitable *a priori* decisions about which pairwise comparisons are important is critical (and this will depend on the aims of your experiment). Of course, by limiting the number of pairwise comparisons you decide to make will reduce the impact of the Bonferroni or Holme correction on the adjusted *p* values following the independent or paired *t*-tests, and so making *a priori* decisions about which pairwise comparisons to make is generally a better strategy to adopt rather than making all possible pairwise comparisons across all groups of data collected.

From an experimental pharmacologist's point of view, ANOVA results that support the Null Hypothesis (i.e. where $p \geq 0.05$) are equally important in identifying significant variation between data sets due to the Main effects of Between or Within-Group Factors or any of the possible interactions between two or more of these factors, and this is where the strategy adopted by an experimental pharmacologist may sometimes differ from that of a pure statistician. Consider the experimental design that includes two Between-Group Factors; for example, the pharmacodynamic interaction between a receptor antagonist and an agonist drug at the same receptor (see Table 17.5). The data from such an experiment would be analysed initially by a two-way ANOVA, producing the following output (with possible pairwise comparisons as summarised in Table 17.14 – see also the following screen shots at the end of this chapter);

- Main effect of Between-Group Factor 1
- Main effect of Between-Group Factor 2
- Interaction between both Between-Group Factors 1 and 2,

If the analysis reveals an interaction between the two main Between-Group Factors, then all possible pairwise comparisons may be performed using one of the standard All Means *post hoc* tests. However, if the analysis only shows one or both of the Main effects, then it is at this point that the strategy to analyse the data further may differ between the pharmacologist and the pure statistician! In this experiment, there are four treatment combinations (see Table 17.24, adapted from Table 17.5), and let us assume there are six subjects per treatment combination; thus,

Table 17.24 Summary of treatment combinations.

| Group no. | Between Factor 2 (Pre-Treatment) | Between Factor 1 (Acute Treatment) | Subject numbers |
|---|---|---|---|
| 1 | Control | Control | 6 |
| 2 | | Agonist drug | 6 |
| 3 | Antagonist drug | Control | 6 |
| 4 | | Agonist drug | 6 |

Let us further assume that the two-way ANOVA revealed a Main effect of acute treatment only. Consequently, there is no significant variation in the data due to the pre-treatment of the subjects. There is a valid statistical argument at this point, adopted by most pure statisticians that I have discussed this with, to collapse the data across pre-treatment factor of the experiment. Thus, the data from treatment combination group 1 (control plus control) would be combined with the data from treatment combination group 3 (antagonist plus control) to produce a group of subjects that received an acute control treatment with $n = 12$. Likewise, the data from treatment combination group 2 (control plus agonist) would be combined with the data from treatment combination group 4 (antagonist plus agonist) to produce a group of subjects that received an acute treatment with the agonist drug and also where $n = 12$.

This collapses the data into two groups, each with $n = 12$, thereby allowing the control group to be compared to the group treated with the agonist drug. Clearly, the pre-treatment factor is ignored in the final pairwise comparison between these groups, although the power of the comparison would be increased due to the increased number of subjects on each group. The decision to collapse data across groups when the Null Hypothesis is accepted is often an approach adopted by the pure statistician and is a perfectly valid strategy!

*But it is not the strategy adopted by the experimental pharmacologist!*

The pharmacologist, however, argues that even though there is no *measurable* difference between the experimental output of the pre-treatment control subjects to those receiving the antagonist drug, these two groups are still different because the control group has drug-vehicle molecules on board, while the other subjects have drug molecules on-board, i.e. these groups are different in some way due to our experimental intervention (i.e. drug treatment) – it is just that the experimental output has failed to identify that difference. Furthermore, demonstrating that a pre-treatment has had no effect on the measured experimental output may be integral to the aims of the experiment. Consequently, the experimental pharmacologist favours maintaining the differentiation and integrity of the various treatment combinations in the experiment.

# Example output from statistical software

## Example data: Two Between-Group Factors = Two-way ANOVA

The following experiment was designed to examine the pharmacodynamic interaction between the 5-HT$_{2C}$ receptor antagonist, mesulergine, and the 5-HT$_{2C}$ receptor agonist, *meta*-chlorophenyl piperazine (*m*CPP) on rodent exploratory locomotor activity. Four groups of eight male Wistar rats per group were treated with saline or mesulergine, followed by either saline or mCPP (cf. Table 17.5) following which exploratory locomotor activity was recorded for 5 min immediately following placing the subjects in activity monitors. Table 17.25 summarises the resulting exploratory locomotor activity counts; these data were previously presented in Figure 1.1 (Chapter 1).

The following screen shots summarise the results of analysis by two-way ANOVA and subsequent *post hoc* analysis according to the different software packages used.

Table 17.25 Effect of mesulergine on *m*CPP-induced reduction in rodent exploratory activity.

| Pre-treatment (1 h) Acute treatment (30 min) | Saline Saline | Saline *m*CPP | Mesulergine Saline | Mesulergine *m*CPP |
|---|---|---|---|---|
| 1 | 583 | 192 | 547 | 495 |
| 2 | 654 | 234 | 624 | 593 |
| 3 | 555 | 96 | 579 | 512 |
| 4 | 590 | 132 | 592 | 535 |
| 5 | 727 | 155 | 745 | 695 |
| 6 | 479 | 67 | 498 | 501 |
| 7 | 614 | 183 | 601 | 584 |
| 8 | 622 | 152 | 624 | 555 |
| Mean | 603.0 | 151.4 | 601.3 | 558.8 |
| Standard Deviation | 72.4 | 53.5 | 71.6 | 66.0 |
| Standard Error of the Mean | 25.6 | 18.9 | 25.3 | 23.4 |

1 hour prior to measurement of locomotor activity, rats were pre-treated with either saline or mesulergine followed 30 min later by acute treatment with either saline of *m*CPP as indicated in the column headings in the table. Values indicate locomotor activity counts for each subject according to treatment combination ($n = 8$ per group). Two-way ANOVA revealed a significant effect of pre-treatment [$F(1, 28) = 74.80$, $p < 0.001$], a significant effect of acute treatment [$F(1, 28) = 111.0$, $p < 0.001$], and a significant pre-treatment × acute treatment interaction [$F(1, 28) = 76.10$, $p < 0.001$]. *Post hoc* analysis (Tukey test) revealed that rats treated with saline plus *m*CPP only exhibited significantly lower exploratory locomotor activity compared to that exhibited by rats in the other treatment combination groups ($p < 0.001$ in all cases).

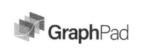 

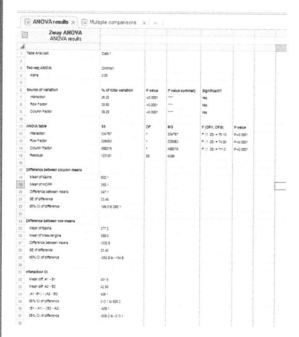

Summary statistical analysis from GraphPad Prism, v8. The left panel shows the summary output following analysis by two-way ANOVA, while the right panel summarises the results of *post hoc* analysis using Tukey's test for multiple comparisons.
*Source*: GraphPad Software.

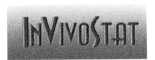

## Analysis of variance (ANOVA) table

| Effect | Sums of squares | Degrees of freedom | Mean square | F-value | p-value |
|--------|-----------------|--------------------|-------------|---------|---------|
| Pre | 329063.281 | 1 | 329063.281 | 74.80 | < 0.0001 |
| Acute | 488319.031 | 1 | 488319.031 | 111.00 | < 0.0001 |
| Pre * Acute | 334766.531 | 1 | 334766.531 | 76.10 | < 0.0001 |
| Residual | 123180.875 | 28 | 4399.317 | | |

Comment: ANOVA table calculated using a Type I model fit, see Armitage et al. (2001).

Conclusion: There is a statistically significant overall difference between the levels of Pre, Acute, Pre:Acute.

Tip: While it is a good idea to consider the overall tests in the ANOVA table, we should not rely on them when deciding whether or not to make pairwise comparisons.

## All pairwise comparisons using Bonferroni's procedure

| Comparison | Difference | Lower 95% CI | Upper 95% CI | Std error | p-value |
|------------|-----------|--------------|--------------|-----------|---------|
| mesulergine Sal - mesulergine mCPP | 42.500 | -25.433 | 110.433 | 33.164 | 1.0000 |
| Sal mCPP - mesulergine mCPP | -407.375 | -475.308 | -339.442 | 33.164 | < 0.0001 |
| Sal Sal - mesulergine mCPP | 44.250 | -23.683 | 112.183 | 33.164 | 1.0000 |
| Sal mCPP - mesulergine Sal | -449.875 | -517.808 | -381.942 | 33.164 | < 0.0001 |
| Sal Sal - mesulergine Sal | 1.750 | -66.183 | 69.683 | 33.164 | 1.0000 |
| Sal Sal - Sal mCPP | 451.625 | 383.692 | 519.558 | 33.164 | < 0.0001 |

Conclusion: The following pairwise tests are statistically significantly different at the 5% level: Sal mCPP - mesulergine mCPP, Sal mCPP - mesulergine Sal, Sal Sal - Sal mCPP.

Warning: This procedure makes an adjustment assuming you want to make all pairwise comparisons. If this is not the case then these tests may be unduly conservative. You may wish to use planned comparisons (using unadjusted p-values) instead, see Snedecor and Cochran (1989), or make a manual adjustment to the unadjusted p-values using the InVivoStat P-value Adjustment module.

Note: The confidence intervals quoted are not adjusted for multiplicity.

## Analysis description

The data were analysed using a 2-way ANOVA approach, with Pre and Acute as the treatment factors. This was followed by all pairwise comparisons between the predicted means of the Pre * Acute interaction using Bonferroni's procedure, Bonferroni (1936).

For more information on the theoretical approaches that are implemented within this module, see Bate and Clark (2014).

Summary statistical analysis from InVivo Stat, v4.0.2. The top panel shows the summary output following analysis by two-way ANOVA, while the bottom panel summarises the results of *post hoc* analysis using Bonferroni's test for multiple comparisons.

*Source*: InVivoStat.

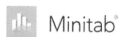

## Analysis of variance

| Source | DF | Adj SS | Adj MS | F-value | P-value |
|---|---|---|---|---|---|
| C1 | 1 | 329 063 | 329 063 | 20.84 | 0.000 |
| C2 | 1 | 488 319 | 488 319 | 30.92 | 0.000 |
| Error | 29 | 457 947 | 15 791 | | |
| Lack-of-fit | 1 | 334 767 | 334 767 | 76.10 | 0.000 |
| Pure error | 28 | 123 181 | 4 399 | | |
| Total | 31 | 1275 330 | | | |

## Grouping information using the Tukey method and 95% confidence

| C4 | N | Mean | Grouping |
|---|---|---|---|
| 1 | 8 | 603.0 | A |
| 3 | 8 | 601.3 | A |
| 4 | 8 | 558.8 | A |
| 2 | 8 | 151.4 | B |

*Means that do not share a letter are significantly different.*

## Grouping information using the Tukey method and 99% confidence

| C4 | N | Mean | Grouping |
|---|---|---|---|
| 1 | 8 | 603.0 | A |
| 3 | 8 | 601.3 | A |
| 4 | 8 | 558.8 | A |
| 2 | 8 | 151.4 | B |

*Means that do not share a letter are significantly different.*

Summary statistical analysis from MiniTab, v18. The top panel shows the summary output following analysis by two-way ANOVA, while the bottom panels summarise the results of *post hoc* analysis using Tukey's test for multiple comparisons at $p < 0.05$ and $p < 0.01$, respectively.

*Source*: Minitab, LLC.

### Tests of Between-Subjects Effects

Dependent Variable: Locomotion

| Source | Type III Sum of Squares | df | Mean Square | F | Sig. |
|---|---|---|---|---|---|
| Corrected Model | 1152148.84[a] | 3 | 384049.615 | 87.298 | .000 |
| Intercept | 7329663.281 | 1 | 7329663.281 | 1666.091 | .000 |
| Antag | 329063.281 | 1 | 329063.281 | 74.799 | .000 |
| Agonist | 488319.031 | 1 | 488319.031 | 110.999 | .000 |
| Antag * Agonist | 334766.531 | 1 | 334766.531 | 76.095 | .000 |
| Error | 123180.875 | 28 | 4399.317 | | |
| Total | 8604993.000 | 32 | | | |
| Corrected Total | 1275329.719 | 31 | | | |

a. R Squared = .903 (Adjusted R Squared = .893)

### Multiple Comparisons

Dependent Variable: Locomotion

Tukey HSD

| (I) VAR00010 | (J) VAR00010 | Mean Difference (I-J) | Std. Error | Sig. | 95% Confidence Interval Lower Bound | Upper Bound |
|---|---|---|---|---|---|---|
| 1.00 | 2.00 | 451.62500* | 33.16367 | .000 | 361.0778 | 542.1722 |
| | 3.00 | 1.75000 | 33.16367 | 1.000 | -88.7972 | 92.2972 |
| | 4.00 | 44.25000 | 33.16367 | .550 | -46.2972 | 134.7972 |
| 2.00 | 1.00 | -451.62500* | 33.16367 | .000 | -542.1722 | -361.0778 |
| | 3.00 | -449.87500* | 33.16367 | .000 | -540.4222 | -359.3278 |
| | 4.00 | -407.37500* | 33.16367 | .000 | -497.9222 | -316.8278 |
| 3.00 | 1.00 | -1.75000 | 33.16367 | 1.000 | -92.2972 | 88.7972 |
| | 2.00 | 449.87500* | 33.16367 | .000 | 359.3278 | 540.4222 |
| | 4.00 | 42.50000 | 33.16367 | .582 | -48.0472 | 133.0472 |
| 4.00 | 1.00 | -44.25000 | 33.16367 | .550 | -134.7972 | 46.2972 |
| | 2.00 | 407.37500* | 33.16367 | .000 | 316.8278 | 497.9222 |
| | 3.00 | -42.50000 | 33.16367 | .582 | -133.0472 | 48.0472 |

*. The mean difference is significant at the 0.05 level.

Summary statistical analysis from SPSS, v27. The left panel shows the summary output following analysis by two-way ANOVA, while the right panel summarises the results of *post hoc* analysis using Tukey's test for multiple comparisons.

*Source*: IBM Corporation.

## Example data: one Between-Group Factor plus one Within-Group Factor = One-way ANOVA with Repeated Measures

The following experiment was designed to examine the effect of increasing doses of amphetamine on rodent locomotor activity.

Four groups of eight male Wistar rats per group were treated with either saline or amphetamine, 0.33, 1.0, or 3.0 mg/kg sc. Thirty min later locomotor activity was recorded every 5 min over a 30-min period immediately following placing the subjects in activity monitors. The tables below summarize the resulting locomotor activity counts for each subject within each treatment group.

**Saline, 2 ml/kg sc**

| Time (5 min time bins) | 0–5 | 5–10 | 10–15 | 15–20 | 20–25 | 25–30 |
|---|---|---|---|---|---|---|
| 1 | 583 | 347 | 200 | 120 | 75 | 72 |
| 2 | 654 | 475 | 325 | 140 | 82 | 60 |
| 3 | 555 | 333 | 203 | 65 | 126 | 78 |
| 4 | 590 | 354 | 110 | 232 | 29 | 57 |
| 5 | 727 | 462 | 210 | 129 | 78 | 128 |
| 6 | 479 | 250 | 115 | 76 | 148 | 55 |
| 7 | 614 | 370 | 229 | 143 | 56 | 20 |
| 8 | 622 | 357 | 300 | 60 | 32 | 121 |
| Mean | 603.0 | 368.5 | 211.5 | 120.6 | 78.3 | 73.9 |
| Standard Deviation | 72.4 | 71.9 | 76.4 | 56.2 | 41.8 | 35.7 |
| Standard Error of the Mean | 25.6 | 25.4 | 27.0 | 19.9 | 14.8 | 12.6 |

**Amphetamine, 0.33 mg/kg sc**

| Time (5 min time bins) | 0–5 | 5–10 | 10–15 | 15–20 | 20–25 | 25–30 |
|---|---|---|---|---|---|---|
| 1 | 383 | 247 | 150 | 80 | 45 | 122 |
| 2 | 454 | 275 | 125 | 70 | 62 | 90 |
| 3 | 355 | 233 | 183 | 55 | 106 | 98 |
| 4 | 390 | 254 | 120 | 132 | 39 | 157 |
| 5 | 527 | 362 | 140 | 109 | 58 | 98 |
| 6 | 379 | 150 | 125 | 85 | 78 | 65 |
| 7 | 414 | 270 | 149 | 113 | 86 | 80 |
| 8 | 422 | 257 | 150 | 90 | 42 | 71 |
| Mean | 415.5 | 256.0 | 142.8 | 91.8 | 64.5 | 97.6 |
| Standard Deviation | 54.3 | 58.1 | 20.4 | 25.0 | 23.8 | 29.9 |
| Standard Error of the Mean | 19.2 | 20.5 | 7.2 | 8.8 | 8.4 | 10.6 |

**Amphetamine, 1.0 mg/kg sc**

| Time (5 min time bins) | 0–5 | 5–10 | 10–15 | 15–20 | 20–25 | 25–30 |
|---|---|---|---|---|---|---|
| 1 | 293 | 177 | 160 | 140 | 175 | 182 |
| 2 | 334 | 195 | 145 | 140 | 162 | 180 |
| 3 | 285 | 193 | 123 | 135 | 186 | 238 |
| 4 | 290 | 244 | 120 | 162 | 129 | 157 |
| 5 | 367 | 192 | 190 | 139 | 128 | 128 |
| 6 | 249 | 220 | 215 | 146 | 148 | 155 |
| 7 | 304 | 190 | 129 | 123 | 106 | 150 |
| 8 | 352 | 187 | 160 | 60 | 102 | 121 |
| Mean | 309.3 | 199.8 | 155.3 | 130.6 | 142.0 | 163.9 |
| Standard Deviation | 39.0 | 21.6 | 33.6 | 30.5 | 31.0 | 36.9 |
| Standard Error of the Mean | 13.8 | 7.6 | 11.9 | 10.8 | 11.0 | 13.0 |

**Amphetamine, 3.0 mg/kg sc**

| Time (5 min time bins) | 0–5 | 5–10 | 10–15 | 15–20 | 20–25 | 25–30 |
|---|---|---|---|---|---|---|
| 1 | 203 | 147 | 180 | 220 | 245 | 272 |
| 2 | 254 | 125 | 155 | 140 | 182 | 200 |
| 3 | 155 | 103 | 123 | 225 | 246 | 258 |
| 4 | 190 | 124 | 130 | 172 | 229 | 247 |
| 5 | 227 | 132 | 160 | 229 | 268 | 288 |
| 6 | 179 | 150 | 145 | 176 | 238 | 255 |
| 7 | 214 | 170 | 159 | 203 | 256 | 220 |
| 8 | 222 | 157 | 130 | 180 | 232 | 221 |
| Mean | 205.5 | 138.5 | 147.8 | 193.1 | 237.0 | 245.1 |
| Standard Deviation | 30.8 | 21.5 | 19.3 | 31.3 | 25.6 | 29.5 |
| Standard Error of the Mean | 10.9 | 7.6 | 6.8 | 11.1 | 9.0 | 10.4 |

30 min prior to measurement of locomotor activity rats were treated with either saline, 2 ml/kg sc, or amphetamine, 0.33, 1.0 or 3.0 mg/kg sc. Values indicate loco-motor activity counts for each subject according to treatment combination ($n = 8$ per group). One-way ANOVA with Repeated Measures revealed a significant effect of Treatment [$F(3, 28) = 14.92$, $p < 0.001$], a significant effect of Time [$F(3.32, 92.95) = 202.8$, $p < 0.001$] (where the Greenhouse–Geisser estimate showed a substantial deviation of sphericity, $\hat{\varepsilon} = 0.6639$) and a significant Treatment × x Time interaction [$F(15, 140) = 50.03$, $p < 0.001$].

The following screen shots summarise the results of analysis by one-way ANOVA with Repeated Measures according to the different software packages used. The results of subsequent *post hoc* analysis have been omitted for brevity.

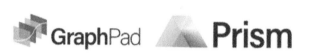

GraphPad Prism

| 1 | Table Analyzed | Data 1 | | | | | |
|---|---|---|---|---|---|---|---|
| 2 | | | | | | | |
| 3 | Two-way RM ANOVA | Matching Across row | | | | | |
| 4 | Assume sphericity? | No | | | | | |
| 5 | Alpha | 0.05 | | | | | |
| 6 | | | | | | | |
| 7 | Source of Variation | % of total variation | P value | P value summary | Significant? | | Geisser-Greenhouse's epsilon |
| 8 | Treatment x Time | 36.84 | <0.0001 | **** | Yes | | |
| 9 | Treatment | 3.990 | <0.0001 | **** | Yes | | |
| 10 | Time | 49.80 | <0.0001 | **** | Yes | | 0.6639 |
| 11 | Subject | 2.496 | 0.0129 | * | Yes | | |
| 12 | | | | | | | |
| 13 | ANOVA table | SS | DF | MS | F (DFn, DFd) | P value | |
| 14 | Treatment x Time | 1153870 | 15 | 76925 | F (15, 140) = 50.03 | P<0.0001 | |
| 15 | Treatment | 124961 | 3 | 41654 | F (3, 28) = 14.92 | P<0.0001 | |
| 16 | Time | 1559485 | 5 | 311897 | F (3.320, 92.95) = 202.8 | P<0.0001 | |
| 17 | Subject | 78179 | 28 | 2792 | F (28, 140) = 1.816 | P=0.0129 | |
| 18 | Residual | 215263 | 140 | 1538 | | | |
| 19 | | | | | | | |
| 20 | Data summary | | | | | | |
| 21 | Number of columns (Time) | 6 | | | | | |
| 22 | Number of rows (Treatment) | 4 | | | | | |
| 23 | Number of subjects (Subject) | 32 | | | | | |
| 24 | Number of missing values | 0 | | | | | |

Summary statistical analysis from GraphPad Prism, v8. The panel shows the summary output following analysis by one-way ANOVA with Repeated Measures; note carefully the values for each degrees of freedom, especially for the main effect of Time following the Greenhouse–Geisser estimate of sphericity.

*Source*: GraphPad Software.

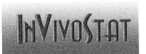

## Table of overall tests of model effects

| Effect | Num. df | Den. df | F-value | p-value |
|---|---|---|---|---|
| Treatment | 3 | 28 | 14.92 | < 0.0001 |
| Time | 5 | 140 | 202.85 | < 0.0001 |
| Treatment * Time | 15 | 140 | 50.03 | < 0.0001 |

Comment: The overall tests in this table are marginal likelihood ratio tests, where the order they appear in the table does not influence the results.

Conclusion: At the 5% level there is a statistically significant overall difference between the levels of Treatment, Time and Treatment * Time.

Tip: While it is a good idea to consider the overall tests in the above table, we should not rely on them when deciding whether or not to make pairwise comparisons.

## Analysis description

The data were analysed using a 2-way repeated measures mixed model approach, with Treatment as the treatment factor and Time as the repeated factor.

The compound symmetric covariance structure was used to model the within-subject correlations. When using this structure we assumed that the variability of the responses was the same at each level of Time and the correlation between responses from any pair of levels of Time is the same.

A full description of mixed model theory, including information on the R nlme package used by InVivoStat, can be found in Venables and Ripley (2003) and Pinheiro and Bates (2002).

For more information on the theoretical approaches that are implemented within this module, see Bate and Clark (2014).

Summary statistical analysis from InVivo Stat, v4.0.2. The panel shows the summary output following analysis by one-way ANOVA with Repeated Measures.

*Source*: InVivoStat.

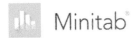

## Analysis of variance

| Source | DF | Adj SS | Adj MS | F-value | P-value |
|---|---|---|---|---|---|
| Treatment | 3 | 124 961 | 41 654 | 14.92 | 0.000 |
| Time | 5 | 1 559 485 | 311 897 | 202.85 | 0.000 |
| Subject (treatment) | 28 | 78 179 | 2792 | 1.82 | 0.013 |
| Treatment*time | 15 | 1 153 870 | 76 925 | 50.03 | 0.000 |
| Error | 140 | 215 263 | 1 538 | | |
| Total | 191 | 3 131 758 | | | |

Summary statistical analysis from MiniTab, v18. The panel shows the summary output following analysis by one-way ANOVA with Repeated Measures.

*Source*: Minitab, LLC.

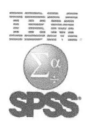

### Tests of Within-Subjects Effects

Measure: Locomotion

| Source | | Type III Sum of Squares | df | Mean Square | F | Sig. |
|---|---|---|---|---|---|---|
| time | Sphericity Assumed | 1559484.651 | 5 | 311896.930 | 202.848 | .000 |
| | Greenhouse-Geisser | 1559484.651 | 3.320 | 469786.279 | 202.848 | .000 |
| | Huynh-Feldt | 1559484.651 | 4.223 | 369281.858 | 202.848 | .000 |
| | Lower-bound | 1559484.651 | 1.000 | 1559484.651 | 202.848 | .000 |
| time * Treatment | Sphericity Assumed | 1153869.870 | 15 | 76924.658 | 50.029 | .000 |
| | Greenhouse-Geisser | 1153869.870 | 9.959 | 115865.677 | 50.029 | .000 |
| | Huynh-Feldt | 1153869.870 | 12.669 | 91077.782 | 50.029 | .000 |
| | Lower-bound | 1153869.870 | 3.000 | 384623.290 | 50.029 | .000 |
| Error(time) | Sphericity Assumed | 215262.646 | 140 | 1537.590 | | |
| | Greenhouse-Geisser | 215262.646 | 92.948 | 2315.954 | | |
| | Huynh-Feldt | 215262.646 | 118.245 | 1820.487 | | |
| | Lower-bound | 215262.646 | 28.000 | 7687.952 | | |

### Tests of Between-Subjects Effects

Measure: Locomotion

Transformed Variable: Average

| Source | Type III Sum of Squares | df | Mean Square | F | Sig. |
|---|---|---|---|---|---|
| Intercept | 7653223.380 | 1 | 7653223.380 | 2741.021 | .000 |
| Treatment | 124961.474 | 3 | 41653.825 | 14.918 | .000 |
| Error | 78178.979 | 28 | 2792.106 | | |

Summary statistical analysis from SPSS, v27. The upper panel shows the summary output following analysis by one-way ANOVA with Repeated Measures involving the Within-Group Factor, Time, while the lower panel summarises the output for the Between-Group Factor, Treatment. In all cases, $p < 0.001$.

*Source*: IBM Corporation.

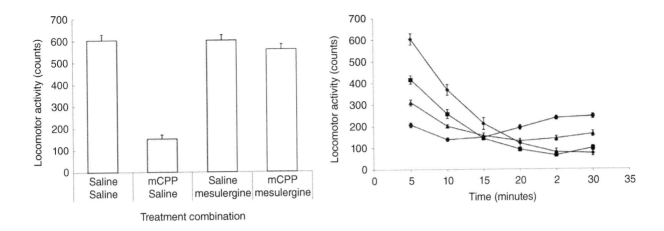

Summary figures: **Left panel** – summary of pharmacodynamic interaction between mesulergine and *m*CPP. *X*-axis indicates treatment combination administered to each group of rats. *Y*-axis indicates locomotor activity counts. Vertical bars indicate mean + S.E.M. exploratory locomotor activity recorded over 0–5 min following introduction into activity monitors (*n* = 8 per group). Raw data analysed by two-way ANOVA with pre-treatment and acute treatment as Between-Group Factors (see screen shots above). **Right panel** – summary time course data of the effect of increasing doses of amphetamine on rodent locomotor activity. *X*-axis indicates sequential 5 min time bins throughout the experiment. *Y*-axis indicates locomotor activity counts. Closed diamonds indicate saline, 2 ml/kg sc, closed squares indicate amphetamine, 0.33 mg/kg sc, closed triangles indicate 1.0 mg/kg sc, closed circles indicate amphetamine, 3.0 mg/kg sc. Raw data analysed by one-way ANOVA with Repeated Measures, with acute treatment as Between-Group Factor and time as Within-Group Factor (see screen shots earlier).

# 18 Non-parametric ANOVA

## Overview

As previously explained, the various ANOVA models described in Chapters 15–17 are only suitable for data sets that are normally distributed; but how do we analyse the data from experiments with more than two Between-Group or Within-Group Factors, where the data sets do not follow a normal distribution? As described at length in Chapter 17 (sorry!), there is an array of complex ANOVA models that we may use to analyse normally distributed data sets arising from quite complicated experimental designs. Unfortunately, there do not appear to be a similar range of non-parametric ANOVA models. In fact, most statistical textbooks only describe two non-parametric ANOVA tests:

- The Kruskal–Wallis test (the non-parametric equivalent of the one-way ANOVA with one Between-Group Factor)
- The Friedman test (the non-parametric equivalent of the Repeated Measures ANOVA with one Within-Group Factor).

In addition, there is the Scheirer–Ray–Hare extension to the Kruskal–Wallis test that allows non-parametric data with two Between-Group Factors to be analysed; i.e. a non-parametric equivalent of the two-way ANOVA.

In this chapter, I shall use the same approach as in the previous chapters describing ANOVA models. First, I shall describe the non-parametric ANOVA models indicated above after which I shall describe methods by which multiple pairwise comparisons may be performed. It should be noted that as with other non-parametric methods the models of non-parametric ANOVA use the ranks of the samples rather than the actual values of each sample. For this reason, such tests are generally lower in power compared to their equivalent parametric ANOVA models and therefore considered to be more conservative.

## Example 18.1 Non-parametric one-way ANOVA: The Kruskal–Wallis test

The Kruskal–Wallis test is the non-parametric equivalent of the one-way ANOVA. Consequently, there is only one Between-Group Factor.

Stimulation of 5-HT$_{2A}$ receptors induces head-shake behaviour in rats, which may be easily counted. Consider the following experiment where 30 male, adult, Wistar rats were divided into three equal groups ($n = 10$ per group), and each group treated subcutaneously with one of the following treatments; 0.9% saline (dose volume 1 ml/kg) or Drug A (a potential 5-HT$_{2A}$ receptor agonist) at either 1 or 3 mg/kg. The occurrence of head shakes was counted by an observer (who was blind to treatment) for each subject for 10 minutes immediately following treatment; the resulting scores are shown in Table 18.1.

Table 18.1 Induction of head-shake behaviour.

| Subject number | 0.9% Saline | Drug A, 1.0 mg/kg | Drug A, 3.0 mg/kg |
|---|---|---|---|
| 1 | 3 | 4 | 7 |
| 2 | 4 | 5 | 8 |
| 3 | 3 | 2 | 7 |
| 4 | 5 | 5 | 11 |
| 5 | 2 | 4 | 24 |
| 6 | 2 | 6 | 13 |
| 7 | 2 | 4 | 15 |
| 8 | 3 | 2 | 14 |
| 9 | 8 | 5 | 11 |
| 10 | 3 | 8 | 19 |
| Median | 3 | 4.5 | 12 |

The Null Hypothesis for the experiment is that there is no difference between the magnitude of head-shake behaviour expressed by the three groups of rats irrespective of treatment. As the data are non-parametric, we would therefore expect to see no difference in the median values for the data sets.

The first step in the Kruskal–Wallis test is to rank the scores from the lowest to the highest irrespective of the treatment group to which each subject belongs, as summarised in Table 18.2. Notice that wherever there are identical head-shake scores then the assigned ranks reflect the average of the ranks originally assigned to that head-shake score; this is known as *tied-ranks* as previously described (see Chapter 13).

Once all the scores have been assigned their rank value then the sum of the ranks for each independent group is calculated; thus,

**Sum of Ranks;**
0.9% saline $\quad \sum R_1 = 88$
Drug A, 1 mg/kg $\quad \sum R_2 = 127$
Drug A, 3 mg/kg $\quad \sum R_3 = 250$

The test statistic, $H$, is then calculated as follows (where $R$ = the sum of ranks for each group, $N$ = total number of observations and $n$ = the number of observations in a particular group);

$$H = \frac{12}{N(N + 1)} \sum \frac{R_i^2}{n_i} - 3(N + 1) \tag{18.1}$$

$$H = \frac{12}{30(31)} \left( \frac{88^2}{10} + \frac{127^2}{10} + \frac{250^2}{10} \right) - 3(31) \tag{18.2}$$

$$H = \frac{12}{930} (774.4 + 1612.9 + 6250.0) - 91 \tag{18.3}$$

$$H = 0.0129(8637.3) - 91 \tag{18.4}$$

*Experimental Design and Statistical Analysis for Pharmacology and the Biomedical Sciences*, First Edition. Paul J. Mitchell.
© 2022 John Wiley & Sons Ltd. Published 2022 by John Wiley & Sons Ltd

Table 18.2 Ranking the head-shake data.

| Head-shake score | Rank | Assigned rank | Treatment |
|---|---|---|---|
| 2 | 1 | 3 | 0.9% saline |
| 2 | 2 | 3 | 0.9% saline |
| 2 | 3 | 3 | 0.9% saline |
| 2 | 4 | 3 | Drug A, 1 mg/kg |
| 2 | 5 | 3 | Drug A, 1 mg/kg |
| 3 | 6 | 7.5 | 0.9% saline |
| 3 | 7 | 7.5 | 0.9% saline |
| 3 | 8 | 7.5 | 0.9% saline |
| 3 | 9 | 7.5 | 0.9% saline |
| 4 | 10 | 11.5 | 0.9% saline |
| 4 | 11 | 11.5 | Drug A, 1 mg/kg |
| 4 | 12 | 11.5 | Drug A, 1 mg/kg |
| 4 | 13 | 11.5 | Drug A, 1 mg/kg |
| 5 | 14 | 15.5 | 0.9% saline |
| 5 | 15 | 15.5 | Drug A, 1 mg/kg |
| 5 | 16 | 15.5 | Drug A, 1 mg/kg |
| 5 | 17 | 15.5 | Drug A, 1 mg/kg |
| 6 | 18 | 18 | Drug A, 1 mg/kg |
| 7 | 19 | 19.5 | Drug A, 3 mg/kg |
| 7 | 20 | 19.5 | Drug A, 3 mg/kg |
| 8 | 21 | 22 | 0.9% saline |
| 8 | 22 | 22 | Drug A, 1 mg/kg |
| 8 | 23 | 22 | Drug A, 3 mg/kg |
| 11 | 24 | 24.5 | Drug A, 3 mg/kg |
| 11 | 25 | 24.5 | Drug A, 3 mg/kg |
| 13 | 26 | 26 | Drug A, 3 mg/kg |
| 14 | 27 | 27 | Drug A, 3 mg/kg |
| 15 | 28 | 28 | Drug A, 3 mg/kg |
| 19 | 29 | 29 | Drug A, 3 mg/kg |
| 24 | 30 | 30 | Drug A, 3 mg/kg |

$$H = 111.42117 - 91 \tag{18.5}$$

$$H = 20.42117 \tag{18.6}$$

The $H$ test statistic has a Chi-square distribution (see Chapter 4, Figure 4.8 and Appendices A.4 and F) which is defined by the degrees of freedom. For the Kruskal–Wallis test, the degrees of freedom is the number of groups −1.

The results of the Kruskal–Wallis test are generally summarized as

$H(\text{df}) = h$ value, $p = p$ value, where df is the degrees of freedom

For these data, $H(2) = 20.42$, $p < 0.001$

The result of the Kruskal–Wallis test indicates the probability of the Null Hypothesis being true is less than 0.001. Consequently, we may reject the Null Hypothesis and conclude that there is sufficient variation between the groups to indicate that one of the groups is different from at least one of the others. However, like the parametric ANOVA models, such a result does not indicate which groups differ. For that we need to perform a series of pairwise comparisons (see Examples 18.4–18.7, below).

## Example 18.2 Non-parametric two-way ANOVA: The Scheirer–Ray–Hare extension

The Scheirer–Ray–Hare extension to the Kruskal–Wallis provides a non-parametric equivalent to the two-way ANOVA, and as such may be used to investigate the Null Hypotheses that neither of the two Between-Group Factors nor their interaction have any effect on the experimental output measured.

Consider the following experiment where the we wish to examine whether pre-treatment with a novel drug exhibits potential antagonist activity at the 5-HT$_{2A}$ receptor subtype. Here forty adult, male Wistar rats are divided into two groups of 20 subjects per group. The first group is treated subcutaneously with 0.9% saline (antagonist control group), and the second group is treated similarly with the potential antagonist drug. Sometime later, each of the groups is further subdivided into two groups of 10 subjects. In each case, the first of these are treated subcutaneously with 0.9% saline (agonist control group), while the second group receives Drug A, 3.0 mg/kg, which the previous example had suggested increased head-shake behaviour in rats. The occurrence of head-shake behaviour was then counted by an independent observer over the following 10 minutes. The experimental design is summarised in Table 18.3 (which the observant amongst you will realise is exactly the same as Table 17.5!), with the resulting scores, as shown in Table 18.4.

Table 18.3 Two Between-Group Factors = two-way ANOVA.

| Between Factor 2 (Pre-treatment) | Between Factor 1 (Acute treatment) | Subject numbers | Measured output (head shakes) |
|---|---|---|---|
| Control | Control | 10 | |
| | Agonist drug | 10 | |
| Antagonist drug | Control | 10 | |
| | Agonist drug | 10 | |

The preliminary stages to perform the two-way ANOVA are the same as previously described for the one-way ANOVA (see Chapter 15). Consequently, we need to calculate the *total variance* of the data, the *Between-Group variance,* and the *Within-Group variance*, but remember for these calculations we are working with the **rank values** of the data rather than the original observations! In each case, the initial calculation determines the appropriate Sum of Squares (SSQ); thus,

### Total Sum of Squares; $SSQ_{total}$

The first step in calculating the Total Sum of Squares ($SSQ_{total}$) is to calculate the Grand Mean of all the assigned rank values (see in the bottom of Table 18.4);

$$\overline{Y}_{\text{Grand}} = \frac{\sum y}{N_{\text{total}}} = \frac{820}{40} = 20.5 \tag{18.7}$$

Next, the differences between each assigned rank value and the Grand Mean of the rank values is calculated and this value is

Table 18.4 Two Between-Group Factors = two-way ANOVA.

| | | Acute treatment | | | | |
|---|---|---|---|---|---|---|
| | | Saline | | Drug A | | |
| Pre-treatment | Subject | Scores | Rank | Scores | Rank | Row mean ranks |
| Saline | 1 | 3 | 13 | 12 | 34.5 | 24.9 |
| | 2 | 4 | 20.5 | 8 | 31 | |
| | 3 | 3 | 13 | 12 | 34.5 | |
| | 4 | 5 | 25.5 | 11 | 32.5 | |
| | 5 | 2 | 5.5 | 24 | 40 | |
| | 6 | 2 | 5.5 | 13 | 36 | |
| | 7 | 2 | 5.5 | 15 | 38 | |
| | 8 | 3 | 13 | 14 | 37 | |
| | 9 | 6 | 28.5 | 11 | 32.5 | |
| | 10 | 3 | 13 | 19 | 39 | |
| Group mean ranks | | | 14.3 | | 35.5 | |
| Antagonist | 1 | 1 | 1.5 | 4 | 20.5 | 16.1 |
| | 2 | 5 | 25.5 | 4 | 20.5 | |
| | 3 | 2 | 5.5 | 4 | 20.5 | |
| | 4 | 7 | 30 | 3 | 13 | |
| | 5 | 3 | 13 | 5 | 25.5 | |
| | 6 | 4 | 20.5 | 5 | 25.5 | |
| | 7 | 1 | 1.5 | 3 | 13 | |
| | 8 | 3 | 13 | 6 | 28.5 | |
| | 9 | 3 | 13 | 2 | 5.5 | |
| | 10 | 2 | 5.5 | 4 | 20.5 | |
| Group mean ranks | | | 12.9 | | 19.3 | |
| Column mean ranks | | | 13.6 | | 27.4 | |
| Grand mean ranks | | | | 20.5 | | |

squared. The squared values are then added together to produce the total SSQ.

$$SSQ_{total} = \sum \left(\overline{Y}_{Grand} - y\right)^2 = 5228.0 \qquad (18.8)$$

The associated degrees of freedom for the total SSQ is the total number of observations – 1; here, the $df_{total}$ is 40 – 1 = 39.

### *Between-Group sum of squares; $SSQ_{Between}$*

The first step in calculating the Between-Group Sum of Squares ($SSQ_{Between}$) is to calculate the mean of the rank values for each treatment combination (see Table 18.4). The difference between each group mean and the Grand mean is then calculated, and this value is squared before multiplying by the number of subjects in the group; thus, for group 1,

$$SSQ_{Between\ 1} = \left(\left(\overline{Y}_{Grand} - \overline{Y}_1\right)^2\right).n_1 \qquad (18.9)$$

The equation shown above is then repeated for each of the four groups in the experiment (see Table 18.5), and the overall $SSQ_{Between}$ calculated by simply adding together the Between-Group SSQ contributions from each group.

The associated degrees of freedom (df) for the overall Between-Group SSQ is the number of groups – 1; here, the $df_{Between}$ is 4 – 1 = 3.

Table 18.5 Between-Group sum of squares; $SSQ_{Between}$.

| Treatment combination | Individual group $SSQ_{Between}$ |
|---|---|
| Saline + saline | 384.4 |
| Saline + Drug A (agonist) | 2250.0 |
| Antagonist + saline | 577.6 |
| Antagonist + Drug A | 14.4 |
| Overall $SSQ_{Between}$ | 3226.4 |

### *Within-Group sum of squares (error term); $SSQ_{Within}$*

The Within-Group Sum of Squares ($SSQ_{Within}$) is initially determined for each group by first calculating the difference for each rank value from its own respective mean rank value (see Table 18.4) for that group. Each difference value is then squared and then the total of the squared differences determined for each group; thus, for group 1,

$$SSQ_{Within\ 1} = \sum \left(\overline{Y}_1 - y\right)^2 \qquad (18.10)$$

This is repeated for each of the four groups (see Table 18.6) and then the overall $SSQ_{Within}$ calculated by simply adding together the Within-Group SSQ contributions from each group.

Table 18.6 Within-Group sum of squares; $SSQ_{Within}$.

| Treatment combination | Individual group $SSQ_{Within}$ |
|---|---|
| Saline + saline | 604.6 |
| Saline + Drug A (agonist) | 81.5 |
| Antagonist + saline | 878.4 |
| Antagonist + Drug A | 437.1 |
| Overall $SSQ_{Within}$ | 2001.6 |

The associated degrees of freedom (df) for the overall Within-Group SSQ is the total number of observations – the number of groups; here the $df_{Within}$ is 40 – 4 = 36.

The preliminary calculations are summarised in Table 18.7

Table 18.7 Between- and Within-Group variances

| Source | SSQ | df | variance |
|---|---|---|---|
| Between | 3226.4 | 3 | 1075.467 |
| Within | 2001.6 | 36 | 55.600 |
| Total | 5228.0 | 39 | |

One component of the preliminary calculations was to calculate the Between-Group SSQ, which reflects the differences between the groups and the Grand Mean of all the assigned ranks. However, this may be partitioned according to each of the Between-Group Factors as shown by the relative rows and columns in Table 18.4. Consequently, the second phase of the non-parametric two-way ANOVA is to determine the Sum of Squares values for each of the Between-Group Factors in the experiment, i.e. for each of the rows and columns in Table 18.4, from which the Sum of

Squares for the interaction between the two Between-Group Factors may be determined.

### Rows sum of squares; $SSQ_{Rows}$

The assigned rank values shown in Table 18.4 may be sub-divided into to two rows according to whether the subjects were treated with either saline or the potential antagonist (irrespective of the subsequent acute treatment with saline or the agonist). The first step is to calculate the row total (i.e. total assigned ranks) for all subjects pre-treated with saline and then divide by the number of subjects to determine the mean rank value for saline-pre-treated subjects; thus,

$$\overline{R}_{\text{row 1}} = \frac{\sum y_{\text{row 1}}}{n_{\text{row 1}}} \qquad (18.11)$$

Next, the square of the difference between the row mean rank value $(\overline{R}_{\text{row1}})$ and the Grand Mean of the rank values $(\overline{Y}_{\text{Grand}})$ is determined and then this value is multiplied by the total number of subjects in the row $(n_{\text{row 1}})$ to give the Sum of Squares for the row. This process is then repeated for the subjects in the second row which were pre-treated with the antagonist. These two SSQ values are then added together to give the overall SSQ values for the rows; thus,

$$SSQ_{\text{rows}} = 774.4 \qquad (18.12)$$

The degrees of freedom of the overall Sum of Squares for the rows equals the number of rows – 1.

### Columns sum of squares; $SSQ_{Columns}$

An almost identical approach is used to determine the overall SSQ for the column data. The assigned rank values shown in Table 18.4 may be sub-divided into two columns according to whether the subjects were treated with either saline or the receptor agonist (irrespective of the pre-treatment with saline or the antagonist). The first step is to calculate the column total (i.e. total assigned ranks) for all subjects treated acutely with saline and then divide by the number of subjects to determine the mean rank value for saline-treated subjects; thus,

$$\overline{C}_{\text{column 1}} = \frac{\sum y_{\text{column 1}}}{n_{\text{column 1}}} \qquad (18.13)$$

Next, the square of the difference between the column mean rank value $(\overline{C}_{\text{column 1}})$ and the Grand Mean of the rank values $(\overline{Y}_{\text{Grand}})$ is determined and then this value is multiplied by the total number of subjects in the column $(n_{\text{column 1}})$ to give the Sum of Squares for the column. This process is then repeated for the subjects in the second column which were treated acutely with Drug A, the receptor agonist. These two SSQ values are then added together to give the overall SSQ values for the columns; thus,

$$SSQ_{\text{columns}} = 1904.4 \qquad (18.14)$$

The degrees of freedom of the overall Sum of Squares for the columns equals the number of columns – 1.

### Interaction sum of squares; $SSQ_{Interaction}$

The Sum of Squares for the interaction between the two Between-Group Factors is equal to the overall Between-Group SSQ minus the total SSQ due to the rows and columns of the data; thus,

$$SSQ_{\text{interaction}} = SSQ_{\text{Between}} - (SSQ_{\text{rows}} + SSQ_{\text{columns}}) \qquad (18.15)$$

$$SSQ_{\text{interaction}} = 3226.4 - (774.4 + 1904.4) = 547.6 \qquad (18.16)$$

The degrees of freedom of the overall Sum of Squares for the interaction equals the (number of rows – 1) multiplied by the (number of columns – 1).

### Total variance

Computation of the total variance (also known as the total Mean Square) in the data may be achieved by either of two methods:

**No tied ranks:**

Total variance $= N(N + 1)/12 = 40(41)/12 = 136.667$, (18.17)

where $N =$ total number of subjects. N.B. this is because the expected variance for $n$ ranks $= n(n + 1)/12$!

**Tied ranks:**

$$SSQ_{\text{total}}/df_{\text{total}} = 5228/39 = 134.05 \qquad (18.18)$$

In our set of data, there are numerous tied ranks (see Table 18.4) so we will use the second method to determine the total variance of the data. The computed $H$ value for each source is determined by each variance divided by the total variance for tied ranks (see above). The probability of H is tested as a $\chi^2$ variable with the degrees of freedom according to the variance being tested and is reported in the same format as for the Kruskal–Wallis test. If the value of $H$ is greater than the critical values of the chi-square distribution (see Appendix F), then the Null Hypothesis may be rejected.

The completed two-way ANOVA table for the assigned rank data values may be summarised as follows (Table 18.8);

Table 18.8 Summary of the two-way ANOVA by ranks.

| Source | SSQ | df | variance | H value | p value |
|---|---|---|---|---|---|
| Pre-treatment (rows) | 774.4 | 1 | 774.40 | 5.7769 | <0.05 |
| Acute treatment (columns) | 1904.4 | 1 | 1904.40 | 14.2065 | <0.001 |
| Interaction | 547.6 | 1 | 547.60 | 4.0850 | <0.05 |
| Within (Error) | 2001.6 | 36 | 55.60 | | |
| Total | 5228.0 | 39 | 134.05 | | |

Consequently, we may conclude that the two-way ANOVA by ranks reveals a significant main effect of pre-treatment [$H$ (1) = 5.776, $p < 0.05$], a significant main effect of acute treatment [$H(1) = 14.2065, p < 0.001$] and a significant interaction between the two Between-Group Factors [$H(1) = 4.085, p < 0.05$].

As with the Kruskal–Wallis test, however, the Scheirer–Ray–Hare extension does not identify which groups are significantly different from each other. Interestingly, the significant interaction allows all possible pairwise comparisons to be performed on the data. Had only the main effects of pre-treatment or acute treatment been identified then the restrictions on the number of allowable pairwise comparisons (as described in Chapter 17 for parametric data sets) would also apply.

## Example 18.3 Non-parametric Repeated Measures ANOVA: The Friedman test

In contrast to the previous two tests described in this chapter, the Friedman's ANOVA examines differences between three or more conditions obtained from the same group of subjects, and as such it is the non-parametric equivalent of the Repeated Measures ANOVA model.

Consider the following data (Table 18.9) where 17 Final year Pharmacology students were asked to judge the quality of a lecture (on a scale 0–100) describing complex ANOVA models according to the number of visual aids used, where None = no visual aids, Few = limited visual aids to explain major points only, and Many = a plethora of visual aids to illustrate every point made.

Table 18.9 Assessment of lecture quality.

| | Visual aids used | | |
|---|---|---|---|
| Student No. | None | Few | Many |
| 1 | 66 | 78 | 68 |
| 2 | 48 | 69 | 30 |
| 3 | 87 | 95 | 92 |
| 4 | 78 | 89 | 64 |
| 5 | 45 | 61 | 57 |
| 6 | 58 | 76 | 46 |
| 7 | 65 | 57 | 40 |
| 8 | 63 | 78 | 67 |
| 9 | 84 | 89 | 95 |
| 10 | 77 | 92 | 71 |
| 11 | 69 | 72 | 64 |
| 12 | 61 | 67 | 54 |
| 13 | 58 | 56 | 48 |
| 14 | 68 | 50 | 62 |
| 15 | 48 | 68 | 54 |
| 16 | 37 | 43 | 30 |
| 17 | 54 | 71 | 75 |

After collecting the assessment of each lecture by each student, the data are then ranked for each student across the three lectures with the lowest score given a rank of 1, the next highest a rank of 2 and so on. The assigned ranks are summarised in Table 18.10.

Following the calculation of the sum of ranks, then the $F_r$ statistic is calculated according to the following equation (where $R$ is the sum of ranks for each group, $N$ = the total number of subjects and $k$ = the number of conditions);

$$F_r = \left[\frac{12}{Nk(k+1)}\sum R_i^2\right] - 3N(k+1) \tag{18.19}$$

$$F_r = \left[\frac{12}{(17 \times 3)(3+1)}\sum R_i^2\right] - (3 \times 17)(3+1) \tag{18.20}$$

$$F_r = \left[\frac{12}{(51)(4)}\left(30^2 + 45^2 + 27^2\right)\right] - (3 \times 17)(3+1) \tag{18.21}$$

$$F_r = \left[\frac{12}{204}(900 + 2025 + 729)\right] - (51)(4) \tag{18.22}$$

$$F_r = [0.0588 \times 3654] - 204 \tag{18.23}$$

$$F_r = 214.855 - 204 \tag{18.24}$$

Table 18.10 Rank data for assessment of lecture quality.

| | Visual aids used | | |
|---|---|---|---|
| Student No. | None | Few | Many |
| 1 | 1 | 3 | 2 |
| 2 | 2 | 3 | 1 |
| 3 | 1 | 3 | 2 |
| 4 | 2 | 3 | 1 |
| 5 | 1 | 3 | 2 |
| 6 | 2 | 3 | 1 |
| 7 | 3 | 2 | 1 |
| 8 | 1 | 3 | 2 |
| 9 | 1 | 2 | 3 |
| 10 | 2 | 3 | 1 |
| 11 | 2 | 3 | 1 |
| 12 | 2 | 3 | 1 |
| 13 | 3 | 2 | 1 |
| 14 | 3 | 1 | 2 |
| 15 | 1 | 3 | 2 |
| 16 | 2 | 3 | 1 |
| 17 | 1 | 2 | 3 |
| Sum of ranks | 30 | 45 | 27 |

$$F_r = 10.855 \tag{18.25}$$

When the number of subjects is greater than 10 then the $F_r$ statistic, just like the H test statistic produced by the Kruskal–Wallis test, also has a chi-square distribution defined by the degrees of freedom (see Appendix F). For the Friedman test, the degrees of freedom is the number of groups −1.

The results of the Friedman test are generally summarised as

$F_r(\text{df}) = F_r$ value, $p = p$ value, where df is the degrees of freedom

For these data, $F_r(2) = 10.855$, $p < 0.01$

The result of the Friedman test indicates the probability of the Null Hypothesis being true is less than 0.01. Consequently, we may reject the Null Hypothesis and conclude that there is sufficient variation between the groups to indicate that one of the groups is different from at least one of the others. However, just like the Kruskal–Wallis test described above, such a result does not indicate which groups differ. For that we need to perform a series of pairwise comparisons (see later).

## Limitations of non-parametric ANOVA models

Before moving on to discuss how multiple pairwise comparison tests may be used following non-parametric ANOVA, it is important here to highlight some of the limitations when the experimenter wishes to analyse multiple data sets where the data do not follow a normal distribution. The non-parametric ANOVA models discussed in this chapter are appropriate for those experimental designs that include one or two Between-Group Factors (the Kruskal–Wallis test and Scheirer–Ray–Hare extension, respectively) or one Within-Group Factor **only**! Chapter 17 described a number of complex ANOVA models (including mixed ANOVA models) for which there are no non-parametric equivalent ANOVA tests. I have spent years searching the literature for such readily accessible tests and only really succeeded in developing a mop of very grey hair (at least it's still my own and no bald patches,...... yet)! If you're confronted by a situation where a complicated experimental design suggests you require a mixed ANOVA model to analyse the data, but where the data sets are clearly non-parametric then I think you have a choice of two strategies;

**1** Transform your data to allow you to use one of the complex parametric ANOVA models described earlier (see Chapter 17).
**2** A less-desirable strategy would be to break your data sets in smaller chunks that allows you to use one of the non-parametric ANOVA models described earlier – but beware, this opens up the very real possibility making a Type 1 or Type 2 error; if you are open and transparent about such an approach, then at least your future readers will know that you are aware of the hidden dangers in such a strategy!

## Multiple pairwise comparisons following non-parametric ANOVA

In Chapters 15–17, I discussed how standard *post hoc* multiple pairwise comparison tests may be used to identify which experimental groups of data differ from other groups of data following different ANOVA models applied to parametric data sets. In some cases, due to the complexity of the experimental design, the experimenter must make *a priori* decisions about which pairwise comparisons are appropriate, and consequently, has no option but to use multiple independent or paired *t*-tests (with Bonferroni correction) to identify which data groups are significantly different from each other. Unfortunately, a similar range of *post hoc* tests are not available to identify differences between experimental groups following the non-parametric models of ANOVA. Consequently, the experimenter has a limited number of options available to him/her to perform multiple pairwise comparisons. These options are limited to the following;

- Repeated use of the Mann–Whitney *U*-test to compare multiple independent non-parametric data sets with Bonferroni correction following the Kruskal–Wallis ANOVA.
- Repeated use of the Wilcoxon Signed-Rank test to compare multiple paired non-parametric data sets with Bonferroni correction following the Freidman ANOVA.
- The use of one of the variants of the Dunn's test for multiple comparisons.

Repeated use of the Mann–Whitney *U*-test or Wilcoxon Signed-Rank test, with Bonferroni correction in both cases, means that the experimenter *has* to make *a priori* decisions about which pairwise comparisons to perform (including whether the experimental design includes a control group or not) and consequently the strategies used in such cases are the same as those following the complex models of parametric ANOVA (especially following mixed ANOVA) described in Chapter 17.

## Multiple pairwise comparisons using the Mann–Whitney *U*-test

It is appropriate to perform multiple pairwise comparisons using the Mann–Whitney *U*-test (see Chapter 13 for description) following either the Kruskal–Wallis test (one-way ANOVA) or the Scheirer–Ray–Hare extension (two-way ANOVA). In both cases, the non-parametric data sets differ in either one or two Between-Group Factors and the data sets may be assumed to be independent (yes, even in the case of a significant interaction between the two Between-Group Factors following the Scheirer–Ray–Hare extension!). Note, however, that the Bonferroni correction must be applied in order to correct for the number of multiple comparisons performed.

## Multiple pairwise comparisons using the Wilcoxon Signed-Rank test

It is appropriate to perform multiple pairwise comparisons using the Wilcoxon Signed-Rank test (see Chapter 14 for description) following the Friedman's test. In this case the non-parametric data sets differ in one Within-Group Factor and the data sets may be assumed to be paired. Note, however, that the Bonferroni correction must be applied in order to correct for the number of multiple comparisons performed.

## Multiple pairwise comparisons using a variant of Dunn's test

As mentioned earlier, there are variants of the Dunn's test, and it is important that the experimenter understands the differences between these in order to choose correctly the appropriate variant to use. These variants differ according to whether the data sets are independent (i.e. appropriate following the Kruska–Wallis ANOVA or the Scheirer–Ray–Hare extension) or paired (i.e. appropriate following Friedman's ANOVA); in both cases, there is a further variant depending on whether the data sets include a control group or not.

The variants of Dunn's test described later compare the absolute differences in the rank values (sum of ranks or mean ranks) of the data sets being compared against a critical value calculated by multiplying a **z score** or equivalent (based on the α value, usually 0.05, and the number of comparisons required) by a factor (calculated according to either the total number of subjects across all groups and/or the number of subjects in the groups being compared and/or the number of comparisons required). In all cases, if the calculated difference in the rank scores is equal to or greater than the calculated critical value, then it may be concluded that the probability of the Null Hypothesis being true is *less* than the α value at which the groups are being compared. Consequently, the Null Hypothesis may be rejected, and the experimenter may conclude that two groups being compared are significantly different.

### Independent Groups (following Kruskal–Wallis ANOVA) (see Example 18.1)

### Example 18.4  Multiple comparisons between all groups

The first variant of the Dunn's test allows pairwise comparison of all independent data groups to each other (so in this respect it is similar to the Tukey or SNK *post hoc* test used for parametric data described in Chapter 15).

The overall equation is summarised as

$$|\overline{R}_u - \overline{R}_v| \geq z_{\alpha/k(k-1)} \sqrt{\frac{N(N+1)}{12}\left(\frac{1}{n_u} + \frac{1}{n_v}\right)} \qquad (18.26)$$

Where $\overline{R}_u$ and $\overline{R}_v$ are the mean rank values of the groups being compared, $N$ is the total number of subjects in the experiment, and $n_u$ and $n_v$ are the respective number of subjects in each group, respectively.

The first stage of the analysis is to calculate the absolute difference between the mean rank values for the two groups that are being compared. Initially, the mean rank value for each group is determined, and then it is a simple matter of calculating the difference in these values according to each pairwise comparison.

As an example, consider the data summarised in Table 18.1 (yes, I know this includes a saline-treated control group, but here we wish to examine whether there is an additional difference between the effect of the two doses of drug used). Table 18.11 (below) summarises the sum of ranks and mean ranks for each data set taken from the assigned rank values (see Table 18.2).

Table 18.11 Sum of ranks and mean ranks of head-shake data.

| Treatment | $n$ | Sum of ranks | Mean ranks |
|---|---|---|---|
| 0.9% saline | $n_1 = 10$ | $R_1 = 88$ | $\bar{R}_1 = 8.8$ |
| Drug A, 1.0 mg/kg | $n_2 = 10$ | $R_2 = 127$ | $\bar{R}_2 = 12.7$ |
| Drug A, 3.0 mg/kg | $n_3 = 10$ | $R_3 = 250$ | $\bar{R}_3 = 25.0$ |

Data taken from assigned rank values to original data as summarised in Table 18.2.

The absolute difference in the mean ranks is then calculated; thus,

$$|\bar{R}_1 - \bar{R}_2| = |8.8 - 12.7| = 3.9 \tag{18.27}$$

$$|\bar{R}_1 - \bar{R}_3| = |8.8 - 25.0| = 16.2 \tag{18.28}$$

$$|\bar{R}_2 - \bar{R}_3| = |12.7 - 25.0| = 12.3 \tag{18.29}$$

The next stage is to calculate the critical value to which the above differences in mean ranks may be compared. This is 2-part process where first the value of $z_{\alpha/k(k-1)}$ is calculated (where $k$ is the total number of groups). For the geeks amongst us (hands up, please), this is the abscissa value taken from the unit normal distribution *above* which is the $\alpha/k(k-1)$ percent of the distribution. This process works because when the sample size is large, then the differences in the mean rank values approximates to a normal distribution.

$$z_{\alpha/k(k-1)} = z_{0.05/3(3-1)} = z_{0.05/6} = z_{0.0083} \tag{18.30}$$

The value of $z$ may be obtained by looking up the table of Standard Normal probabilities summarised in Appendix B. If you search for the $z$ value for $p = 0.0083$, then the closest is $p = 0.0084$ where $z = 2.39$.

Alternatively, an easier method to determine the $z$ value is provided by the Table G.1 (see Appendix G), which summarises the appropriate values from the standard normal distribution that have been listed so that $z$ values may be obtained easily depending on the value of $\alpha$ and the number of comparisons being performed, where there are k groups then there are $k(k-1)/2$ possible comparisons. This is the point on the standard normal distribution where the upper-tail probability is equal to

$$\frac{1}{2}\alpha / (k(k-1)/2). \tag{18.31}$$

Thus, in the example described here

$$k(k-1)/2 = 3(2)/2 = 3 \tag{18.32}$$

Consequently, the z value taken from Table G.1 (see Appendix G) for a two-tailed test with $\alpha = 0.05$ and three comparisons = 2.394

(compare this value to the 2.39 obtained from Appendix B, see above).

Of course, the $z$ value may also be calculated for $\alpha = 0.01$ (from Appendix B); thus,

$$z_{\alpha/k(k-1)} = z_{0.01/3(3-1)} = z_{0.01/6} = z_{0.00167} = 2.94 \tag{18.33}$$

The second stage to determine the critical value is to calculate the factor by which the $z$ score is multiplied; thus,

$$\sqrt{\frac{N(N+1)}{12}\left(\frac{1}{n_u} + \frac{1}{n_v}\right)} \tag{18.34}$$

where $N$ = total number of subjects and $n$ = number of subjects in the appropriate groups being compared. So,

$$\sqrt{\frac{N(N+1)}{12}\left(\frac{1}{n_u} + \frac{1}{n_v}\right)} = \sqrt{\frac{30(30+1)}{12}\left(\frac{1}{10} + \frac{1}{10}\right)} \tag{18.35}$$

$$\sqrt{\frac{30(31)}{12}\left(\frac{1}{10} + \frac{1}{10}\right)} = \sqrt{\frac{930}{12}(0.1 + 0.1)} = \sqrt{77.5\,(0.2)} \tag{18.36}$$

$$\sqrt{77.5\,(0.2)} = \sqrt{15.5} = 3.937 \tag{18.37}$$

Consequently, the critical value equals
For $\alpha = 0.05$

$$z_{\alpha/k(k-1)}\sqrt{\frac{N(N+1)}{12}\left(\frac{1}{n_u} + \frac{1}{n_v}\right)} = 2.394 \times 3.937 = 9.425 \tag{18.38}$$

For $\alpha = 0.01$

$$z_{\alpha/k(k-1)}\sqrt{\frac{N(N+1)}{12}\left(\frac{1}{n_u} + \frac{1}{n_v}\right)} = 2.94 \times 3.937 = 11.575 \tag{18.39}$$

We now need to compare the absolute difference in the mean ranks for each pairwise comparison to this critical value as summarised in Table 18.12.

Table 18.12 Multiple comparisons between all groups using Dunn's test.

| Compared groups | Difference in mean ranks | Critical value $\alpha = 0.05$ $\alpha = 0.01$ | $p$ value |
|---|---|---|---|
| 0.9% saline v Drug A, 1.0 mg/kg | 3.9 | 9.425 | $p > 0.05$ |
| 0.9% saline v Drug A, 3.0 mg/kg | 16.2 | 11.575 | $p < 0.01$ |
| Drug A, 1.0 mg/kg v Drug A, 3.0 mg/kg | 12.3 | | $p < 0.01$ |

The results of the Dunn's test show that there was no significant difference in the number of head shakes exhibited by rats treated with saline or Drug A, 1.0 mg/kg. However, rats treated with Drug A, 3.0 mg/kg, exhibited a greater number of head shakes than rats treated with either of the other two treatments ($p < 0.01$ in both cases).

But what would we conclude had we performed multiple pairwise comparisons using the Mann–Whitney $U$-test with Bonferroni correction instead of the Dunn's test? The results of repeated comparisons using the Mann–Whitney $U$-test with Bonferroni correction are summarised in Table 18.13.

**Table 18.13** Multiple comparisons between all groups using Mann–Whitney $U$-test with Bonferroni correction.

| Compared groups | Mann–Whitney $U$-test | Calculated uncorrected $p$ value |
|---|---|---|
| 0.9% saline v Drug A, 1.0 mg/kg | 30.5 | $p = 0.162$ |
| 0.9% saline v Drug A, 3.0 mg/kg | 2.5 | $p < 0.001**$ |
| Drug A, 1.0 mg/kg v Drug A, 3.0 mg/kg | 2.5 | $p < 0.001**$ |

The critical values for $U$ for $n_1 = 10$ and $n_2 = 10$ for a two-tailed test and $p = 0.05$ are 23 and 77, and for $p = 0.01$ are 16 and 84 (see Appendix D, Tables D.3 and D.4). The calculated $U$ values for the second and third comparisons are both less than the lower critical value when $p = 0.001$; thus, $p < 0.001$ in both cases. The exact uncorrected calculated $p$ values for each comparison quoted above were determined using GraphPad Prism. Corrected $p$ values; $* p < 0.05$, $** p < 0.01$. The Bonferroni-corrected $p$ value for a family error rate <0.05 with three pairwise comparisons equals $0.05/3 = 0.0167$. Similarly, for family error rates of 0.01 and 0.001, then Bonferroni-corrected $p$ values are $0.01/3 = 0.0033$ and $0.001/3 = 0.00033$, respectively.

The results of the Dunn's test are in good agreement with the Bonferroni corrected $p$ values determined by repeated comparisons using the Mann–Whitney $U$-test (compare Tables 18.12 and 18.13). So, our conclusions would be the same regardless of which test was used to perform the multiple pairwise comparisons!

## Example 18.5 Multiple comparisons between a control group and test groups

Of course, the experimental design giving rise to the head-shake data summarised in Tables 18.1 and 18.2 clearly provides a control group (i.e. those rats treated with 0.9% saline). In situations where we are only interested in multiple comparisons to a control group then, under two-tailed conditions, the following variant of the Dunn's test is used (so in this respect this variant is similar to the Dunnett's *post hoc* test used for parametric data).

$$\left|\overline{R}_c - \overline{R}_u\right| \geq z_{\alpha/2(k-1)} \sqrt{\frac{N(N+1)}{12}\left(\frac{1}{n_c} + \frac{1}{n_u}\right)} \quad (18.40)$$

where $\overline{R}_c$ and $\overline{R}_u$ are the mean rank values of the control and test groups concerned, respectively, $N$ equals the total number of subjects in the experiment, and $n_c$ and $n_u$ are the respective number of subjects in the control and test groups, respectively.

In this variant we are only interested in the comparison of the control group with the two drug-treated groups. As before the absolute difference in the mean ranks for both comparisons (see Table 18.11) are calculated; thus,

$$\left|\overline{R}_1 - \overline{R}_2\right| = |8.8 - 12.7| = 3.9 \quad (18.41)$$

$$\left|\overline{R}_1 - \overline{R}_3\right| = |8.8 - 25.0| = 16.2 \quad (18.42)$$

As in the earlier example, the next stage is to calculate the critical value to which the above differences in mean ranks may be compared, which is the product of the appropriate $z$ value and a factor dependent on the total number of subjects and the number of subjects in each group. Notice, however, the difference in the subscript for the $z$ value (i.e. $z_{\alpha/2(k-1)}$), resulting in a different $z$ value to that used in the all groups variant, while the factor by which the $z$ value is multiplied remains the same. Again, the value of $z$ is obtained by consulting Appendix B or Table G.1 (see Appendix G).

For $\alpha = 0.05$ (from Appendix B)

$$z_{\alpha/2(k-1)} = z_{0.05/2(3-1)} = z_{0.0125} = 2.24 \quad (18.43)$$

For $\alpha = 0.01$ (from Appendix B)

$$z_{\alpha/2(k-1)} = z_{0.01/2(3-1)} = z_{0.0025} = 2.81 \quad (18.44)$$

An additional point to note here is that if the number of subjects in *all* groups is the same, then a better approximation for $z$ is obtained by consulting Table G.2 in Appendix G (where for a two-tailed test with two comparisons and $\alpha = 0.05$, $z = 2.21$, while for $\alpha = 0.01$, $z = 2.79$). In the experiment described here, there are an equal number of subjects in each group so Table G.2 (see Appendix G) is appropriate here.

Consequently, for $\alpha = 0.05$ the critical value equals

$$z_{\alpha/2(k-1)} \sqrt{\frac{N(N+1)}{12}\left(\frac{1}{n_c} + \frac{1}{n_u}\right)} = 2.21 \times 3.937 = 8.701$$

$$(18.45)$$

while for $\alpha = 0.01$ the critical value equals

$$z_{\alpha/2(k-1)} \sqrt{\frac{N(N+1)}{12}\left(\frac{1}{n_c} + \frac{1}{n_u}\right)} = 2.79 \times 3.937 = 10.984$$

$$(18.46)$$

[Note, if Appendix B or Table G.1 is used then the critical value for $\alpha = 0.05$ equals $2.241 \times 3.937 = 8.823$, while for $\alpha = 0.01$ equals $2.81 \times 3.937 = 11.063$.]

Quite clearly, therefore, Dunn's test strongly suggests no significance between the number of head shakes exhibited by the control, saline-treated, rats and the lowest dose of Drug A (where the difference in the mean rank values is less than the critical value for $\alpha = 0.05$), but a significant increase in head-shake behaviour when the rats were treated with the higher dose of Drug A (where the difference in the mean rank values is greater than the critical value for $\alpha = 0.01$). Satisfyingly, very similar results are obtained if the Mann–Whitney $U$-test with Bonferroni correction is used to perform the two pairwise comparisons (refer to Table 18.13, above, but recalculate the Bonferroni corrected $p$ values for just two comparisons).

The discussion in this section has been focused on **two-tailed** comparisons using the variant of Dunn's test. If, however, the experimenter wished to perform this variant under **one-tailed** conditions then the following equation should be used that utilises different $z$ values derived from Appendix B, Table G.1, or Table G.2 as appropriate.

$$\left| \overline{R}_c - \overline{R}_u \right| \geq z_{\alpha/(k-1)} \sqrt{\frac{N(N+1)}{12} \left( \frac{1}{n_c} + \frac{1}{n_u} \right)} \qquad (18.47)$$

## Paired Groups (following Friedman's ANOVA) (see Example 18.3)

## Example 18.6  Multiple comparisons between all groups

The next variant of the Dunn's test allows multiple pairwise comparisons of all paired data groups to each other.

The overall equation is summarised as:

$$\left| R_u - R_v \right| \geq z_{\alpha/k(k-1)} \sqrt{\frac{Nk(k+1)}{6}} \qquad (18.48)$$

where $R_u$ and $R_v$ are the sum of the ranks for each of the two conditions being compared, $N$ is the total number of subjects in the experiment, and $k$ is the number of conditions.

Consider the analysis of lecture quality data summarised in Tables 18.9 (original scores) and 18.10 (assigned rank values).

The differences in the sum of ranks between each condition for every pairwise comparison are summarised in Table 18.14; thus,

**Table 18.14**  Differences in sum of ranks.

| Comparison | $\left\| R_u - R_v \right\|$ | Difference in sum of ranks |
|---|---|---|
| None v Few | $\|30 - 45\|$ | 15 |
| None v Many | $\|30 - 27\|$ | 3 |
| Few v Many | $\|45 - 27\|$ | 18 |

The next stage is to calculate the critical value to which the above differences in the sum of ranks may be compared. As for the previous description of the Dunn's test for independent groups this is a 2-part process where the first value of $z_{\alpha/k(k-1)}$ is calculated (where $k$ is the total number of conditions in the experiment); note that this is the same value of $z$ as used in the earlier variant of Dunn's test used to compare all independent groups to each other! Thus,

$$z_{\alpha/k(k-1)} = z_{0.05/3(3-1)} = z_{0.05/6} = z_{0.0083} \qquad (18.49)$$

As we saw before, the value of $z$ may be obtained from the table in Appendix B where the closest estimate of $z$ is where $p = 0.0084$. Thus, $z = 2.39$.

Also, if $\alpha = 0.01$ (from Appendix B), then

$$z_{\alpha/k(k-1)} = z_{0.01/3(3-1)} = z_{0.01/6} = z_{0.00167} = 2.94 \qquad (18.50)$$

The second stage is to determine the critical value is to calculate the factor by which the $z$ score is multiplied, thus (notice that this factor is very different from that used for comparison of independent data sets):

$$\sqrt{\frac{Nk(k+1)}{6}} \qquad (18.51)$$

where N = total number of subjects and $k$ the number of conditions. So, for the data in Table 18.10;

$$\sqrt{\frac{Nk(k+1)}{6}} = \sqrt{\frac{17 \times 3(3+1)}{6}} = \sqrt{\frac{17 \times 12}{6}} = \sqrt{34} = 5.831 \qquad (18.52)$$

Consequently, the critical value equals
For $\alpha = 0.05$

$$z_{\alpha/k(k-1)} \sqrt{\frac{Nk(k+1)}{6}} = 2.39 \times 5.831 = 13.936 \qquad (18.53)$$

For $\alpha = 0.01$

$$z_{\alpha/k(k-1)} \sqrt{\frac{Nk(k+1)}{6}} = 2.94 \times 5.831 = 17.143 \qquad (18.54)$$

We now need to compare the absolute difference in the sum of ranks for each pairwise comparison to this critical value as summarised in Table 18.15.

**Table 18.15**  Multiple comparisons between all groups using Dunn's test.

| Compared groups | Difference in sum of ranks | Critical value $\alpha = 0.05$ $\alpha = 0.01$ | p value |
|---|---|---|---|
| None v Few | 15 | 13.936 | $p < 0.05$ |
| None v Many | 3 | | $p > 0.05$ |
| Few v Many | 18 | 17.143 | $p < 0.01$ |

Difference in sum of rank data from Table 18.14

Consequently, the results of the Dunn's test indicate that there was no significant difference between the assessed quality of the lectures when no or many visual aids were used, but there was a significant difference when few visual aids were used compared to both of the other conditions.

An alternative method to this variant of the Dunn's test is to use the absolute difference in the mean ranks of the two groups being compared, and the overall equation may be summarised as follows:

$$\left| \overline{R}_u - \overline{R}_v \right| \geq z_{\alpha/k(k-1)} \sqrt{\frac{k(k+1)}{6N}} \qquad (18.55)$$

Note the difference in the factor by which the $z$ score is multiplied, i.e.

$$\sqrt{\frac{k(k+1)}{6N}} = \sqrt{\frac{12}{6 \times 17}} = \sqrt{\frac{12}{102}} = \sqrt{0.1176} = 0.343 \qquad (18.56)$$

If we use this variant of Dunn's test, then the critical values are
For $\alpha = 0.05$

$$z_{\alpha/k(k-1)} \sqrt{\frac{k(k+1)}{6N}} = 2.39 \times 0.343 = 0.82 \qquad (18.57)$$

For $\alpha = 0.01$

$$z_{\alpha/k(k-1)}\sqrt{\frac{k(k+1)}{6N}} = 2.94 \times 0.343 = 1.01 \qquad (18.58)$$

If we compare Tables 18.15 and 18.16, then clearly the $p$ values for each pairwise comparison agree regardless of whether we use the critical values appropriate for either the difference in the sum of ranks or the difference in the respective mean ranks (phew!).

Table 18.16 Multiple comparisons between all groups using Dunn's test.

| Compared groups | $\lvert\overline{R}_u - \overline{R}_v\rvert$ | Difference in mean ranks | Critical value $\alpha = 0.05$ $\alpha = 0.01$ | $p$ value |
|---|---|---|---|---|
| None v Few | $\lvert 1.765 - 2.647 \rvert$ | 0.882 | 0.82 | $p < 0.05$ |
| None v Many | $\lvert 1.765 - 1.588 \rvert$ | 0.177 | 1.01 | $p > 0.05$ |
| Few v Many | $\lvert 2.647 - 1.588 \rvert$ | 1.059 | | $p < 0.01$ |

Mean rank values calculated from Table 18.10

But what would we conclude had we performed multiple pairwise comparisons using the Wilcoxon Signed-Rank test with Bonferroni correction instead of the Dunn's test? The results of which are summarised in Table 18.17.

Table 18.17 Multiple comparisons between all groups using Wilcoxon Signed-Rank test with Bonferroni correction.

| Compared groups | Sum of signed ranks ($W$) | Calculated uncorrected $p$ value |
|---|---|---|
| None v Few | 109 | $p = 0.0076*$ |
| None v Many | −49 | $p = 0.2576$ |
| Few v Many | −122 | $p = 0.0022**$ |

The exact uncorrected calculated p values for each comparison quoted above were determined using GraphPad Prism. Corrected $p$ values; $*$ $p < 0.05$, $**$ $p < 0.01$. The Bonferroni-corrected $p$ value for a family error rate <0.05 with three pairwise comparisons equals 0.05/3 = 0.0167. Similarly, for family error rates of 0.01 and 0.001 then Bonferroni-corrected $p$ values are 0.01/3 = 0.0033 and 0.001/3 = 0.00033, respectively.

Consequently, the results of the Dunn's test are in complete agreement with the Bonferroni-corrected $p$ values determined by repeated comparisons using the Wilcoxon Signed-Rank test. So, as we saw with the repeated analysis of independent data sets using the Mann–Whitney $U$-test described earlier in this chapter, our conclusions would be the same regardless of which test was used to perform the multiple pairwise comparisons for paired data sets!

## Example 18.7  Multiple comparisons between a control group and test groups

Of course, some experimental designs may clearly include a control group and in such situations we would only be interested in multiple comparisons to that control group. The final variant of the Dunn's test provides for multiple pairwise comparisons for paired data sets to a control group. As for the previous example, the overall equation used depends on whether the data sets are expressed as either the sum of ranks or the mean rank for each condition. Thus, the equation for sum of ranks for each condition is;

$$\lvert R_1 - R_u \rvert \geq q(\alpha, \#c)\sqrt{\frac{Nk(k+1)}{6}} \qquad (18.59)$$

The equation for mean ranks for each condition is

$$\lvert \overline{R}_1 - \overline{R}_u \rvert \geq q(\alpha, \#c)\sqrt{\frac{k(k+1)}{6N}} \qquad (18.60)$$

In these equations, $R_1$ or $\overline{R}_1$ indicate the sum of ranks or the mean rank value, respectively, for the control group. In addition, $q$ indicates the alternate estimated value of $z$ at a given value of $\alpha$ (usually 0.05 or 0.01) and for the number of comparisons (denoted by $\#c$, where $\#c = k - 1$ and $k$ indicates the total number of conditions) as listed in Appendix G, Table G.2.

As above, consider the lecture quality data in Table 18.9 and the associated rank data in Table 18.10. In addition, we shall assume that the lecture condition with no visual aids is the control group. We are therefore only interested in two comparisons, i.e. none compared to few and none compared to many. Consequently, the alternate 2-tailed estimates of $z$ for $\alpha = 0.05$ or 0.01 and for two comparisons taken from Appendix G, Table G.2 are as follows:

For $\alpha = 0.05$, $z = 2.21$
For $\alpha = 0.01$, $z = 2.79$

Furthermore, the constant by which the $z$ estimate is multiplied by for where the data are expressed as either the sum of ranks or mean ranks are;

For sum of ranks,

$$\sqrt{\frac{Nk(k+1)}{6}} = 5.831 \qquad (18.61)$$

For mean ranks,

$$\sqrt{\frac{k(k+1)}{6N}} = 0.343 \qquad (18.62)$$

The critical values may therefore be summarised as

For sum of rank data

where $\alpha = 0.05$, critical value = $2.21 \times 5.831 = 12.887$ (18.63)

where $\alpha = 0.01$, critical value = $2.79 \times 5.831 = 16.268$ (18.64)

For mean rank data

where $\alpha = 0.05$, critical value $= 2.21 \times 0.343 = 0.758$  (18.65)

where $\alpha = 0.01$, critical value $= 2.79 \times 0.343 = 0.957$  (18.66)

The final data analysis is summarised in Table 18.18.

Clearly, the results of Dunn's test show that there is no difference in the assessment lecture quality when no or many visual aids are used, but there is a difference in assessed lecture quality between none and few visual aids, regardless of whether the sum of ranks or mean rank values are used.

Again, the pairwise comparisons by repeated Wilcoxon Signed-Rank test with Bonferroni correction are consistent with the variant of Dunn's test (see Table 18.19).

**Table 18.18** Multiple comparisons to control data using Dunn's test.

| Compared groups | Difference in sum of ranks | Difference in mean ranks | p value |
|---|---|---|---|
| None v Few | 15 | | $p < 0.05$ |
| None v Many | 3 | | $p > 0.05$ |
| None v Few | | 0.882 | $p < 0.05$ |
| None v Many | | 0.177 | $p > 0.05$ |

Difference in sum of rank data from Table 18.14. Differences in mean rank data from Table 18.16.

**Table 18.19** Multiple comparisons between all groups using Wilcoxon Signed-Rank test with Bonferroni correction.

| Compared groups | Sum of signed ranks ($W$) | Calculated p value |
|---|---|---|
| None v Few | 109 | $p = 0.0076*$ |
| None v Many | −49 | $p = 0.2576$ |

The exact uncorrected calculated $p$ values for each comparison quoted above were determined using GraphPad Prism. Corrected $p$ values; $* p < 0.05$. The Bonferroni-corrected $p$ value for a family error rate <0.05 with two pairwise comparisons equals $0.05/2 = 0.025$. Similarly, for family error rates of 0.01 and 0.001, then Bonferroni-corrected $p$ values are $0.01/2 = 0.005$ and $0.001/2 = 0.0005$, respectively.

# Example output from statistical software

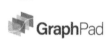 

**A**

**B**

Summary statistical analysis from GraphPad Prism, v8. Panel A shows the summary of the descriptive statistics of the rodent head-shake data from Table 18.1, together with the results of the Kruskal–Wallis ANOVA and the results of the *post hoc* Dunn's multiple comparison tests (compare to Tables 18.11 and 18.12). Panel B shows the summary of the descriptive statistics of the lecture quality data from Table 18.9, together with the results of the Friedman Repeated Measures ANOVA and the results of the *post hoc* Dunn's multiple comparison tests (compare to Tables 18.14 and 18.15).

*Source*: GraphPad Software.

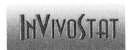

## A

View Analysis Log  Export to Html  Export Images

## InVivoStat Summary Statistics

### Variable selection

Response HS is analysed in this module, with results categorised by factor subs.

### Summary statistics for HS categorised by subs

| Categorisation Factor levels | N | Min | Max | Median | Lower quartile | Upper quartile |
|---|---|---|---|---|---|---|
| 1 | 10 | 2.0000 | 8.0000 | 3.0000 | 2.0000 | 4.0000 |
| 2 | 10 | 2.0000 | 8.0000 | 4.5000 | 4.0000 | 5.0000 |
| 3 | 10 | 7.0000 | 24.0000 | 12.0000 | 8.0000 | 15.0000 |

### Kruskal-Wallis test

| | Test statistic | Degrees of freedom | p-value |
|---|---|---|---|
| Test result | 18.68 | 2 | < 0.0001 |

### All pairwise comparisons - Mann-Whitney tests

| Comparison Number | Gp 1 | vs. | Gp 2 | p-value | p-value type |
|---|---|---|---|---|---|
| 1 | 1 | vs. | 2 | 0.1430 | Asymptotic |
| 2 | 1 | vs. | 3 | 0.0003 | Asymptotic |
| 3 | 2 | vs. | 3 | 0.0004 | Asymptotic |

As there are ties in some of the responses, and/or some of the groups have more than 50 responses, the asymptotic Mann-Whitney test results has been calculated in these cases.

## B

View Analysis Log  Export to Html  Export Images

## InVivoStat Summary Statistics

### Variable selection

Response Visual Aid score is analysed in this module, with results categorised by factor subs2.

### Summary statistics for Visual Aid score categorised by subs2

| Categorisation Factor levels | Mean | N | Std dev | Lower 95% CI | Upper 95% CI | Median | Lower quartile | Upper quartile |
|---|---|---|---|---|---|---|---|---|
| 1 | 62.7059 | 17 | 13.9094 | 55.5543 | 69.8574 | 63.0000 | 54.0000 | 69.0000 |
| 2 | 71.2353 | 17 | 14.9228 | 63.5627 | 78.9079 | 71.0000 | 61.0000 | 78.0000 |
| 3 | 59.8235 | 17 | 18.3106 | 50.4091 | 69.2380 | 62.0000 | 48.0000 | 68.0000 |

### Friedman Rank Sum test

| | Test statistic | Degrees of freedom | p-value |
|---|---|---|---|
| Test result | 10.94 | 2 | 0.0042 |

### All pairwise comparisons - Wilcoxon Signed Rank tests

| Comparison Number | Gp 1 | vs. | Gp 2 | p-value | p-value type |
|---|---|---|---|---|---|
| 1 | 1 | vs. | 2 | 0.0098 | Asymptotic |
| 2 | 1 | vs. | 3 | 0.2457 | Asymptotic |
| 3 | 2 | vs. | 3 | 0.0039 | Asymptotic |

As there are ties in some of the response differences, and/or some of the groups have more than 20 responses, the asymptotic test result has been calculated in these cases.

Summary statistical analysis from InVivoStat, v4.0.2. Panel A shows the summary of the descriptive statistics of the rodent head-shake data from Table 18.1, together with the results of the Kruskal–Wallis ANOVA and the results of repeated Mann–Whitney *U*-tests prior to applying Bonferroni correction (compare to Table 18.13). Panel B shows the summary of the descriptive statistics of the lecture quality data from Table 18.9, together with the results of the Friedman Repeated Measures ANOVA and the results of repeated Wilcoxon Signed-Rank tests prior to applying Bonferroni correction (compare to Table 18.17).

*Source*: InVivoStat.

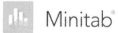 Minitab

## A

### Descriptive statistics

| subs | N | Median | Mean rank | Z-value |
|------|----|--------|-----------|---------|
| 1 | 10 | 3.0 | 8.8 | −2.95 |
| 2 | 10 | 4.5 | 12.7 | −1.23 |
| 3 | 10 | 12.0 | 25.0 | 4.18 |
| Overall | 30 | | 15.5 | |

### Test

| Null hypothesis | $H_0$: All medians are equal |
|---|---|
| Alternative hypothesis | $H_1$: At least one median is different |

| Method | DF | H-value | P-value |
|--------|----|---------|---------|
| Not adjusted for ties | 2 | 18.45 | 0.000 |
| Adjusted for ties | 2 | 18.68 | 0.000 |

## B

### Descriptive statistics

| subs2 | N | Median | Sum of ranks |
|-------|----|--------|--------------|
| 1 | 17 | 62.0000 | 30.0 |
| 2 | 17 | 71.0000 | 45.0 |
| 3 | 17 | 58.0000 | 27.0 |
| Overall | 51 | 63.6667 | |

### Test

| Null hypothesis | $H_0$: All treatment effects are zero |
|---|---|
| Alternative hypothesis | $H_1$: Not all treatment effects are zero |

| DF | Chi-square | P-value |
|----|-----------|---------|
| 2 | 10.94 | 0.004 |

Summary statistical analysis from MiniTab, v19. Panel A shows the summary of the descriptive statistics of the rodent head-shake data from Table 18.1, together with the results of the Kruskal–Wallis ANOVA and the results of repeated Mann–Whitney $U$-tests prior to applying Bonferroni correction (compare to Table 18.13). Panel B shows the summary of the descriptive statistics of the lecture quality data from Table 18.9, together with the results of the Friedman repeated measures ANOVA and the results of repeated Wilcoxon Signed-Rank tests prior to applying Bonferroni correction (compare to Table 18.17).

*Source*: Minitab, LLC.

**A**

**Descriptive Statistics**

| | N | Percentiles 25th | 50th (Median) | 75th |
|---|---|---|---|---|
| HS | 30 | 3.0000 | 5.0000 | 8.7500 |
| subs | 30 | 1.0000 | 2.0000 | 3.0000 |

**Kruskal-Wallis Test**

**Ranks**

| | subs | N | Mean Rank |
|---|---|---|---|
| HS | 1.00 | 10 | 8.80 |
| | 2.00 | 10 | 12.70 |
| | 3.00 | 10 | 25.00 |
| | Total | 30 | |

**Test Statistics[a,b]**

| | HS |
|---|---|
| Kruskal-Wallis H | 16.682 |
| df | 2 |
| Asymp. Sig. | .000 |

a. Kruskal Wallis Test
b. Grouping Variable: subs

**Mann-Whitney Test**

**Ranks**

| | HS_Factors | N | Mean Rank | Sum of Ranks |
|---|---|---|---|---|
| HS_Sal_DrgA1 | 1.00 | 10 | 8.55 | 85.50 |
| | 2.00 | 10 | 12.45 | 124.50 |
| | Total | 20 | | |

**Test Statistics[a]**

| | HS_Sal_DrgA1 |
|---|---|
| Mann-Whitney U | 30.500 |
| Wilcoxon W | 85.500 |
| Z | -1.503 |
| Asymp. Sig. (2-tailed) | .133 |
| Exact Sig. [2*(1-tailed Sig.)] | .143[b] |

a. Grouping Variable: HS_Factors
b. Not corrected for ties

**Mann-Whitney Test**

**Ranks**

| | HS_Factors | N | Mean Rank | Sum of Ranks |
|---|---|---|---|---|
| HS_Sal_Drg_B | 1.00 | 10 | 5.75 | 57.50 |
| | 2.00 | 10 | 15.25 | 152.50 |
| | Total | 20 | | |

**Test Statistics[a]**

| | HS_Sal_Drg_B |
|---|---|
| Mann-Whitney U | 2.500 |
| Wilcoxon W | 57.500 |
| Z | -3.614 |
| Asymp. Sig. (2-tailed) | .000 |
| Exact Sig. [2*(1-tailed Sig.)] | .000[b] |

a. Grouping Variable: HS_Factors
b. Not corrected for ties

**Mann-Whitney Test**

**Ranks**

| | HS_DrgA.DrgB | N | Mean Rank | Sum of Ranks |
|---|---|---|---|---|
| HS_DrgA_DrgB | 1.00 | 10 | 5.75 | 57.50 |
| | 2.00 | 10 | 15.25 | 152.50 |
| | Total | 20 | | |

**Test Statistics[a]**

| | HS_DrgA_DrgB |
|---|---|
| Mann-Whitney U | 2.500 |
| Wilcoxon W | 57.500 |
| Z | -3.607 |
| Asymp. Sig. (2-tailed) | .000 |
| Exact Sig. [2*(1-tailed Sig.)] | .000[b] |

a. Grouping Variable: HS_Factors
b. Not corrected for ties

**B**

**Descriptive Statistics**

| | N | Percentiles 25th | 50th (Median) | 75th |
|---|---|---|---|---|
| None | 17 | 51.0000 | 63.0000 | 73.0000 |
| Few | 17 | 59.0000 | 71.0000 | 83.5000 |
| Many | 17 | 47.0000 | 62.0000 | 69.5000 |

**Friedman Test**

**Ranks**

| | Mean Rank |
|---|---|
| None | 1.76 |
| Few | 2.65 |
| Many | 1.59 |

**Test Statistics[a]**

| N | 17 |
|---|---|
| Chi-Square | 10.941 |
| df | 2 |
| Asymp. Sig. | .004 |

a. Friedman Test

**Wilcoxon Signed Ranks Test**

**Ranks**

| | | N | Mean Rank | Sum of Ranks |
|---|---|---|---|---|
| Few - None | Negative Ranks | 3[a] | 7.33 | 22.00 |
| | Positive Ranks | 14[b] | 9.36 | 131.00 |
| | Ties | 0[c] | | |
| | Total | 17 | | |

a. Few < None
b. Few > None
c. Few = None

**Test Statistics[a]**

| | Few - None |
|---|---|
| Z | -2.581[b] |
| Asymp. Sig. (2-tailed) | .010 |

a. Wilcoxon Signed Ranks Test
b. Based on negative ranks.

**Wilcoxon Signed Ranks Test**

**Ranks**

| | | N | Mean Rank | Sum of Ranks |
|---|---|---|---|---|
| Few - None | Negative Ranks | 3[a] | 7.33 | 22.00 |
| | Positive Ranks | 14[b] | 9.36 | 131.00 |
| | Ties | 0[c] | | |
| | Total | 17 | | |

a. Few < None
b. Few > None
c. Few = None

**Test Statistics[a]**

| | Few - None |
|---|---|
| Z | -2.581[b] |
| Asymp. Sig. (2-tailed) | .010 |

a. Wilcoxon Signed Ranks Test
b. Based on negative ranks.

**Wilcoxon Signed Ranks Test**

**Ranks**

| | | N | Mean Rank | Sum of Ranks |
|---|---|---|---|---|
| Many - Few | Negative Ranks | 14[a] | 9.82 | 137.50 |
| | Positive Ranks | 3[b] | 5.17 | 15.50 |
| | Ties | 0[c] | | |
| | Total | 17 | | |

a. Many < Few
b. Many > Few
c. Many = Few

**Test Statistics[a]**

| | Many - Few |
|---|---|
| Z | -2.889[b] |
| Asymp. Sig. (2-tailed) | .004 |

a. Wilcoxon Signed Ranks Test
b. Based on positive ranks.

Summary statistical analysis from SPSS, v27. Panel A shows the summary of the descriptive statistics of the rodent head-shake data from Table 18.1, together with the results of the Kruskal–Wallis ANOVA and the results of repeated Mann–Whitney U-tests prior to applying Bonferroni correction (compare to Table 18.13). Panel B shows the summary of the descriptive statistics of the lecture quality data from Table 18.9, together with the results of the Friedman repeated measures ANOVA and the results of repeated Wilcoxon Signed-Rank tests prior to applying Bonferroni correction (compare to Table 18.17).

*Source*: IBM Corporation.

**Decision Flowchart 2: Inferential Statistics – Single and multiple pairwise comparisons**

| Test type and data distribution | Group type | Number of groups = 2 ONLY! | Grouping factors(s) | Number of Groups > 2 — ANOVA model | Post hoc multiple comparisons |
|---|---|---|---|---|---|
| Parametric (Normal or distribution) | Independent | Independent t-test (Chapter 11) | 1 Between Group | One-way ANOVA (Chapter 15) | • All Means comparisons or<br>• Control group comparisons (Chapter 15; Table 15.13) |
| | | | 2 Between Groups | Two-way ANOVA (Chapter 17) | As above or multiple Independent t-tests with Bonferroni or Holme correction, as appropriate (Chapter 17) |
| | | | 3 Between Groups | Three-way ANOVA (Chapter 17) | |
| | Paired | Paired t-test (Chapter 12) | 1 Within Group | Repeated Measures ANOVA (Chapter 16) | • Turkey, Games-Howell.<br>• Turkey with Bonferroni or Sidak correction<br>• Multiple paired t-tests with Bonferroni or Holme correction (Chapter 16) |
| | Mixed Independent and Paired | | 1 Between Group + 1 Within Group | One-way ANOVA with Repeated Measures (Chapter 17) | Multiple Independent and Paired t-tests with Bonferroni correction as justified by each Main effect of the Grouping Factors and interaction(s) therein (Chapter 17) |
| | | | 2 Between Groups + 1 Within Group | Two-way ANOVA with Repeated Measures (Chapter 17) | |

| | Group type | Number of groups = 2 ONLY! | Grouping factors(s) | Number of Groups > 2 | Post hoc multiple comparisons |
|---|---|---|---|---|---|
| Non-parametric (Non-normal or distribution unknown) | Independent | Wilcoxon Rank Sum test or Mann-Whitney U-test (Chapter 13) | 1 Between Group | Kruskal-Wallis test (Chapter 18) | Multiple Mann-Whitney U-test with Bonferroni or Holme correction or independent variant of Dunn's test Chapter 18 |
| | | | 2 Between Groups | Scheirer-Ray-Hare extension (Chapter 18) | |
| | Paired | Wilcoxon Signed Rank test (Chapter 14) | 1 Within Group | Friedman test (Chapter 18) | Multiple Mann-Whitney U-test with Bonferroni or Holme correction or paired variant of Dunn's test (Chapter 18) |

# 19 Correlation analysis

Throughout my career as a Lecturer at a British University, I often feel the need to emphasise to my students the importance of attending formal teaching sessions (lectures, workshops, practical sessions, etc.) and I, like many of my colleagues across the sector, repeatedly say something along the lines of 'Well, as I'm sure you're aware, there is a clear relationship between your attendance at lectures and your final degree classification!.' Of course, such statements fail to say exactly *what* the relationship is, but the implication is that the *higher* a student's attendance is, the *better* they will perform during their assessments and so will achieve a better degree classification at the culmination of their undergraduate programme. So quite clearly, I'm inferring that there is a clear, direct *association* or *relationship* between two very different variables, i.e. the number or hours of attendance at formal teaching sessions on one hand, and assessment performance on the other. From a statistical point of view, my statement above suggests that there is a **correlation** between the two variables. Of course, I always omit to show the appropriate data since the sole purpose of such a statement is to scare the conscientious student(s) into attending my boring statistics lectures, while those that have no interest simply go back to sleep – assuming that they were awake in the first place to hear my enlightened statement – which is doubtful!

## Bivariate correlation analysis of parametric data

To use simple language, if two apparently unrelated, *independent*, variables are indeed related in some way, then changes in the absolute value of one variable should be reflected by *concomitant* changes in the absolute value of the other variable. Furthermore, the *magnitude* of the change seen in both variables should be related and proportional in some distinct way. This is not to say that the respective changes of both variables should be in the same direction; indeed, as the value of one variable increases, then the values associated with the second may increase or decrease but in a consistent manner.

### Example 19.1 Positive correlation

Consider the following set of data summarised in Table 19.1. Here, the levels of two enzymes in blood plasma from nine different subjects were measured.

Table 19.1 Blood enzyme levels.

| Subject | Enzyme A (ng/ml) Observation | $(x-\bar{x})$ | Enzyme B (ng/ml) Observation | $(y-\bar{y})$ | $(x-\bar{x})(y-\bar{y})$ |
|---|---|---|---|---|---|
| 1 | 5.85 | −0.418 | 2.50 | −0.128 | 0.05338 |
| 2 | 5.91 | −0.358 | 2.19 | −0.438 | 0.15663 |
| 3 | 6.39 | 0.122 | 2.86 | 0.232 | 0.02838 |
| 4 | 6.63 | 0.362 | 2.86 | 0.232 | 0.08412 |
| 5 | 6.64 | 0.372 | 2.91 | 0.282 | 0.10505 |
| 6 | 6.10 | −0.168 | 2.36 | −0.268 | 0.04493 |
| 7 | 6.29 | 0.022 | 2.63 | 0.002 | 0.00004 |
| 8 | 6.19 | −0.078 | 2.60 | −0.028 | 0.00216 |
| 9 | 6.41 | 0.142 | 2.74 | 0.112 | 0.01596 |
| Mean | 6.268 | | 2.628 | | |
| St Dev | 0.2833 | | 0.2450 | | |
| $\Sigma$ | | | | | 0.49066 |

For each set of enzyme data, the second column indicates the difference of each observation from the group mean. The final column indicates the cross-product deviations that each data pair contribute to the covariance.

By far, the best way to appreciate the relationship between two sets of data is to produce a scatterplot of the individual values. The resultant scatterplot of the data for enzyme A and enzyme B from Table 19.1 is shown in Figure 19.1. Notice that when producing scatterplots summarising the relative spread of each set of data, it is imperative that the pairs of values for each subject are kept together (see Table 19.1). The first thing to notice about the scatterplot is that distribution of the data for both variables appears to be the similar. Thus, four of the data points sit <u>below</u> the mean values for *both* Enzyme A and Enzyme B, four data points lie <u>above</u> the respective mean values for *both* enzymes, while the remaining data point sits almost on the mean of *both* enzyme levels. Clearly, the scatterplot suggests that there is a relationship between the respective levels of these two enzymes; as the level of one enzyme increases, so does the level of the other enzyme. But, how may the similarity (or dissimilarity) be quantified statistically?

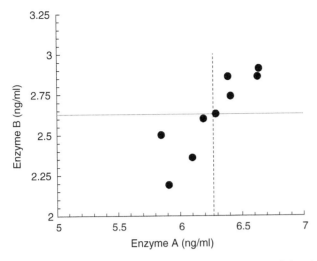

**Figure 19.1** **Scatterplot of the levels of Enzyme A and Enzyme B for nine subjects**. The vertical dashed line indicates the mean concentration of Enzyme A (6.268 ng/ml), while the horizontal dotted line indicates the mean concentration of Enzyme B (2.628 ng/ml).

$$\text{Covariance } (x, y) = \frac{\sum (x - \bar{x})(y - \bar{y})}{N - 1} = \frac{0.49066}{8} = 0.06133$$

$$(19.1)$$

Thus, a positive covariance indicates that both variables deviate from their respective mean values in the same direction (either both positive or both negative). In contrast, a negative covariance indicates that as one variable deviates in one direction, then the other deviates in the opposite direction.

However, the covariance is not a standardised measure and depends on the scale of measurement used. In the example here, the level of each enzyme in the blood plasma was expressed as ng/ml; consequently, the unit of covariance is ng/ml squared (or $(ng/ml)^2$ if you prefer). Such expression of the covariance unit only applies when the two sets of data are measured in the same units. This becomes an even bigger issue when the two variables have different units of measurement. To circumvent this issue, it is necessary to standardise the covariance and to do this, we use the standard deviation associated with each variable. In Chapter 7, I discussed how a normal distribution may be expressed as a Standard Normal Distribution with mean = 0 and standard deviation = 1 and later in Chapter 10, how the standard deviation may be expressed as a $z$ score. The standard deviation of a data set allows the estimation of the average deviation (i.e. spread of data) around the mean, and $z$ scores are simply multiples of the standard deviation. If any observation in a data set is divided by the standard deviation, then we obtain a measure of the distance of that observation from the mean in standard deviation units (i.e. the $z$ score!). Consequently, dividing the covariance by the standard deviation expresses the covariance in a standard unit of measurement. However, in the situation described here, there are two variables, each with a standard deviation. Furthermore, the covariance was determined by multiplying the two deviations. A similar method is used to standardise the covariance; the standard deviation scores are multiplied together (known as the pooled standard deviation). The covariance is then divided by the pooled standard deviation, as shown in the equation below.

$$\frac{\sum (x - \bar{x})(y - \bar{y})}{(N - 1).s_x.s_y} = \frac{\text{cov}_{xy}}{s_x.s_y} = r \qquad (19.2)$$

where $s_x$ and $s_y$ are the standard deviation scores for the first and second variables, respectively.

This standardised covariance is known as the correlation coefficient (aka the **Pearson product-moment correlation coefficient** or, simply, **Pearson's correlation coefficient**) and denoted by $r$ (pronounced 'rho').

If we apply this process to the enzyme data described in Table 19.1,

$$r = \frac{\sum (x - \bar{x})(y - \bar{y})}{(N - 1).s_x.s_y} = \frac{0.06133}{0.2833 \times 0.2450}$$

$$= \frac{0.06133}{0.06941} = 0.8835 \qquad (19.3)$$

Way back in Chapter 5, I discussed how Descriptive Statistics could be used to summarise a group of data and a similar approach may be used here. One possible method would be to calculate the difference of our observations from the mean value for the data set, but we know from experience that the positive and negative differences would simply cancel each other out! For a single data set, we got around this problem by simply squaring the differences of each observation from the mean to produce an array of positive values, the sum of which we called the Sum of Squares, and from there, it was a simple process to determine the variance and Standard Deviation of the data. These descriptive measures allowed us to appreciate the distribution of a single data set, but such an approach if used here would not reveal anything about the relationship between pairs of data from two variables. Instead when there are two variables, we can simply multiply the deviations from the group mean for all the observations of one variable by the deviations from the respective group mean for all the observations of the second variable; these values are also summarised in Table 19.1. If *both* deviations arising from a single subject are positive or negative, then multiplying these values together will produce a **positive value** showing that the deviations are commonly either greater or less than the respective group means; this relates to the lower left and upper right areas of Figure 19.1, as divided by the mean values of the two variables. However, a **negative value** will result if one deviation is positive and the other negative (i.e. the upper left and lower right areas as divided by the variable means), showing that the observations are heading in opposite directions (an example of this will be discussed later).

Multiplying the deviations from the mean value of one variable by the deviations from the mean value of the second variable and adding these values together produce the **cross-product deviations** as shown in the final column of Table 19.1. Back in Chapter 5, the variance was calculated by dividing the Sum of Squares (SSQ) by the degrees of freedom for the single set of data. Similarly, we can obtain an average of the combined deviations for the two variables by dividing the sum of the cross-product deviations by the degrees of freedom for the number of pairs of data (i.e. $N - 1$), and this value is termed the **covariance**; thus,

For data sets where the covariance is a positive value, then the standardisation process produces a correlation coefficient that lies between 0 and +1 and the closer the correlation coefficient approaches +1, the greater the positive correlation between the two variables. It should be appreciated here that a close relationship between two variables does not imply a cause and effect association between the two, simply that the direction of change in the magnitude of the two variables is the same (that is not to say that there is not an underlying mechanism that underpins the change in the levels of the two enzymes – this, indeed, may be the case but the correlation analysis alone should not be used as evidence of cause and effect!).

But how useful is the correlation coefficient in terms of hypothesis testing? The Null Hypothesis for correlation analysis is that the correlation coefficient is **not** different from zero. But, how do we determine the probability that the Null Hypothesis is correct?

There are two procedures to determine the probability of the Null Hypothesis. The first method determines the $t$-statistic with $N - 2$ degrees of freedom and is directly calculated using correlation coefficient, $r$, according to the following equation,

$$t_r = \frac{r\sqrt{N-2}}{\sqrt{1-r^2}} \tag{19.4}$$

So, for the enzyme data in Table 19.1,

$$t_r = \frac{0.8835\sqrt{9-2}}{\sqrt{1-0.8835^2}} = \frac{0.8835 \cdot 2.645}{\sqrt{1-0.8835^2}} \tag{19.5}$$
$$= \frac{2.3369}{\sqrt{1-0.7806}}$$

$$t_r = \frac{2.3369}{\sqrt{0.2194}} = \frac{2.3369}{0.4684} = 4.9891 \tag{19.6}$$

The corresponding $p$ value may then be determined by using the critical values of the $t$-distribution summarised in Appendix C. The table shows that the critical value of $t$ with 7 degrees of freedom for $p = 0.01$ is $t_{crit} = 3.499$, while for $p = 0.001$, $t_{crit} = 5.408$. Consequently, the probability of the Null Hypothesis being true lies between 0.01 and 0.001. This may be summarised as;

$$t_r(7) = 4.9891, p < 0.01 \tag{19.7}$$

The second method of determining $p$ uses the $z$-scores. On the face of it, this is a useful method since $z$-scores are related to the normal distribution (see discussion above and especially Chapter 10). Unfortunately, the sampling distribution of $r$ does not follow a normal distribution. All is not lost, however, since $r$ may be adjusted so that its sampling distribution is normal by using the following equation,

$$z_r = \frac{1}{2}\log_e\left(\frac{1+r}{1-r}\right) \tag{19.8}$$

with a standard error according to,

$$SE_{z_r} = \frac{1}{\sqrt{N-3}} \tag{19.9}$$

For the data from Table 19.1,

$$z_r = \frac{1}{2}\log_e\left(\frac{1+0.8835}{1-0.8835}\right)$$
$$= \frac{1}{2}\log_e\left(\frac{1.8835}{0.1165}\right) = \frac{1}{2}\log_e(16.167) \tag{19.10}$$

$$z_r = \frac{1}{2}(2.783) = 1.391 \tag{19.11}$$

$$\text{while; } SE_{z_r} = \frac{1}{\sqrt{N-3}} = \frac{1}{\sqrt{6}} = \frac{1}{2.449} = 0.408 \tag{19.12}$$

Consequently, the correlation coefficient, $r = 0.8835$, is adjusted to $z_r = 1.391$ with a standard error of 0.408. The adjusted value may now be expressed as a $z$-score simply by dividing $z_r$ by its standard error, $SE_{z_r}$. Thus,

$$z = \frac{z_r}{SE_{z_r}} = \frac{1.3915}{0.4083} = 3.41 \tag{19.13}$$

If we consult the list of Standard Normal Distribution probabilities (see Appendix B), then the one-tailed probability of $z(3.41)$ is 0.0003 (examine the smaller proportion in Appendix B and ignore the sign). Consequently, the two-tailed probability of the Null Hypothesis being true is $2 \times 0.0003 = 0.0006$.

Regardless of which method we use ($t$-statistic or $z$-score), the resulting probability that the Null Hypothesis is true is <0.01. Consequently, we may reject the Null Hypothesis in favour of the alternate hypothesis and conclude that the correlation is significant.

Alternatively, the corresponding $p$ value for the Pearson correlation coefficient may be determined by consulting the critical values of $r$ (according to the number of data pairs) provided in Appendix H, Table H.1. This table indicates that for nine pairs of data ($N$), the critical value of $r$ for $p = 0.05$ is $r_{crit} = 0.602$, while for $p = 0.01$, $r_{crit} = 0.735$. Thus, the correlation coefficient for the current example is 0.8835 exceeds the critical value of $r$ for $p = 0.01$, which agrees with the earlier methods of determining the probability in support of the Null Hypothesis.

The correlation analysis may therefore be summarised as,

$$r = 0.8835, p < 0.01 \tag{19.14}$$

## Example 19.2 Negative correlation

Now consider the set of data summarised in Table 19.2 resulting from a study which examined if there was a relationship between birth weight (in kg) and diastolic blood pressure (in mm Hg) once the subjects had reached adulthood.

Table 19.2 Birth weight and adult diastolic blood pressure.

| Subject | Birth weight (kg) Observation | $(x-\bar{x})$ | Adult DBP (mm Hg) Observation | $(y-\bar{y})$ | $(x-\bar{x})(y-\bar{y})$ |
|---|---|---|---|---|---|
| 1 | 2.5 | −0.442 | 110 | 8.857 | −3.915 |
| 2 | 3.2 | 0.257 | 90 | −11.143 | −2.864 |
| 3 | 2.0 | −0.943 | 126 | 24.857 | −23.440 |
| 4 | 3.5 | 0.557 | 80 | −21.143 | −11.777 |
| 5 | 2.1 | −0.843 | 115 | 13.857 | −11.640 |
| 6 | 4.2 | 1.257 | 85 | −16.143 | −20.292 |
| 7 | 3.1 | 0.157 | 102 | 0.857 | 0.135 |
| Mean | 2.942 | | 101.143 | | |
| St Dev | 0.793 | | 16.935 | | |
| $\Sigma$ | | | | | −73.793 |

For each set of data, the second column indicates the difference of each observation from the group mean. The final column indicates the contribution of each paired data set to the covariance.

The scatterplot of the birth weight data against diastolic blood pressure (DBP) in adulthood from Table 19.2 is shown in Figure 19.2. The first point to notice is that the distribution of the data for both variables is dissimilar. Thus, when the birth weight values are <u>greater</u> than the group mean, then the DBP values are generally equal to or <u>less</u> than the respective group mean.

Similarly, when the DBP values are <u>greater</u> than the group mean, then the corresponding birth weight values are <u>less</u> than the respective group mean.

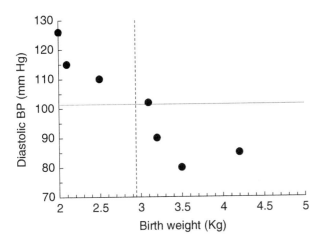

**Figure 19.2** **Scatterplot of birth weight and adult diastolic blood pressure in 7 healthy subjects**. The vertical dashed line indicates the mean concentration of birth weight (2.943 kg), while the horizontal dotted line indicates the mean diastolic blood pressure (101.14 mm Hg).

This implies an *inverse* or *indirect* relationship between the two variables. Indeed, for this set of data, all bar one of the calculated cross-product deviations are negative, indicating that when the deviation of one observation from its respective group mean is positive, then the deviation of the other paired observation is negative; clearly, this suggests the observations are heading in opposite directions (thus, the scatterplot in Figure 19.2 shows the data points limited to the upper left and lower right areas as divided by the variable means; cf. Figure 19.1).

As in the earlier example, the covariance may be obtained by dividing the sum of the cross-product deviations by the degrees of freedom, thus,

$$\text{Covariance}(x, y) = \frac{\sum(x - \bar{x})(y - \bar{y})}{N - 1}$$

$$= \frac{-73.793}{6} = -12.3071$$

(19.15)

The negative covariance indicates that the variables deviate from their respective group means in opposite directions.

The next step is to standardise the covariance by dividing by the pooled standard deviation to calculate Pearson's correlation coefficient, $r$, thus,

$$\frac{\sum(x - \bar{x})(y - \bar{y})}{(N - 1).s_x.s_y} = \frac{\text{cov}_{xy}}{s_x.s_y} = \frac{-12.307}{0.793 \times 16.935}$$

$$= \frac{-12.307}{13.429} = -0.916 = r$$

(19.16)

For data sets where the covariance is a negative value, then the standardisation process produces a correlation coefficient that lies between 0 and −1 and the closer the correlation coefficient approaches −1, then the greater the negative correlation between the two variables.

The important point to note here, and as demonstrated by the two examples used so far in this chapter, is that the correlation coefficient falls within the range of −1 through 0 to +1 and consequently contains two important pieces of information,

**1** The sign (− or +) indicates the quality of the correlation, either negative or positive
**2** The value indicates the degree of association between the two variables.

The third piece of information required is the probability that the Null Hypothesis (that the correlation coefficient is not different from zero) is true. As described above, there are two methods by which the probability may be calculated. For the sake of brevity, and also for the fact that most statistical packages use this method, I will only calculate the $t$-statistic with $N - 2$ degrees of freedom. Thus,

$$t_r = \frac{r\sqrt{N - 2}}{\sqrt{1 - r^2}}$$

(19.17)

where $r^2$ is known as the **coefficient of determination**.
So, for the birth weight/DBP data in Table 19.2,

$$t_r = \frac{-0.916\sqrt{7 - 2}}{\sqrt{1 - (-0.916^2)}} = \frac{-0.916 \times 2.236}{\sqrt{1 - 0.839}}$$

$$= \frac{-2.048}{\sqrt{0.161}}$$

(19.18)

$$t_r = \frac{-2.048}{0.401} = -5.107$$

(19.19)

The corresponding $p$ value may then be determined by using the critical values of the $t$-distribution summarised in Appendix C. The table shows that the absolute critical value of $t$ with 5 degrees of freedom for $p = 0.01$ is $t_{\text{crit}} = 4.032$ (notice that the sign of the $t$ value is ignored), while for $p = 0.001$, $t_{\text{crit}} = 6.869$. Consequently, the probability of the Null Hypothesis being true lies between 0.01 and 0.001. This may be summarised as,

$$t_r(5) = -5.107, p < 0.01$$

(19.20)

Additionally, the critical value of $r$ for $p = 0.01$ from Appendix H, Table H.1, for $N = 7$ pairs of data, is $r_{\text{crit}} = 0.798$. Since the calculated value of the correlation coefficient for this example exceeds the appropriate critical value (again, ignoring the sign of the calculated correlation coefficient), then it may be concluded that $p < 0.01$.

Correlation analysis of the birth weight and diastolic blood pressure data may therefore be summarised as,

$$r = -0.916, p < 0.01$$

(19.21)

indicating a significant negative, or inverse, correlation between these two variables. It may be concluded, therefore, that relatively high birth weight may indicate a lower diastolic blood pressure in adulthood.

## Example 19.3 Mixed correlation

Of course, any apparent relationship or association between two variables may not be as clear cut in terms of a direct or inverse relationship. Consider the data in Table 19.3, below, which summarises the measured lung function (measured as peak expiratory flow rate, PEFR) in 16 healthy adults between the ages of 18 and 75 years.

**Table 19.3** Lung function and age (18–75 years).

| Subject | PEFR (l/min) Observation | $(x-\bar{x})$ | Age (years) Observation | $(y-\bar{y})$ | $(x-\bar{x})(y-\bar{y})$ |
|---|---|---|---|---|---|
| 1 | 2.1 | −1.51 | 18 | −16.69 | 25.240 |
| 2 | 1.4 | −2.21 | 19 | −15.69 | 34.709 |
| 3 | 3.5 | −0.11 | 19 | −15.69 | 1.765 |
| 4 | 3.4 | −0.21 | 20 | −14.69 | 3.121 |
| 5 | 3.9 | 0.29 | 22 | −12.69 | −3.648 |
| 6 | 4.8 | 1.19 | 24 | −10.69 | −12.691 |
| 7 | 4.3 | 0.69 | 25 | −9.69 | −6.660 |
| 8 | 4.1 | 0.49 | 27 | −7.69 | −3.748 |
| 9 | 5.9 | 2.29 | 30 | −4.69 | −10.723 |
| 10 | 4.8 | 1.19 | 32 | −2.69 | −3.191 |
| 11 | 4.1 | 0.49 | 35 | 0.31 | 0.152 |
| 12 | 3.8 | 0.19 | 40 | 5.31 | 0.996 |
| 13 | 3.9 | 0.29 | 43 | 8.31 | 2.390 |
| 14 | 3.1 | −0.51 | 54 | 19.31 | −9.898 |
| 15 | 2.5 | −1.11 | 72 | 37.31 | −41.510 |
| 16 | 2.2 | −1.41 | 75 | 40.31 | −56.941 |
| Mean | 3.61 | | 34.69 | | |
| St Dev | 1.153 | | 18.132 | | |
| $\Sigma$ | | | | | −80.638 |

For each set of data, the second column indicates the difference of each observation from the respective group mean indicated at the bottom of the previous column. The final column indicates the contribution of each paired data set to the covariance.

Inspection of the scatterplot of these data (see Figure 19.3) appears to suggest an increase in PEFR with age from 18 to about 30 and then a subsequent reduction in lung function through to about 70 years of age. The full correlation analysis, using the equations indicated throughout this chapter and applied to the data in Table 19.3, is summarised in Table 19.4.

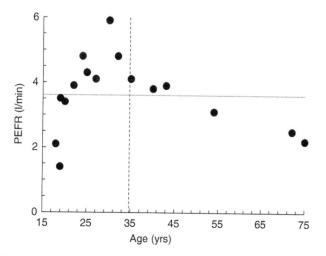

**Figure 19.3 Scatterplot of age and lung function in 16 healthy subjects.** The vertical dashed line indicates the mean age of the subjects (34.69 years), while the horizontal dotted line indicates the mean peak expiratory flow rate (3.61 l/min).

**Table 19.4** Correlation analysis of age and lung function (18–75 years).

| Item | Value |
|---|---|
| Sum of cross-product deviations | −80.638 |
| Degrees of freedom $(N-1)$ | 15 |
| Covariance | −5.376 |
| Pooled standard deviation | 20.904 |
| Correlation coefficient, $r$ | −0.257 |
| $t$-statistic | 0.996 |
| Degrees of freedom $(N-2)$ | 14 |
| $p$ value | $p > 0.10$ |

The correlation analysis of the complete data set, perhaps unsurprisingly (since there are data points in all four quadrants of the scatterplot), fails to identify a clear, statistical, correlation between the two variables. The $t$-statistic of the correlation is 0.996 with 14 degrees of freedom, and the corresponding $p$ value may be determined by using the critical values of the $t$-distribution summarised in Appendix C. The table shows that the critical value of $t$ with 14 degrees of freedom for $p = 0.10$ is $t_{crit} = 1.761$, which is greater than the calculated $t$-value; therefore $p > 0.10$.

In addition, Appendix H, Table H.1, indicates that the calculated value of $r$ for the complete lung function and age data, i.e. −0.257, is less than the critical value of $r$ for $p = 0.05$ with 16 pairs of data, i.e. 0.468. Consequently, $p > 0.05$ in support of the Null Hypothesis.

The overall correlation analysis for the total lung function and age data may be summarised as,

$$r = -0.257, p > 0.10 \qquad (19.22)$$

and consequently, the Null Hypothesis (that the correlation coefficient is not different from 0) must be accepted.

*However, this is not the end of the story!*

As already stated, the visual inspection of the scatterplot suggests that the complete data set may be subdivided into two phases; a rising phase in lung function between the ages of 18 and 30, after which the PEFR values decline as age increases. It is important to recognise that correlation analysis allows the data to be *divided* into bite-sized chunks which may reveal hitherto hidden relationships between the two variables. So, let us examine these two sections of the data separately.

Tables 19.5 and 19.6 summarise the lung function and age data according to the subdivision of 18–27 and 30–75 years of age, respectively.

**Table 19.5** Lung function and age (18–27 years).

| Subject | PEFR (l/min) Observation | $(x-\bar{x})$ | Age (years) Observation | $(y-\bar{y})$ | $(x-\bar{x})(y-\bar{y})$ |
|---|---|---|---|---|---|
| 1 | 2.1 | −1.34 | 18 | −3.75 | 5.025 |
| 2 | 1.4 | −2.04 | 19 | −2.75 | 5.610 |
| 3 | 3.5 | 0.06 | 19 | −2.75 | −0.165 |
| 4 | 3.4 | −0.04 | 20 | −1.75 | 0.070 |
| 5 | 3.9 | 0.46 | 22 | 0.25 | 0.115 |
| 6 | 4.8 | 1.36 | 24 | 2.25 | 3.060 |
| 7 | 4.3 | 0.86 | 25 | 3.25 | 2.795 |
| 8 | 4.1 | 0.66 | 27 | 5.25 | 3.465 |
| Mean | 3.44 | | 21.75 | | |
| St Dev | 1.146 | | 3.284 | | |
| $\Sigma$ | | | | | 19.975 |

For each set of data, the second column indicates the difference of each observation from the respective group mean indicated at the bottom of the previous column. The final column indicates the contribution of each paired data set to the covariance.

**Table 19.6** Lung function and age (30–75 years).

| Subject | PEFR (l/min) Observation | $(x-\bar{x})$ | Age (years) Observation | $(y-\bar{y})$ | $(x-\bar{x})(y-\bar{y})$ |
|---|---|---|---|---|---|
| 1 | 5.9 | 2.11 | 30 | −17.625 | −37.189 |
| 2 | 4.8 | 1.01 | 32 | −15.625 | −15.781 |
| 3 | 4.1 | 0.31 | 35 | −12.625 | −3.914 |
| 4 | 3.8 | 0.01 | 40 | −7.625 | −0.076 |
| 5 | 3.9 | 0.11 | 43 | −4.625 | −0.509 |
| 6 | 3.1 | −0.69 | 54 | 6.375 | −4.399 |
| 7 | 2.5 | −1.29 | 72 | 24.375 | −31.444 |
| 8 | 2.2 | −1.59 | 75 | 27.375 | −43.526 |
| Mean | 3.79 | | 47.625 | | |
| St Dev | 1.210 | | 17.639 | | |
| $\Sigma$ | | | | | −136.838 |

For each set of data, the second column indicates the difference of each observation from the respective group mean indicated at the bottom of the previous column. The final column indicates the contribution of each paired data set to the covariance.

Figure 19.4 shows the same scatterplot of the lung function data, but which has been divided into two sections according to age group. The first section includes the data from 18 to 27 years of age only (solid circles) where the horizontal dotted line indicates the appropriate mean PEFR of 3.61 l/min at an average age of 21.75 years (vertical dashed line). Clearly, most of the data points in the scatterplot lie within the bottom left and top right sectors, suggesting a direct relationship between lung function and age. In contrast, the second section includes the data from 30 to 75 years only (open circles) where the horizontal dotted line indicates the respective mean PEFR of 3.79 l/min at an average age of 47.63 years (vertical dashed line). Here, all data points in the scatterplot lie within the top left or bottom right sectors, indicating an inverse relationship between lung function and age.

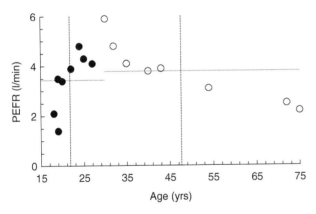

**Figure 19.4 Scatterplot of age and lung function in 16 healthy subjects subdivided according to age.** Solid circles, 18–27 years; open circles, 30–75 years. For both age groups, the horizontal dotted line indicates the mean PEFR (3.44 l/min and 3.79 l/min, respectively), while the vertical dashed line indicates the mean age of the subjects in each group (21.75 and 47.63 years of age, respectively) see Tables 19.5 and 19.6 for summary data, respectively.

The full correlation analysis of both subsets of lung function data is summarised in Table 19.7. The first point to notice is that the covariance (and subsequently the correlation coefficient, $r$) for the youngest age group is positive, while those of the older age group are negative.

**Table 19.7** Correlation analysis of age and lung function according to age subset.

| Item | Age group 18–27 | Age group 30–75 |
|---|---|---|
| Sum of cross-product deviations | 19.98 | −136.84 |
| Degrees of freedom $(N-1)$ | 7 | 7 |
| Covariance | 2.854 | −19.548 |
| Pooled standard deviation | 3.763 | 21.343 |
| Correlation coefficient, $r$ | 0.758 | −0.916 |
| $t$-statistic | 2.847 | 5.594 |
| Degrees of freedom $(N-2)$ | 6 | 6 |
| $p$ value | <0.05 | <0.01 |

As before the corresponding $p$ values for the correlation coefficients may be determined by using the critical values of the $t$-distribution summarised in Appendix C. The table shows that the critical value of $t$ with 6 degrees of freedom for $p = 0.05$ is $t_{crit} = 2.447$, for $p = 0.01$, $t_{crit} = 3.707$ while that for $p = 0.001$, $t_{crit} = 5.959$.

Consequently, the probability of the Null Hypothesis being true for both subsets of lung function data may be summarised as follows,

Age group 18–27 years:  $t_r(6) = 2.847, p < 0.05$
Age group 30–75 years:  $t_r(6) = -5.594, p < 0.01$

Correlation analysis of the lung function data according to age group may therefore be summarised as,

Age group 18–27 years:  $r = 0.758, p < 0.05$
Age group 30–75 years:  $r = -0.916, p < 0.01$

indicating a significant positive correlation between the two variables for the younger age group (suggesting that lung function improves with age) but a negative, or inverse, correlation between these two variables for the older age group (indicating that lung function most likely deteriorates with age).

In both cases, the calculated probability values in support of the Null Hypothesis may also be obtained from Appendix H, Table H.1. This table indicates that the critical value of $r$ for $p = 0.05$ with 8 pairs of data is $r_{crit} = 0.632$, while for $p = 0.01$, $r_{crit} = 0.765$. Consequently, the calculated $r$ value for the lower age range, i.e. 0.758 (see Table 19.7), exceeds the critical value of $r$ for $p = 0.05$ (but not $p = 0.01$), while the calculated $r$ value for the upper age range, i.e. −0.916 (see Table 19.7), exceeds the critical value of $r$ for $p = 0.01$. Again, the probability values from Appendix H, Table H.1, agree with the calculated values from the $t$-distribution.

The important point to note here is that such conclusions may only be drawn following division of the complete data set into appropriate smaller bite-sized subsets following initial visual inspection. Such an approach may be especially useful where observation may naturally fluctuate over time; for example, in circadian rhythm research.

All of the examples discussed so far have concentrated on data sets that follow a normal distribution. However, in pharmacology, as we have already seen, not all data obtained through experimentation and observation follow a normal distribution.

158

Experimental Design and Statistical Analysis for Pharmacology and the Biomedical Sc...

# Correlation analysis of non-parametric data

## Example 19.4 Non-parametric correlation with tied ranks

Consider the following data set from arthritic patients where the level of C-reactive protein in the serum was compared to the subjective joint pain scores reported by the patients (see Table 19.8).

Table 19.8 Serum C-reactive protein and pain.

| Subject | Serum C-reactive protein (µg/ml) | Pain score (0–5) |
|---------|----------------------------------|------------------|
| 1 | 34 | 2 |
| 2 | 7 | 2 |
| 3 | 98 | 5 |
| 4 | 23 | 3 |
| 5 | 14 | 1 |
| 6 | 71 | 4 |
| 7 | 90 | 5 |
| 8 | 85 | 4 |

The resulting scatterplot comparing the data for each variable is summarised in Figure 19.5, below. The first thing to notice about the arrangement of the scatterplot is the way that some points stack according to the pain score (see Figure 19.5; pain scores 2, 4 and 5). This results from the patients being required to **rank** their subjective pain according to a scale of 0–5; the ranking of these scores clearly indicates that the resulting data are non-parametric.

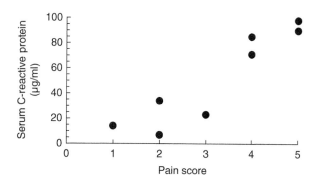

**Figure 19.5** Comparison of serum C-reactive protein levels and subjective pain scores in arthritic patients.

Consequently, it is inappropriate to perform the correlation analysis on the raw data values in the manner previously described in this chapter since ranking the pain scores would violate the assumptions of data that is normally distributed. In such circumstances, a non-parametric version of the correlation analysis is performed, known as **Spearman's Rank Correlation** analysis.

Spearman's correlation coefficient is a non-parametric statistic and denoted by the symbol $r_s$ to differentiate it from the parametric Pearson's correlation coefficient, $r$. Spearman's $r_s$ is determined by applying the appropriate equation (see conditions below) for the correlation coefficient applied to the **rank values** of the data sets for *both* variables (even if one of these may be normally distributed). So, the first step in the analysis is to rank the data values from Table 19.8 and to plot these data as a suitable scatterplot (see Table 19.9 and Figure 19.6).

Table 19.9 Serum C-reactive protein and pain – rank values.

| Subject | Serum C-reactive protein (µg/ml) Value | Serum C-reactive protein (µg/ml) Rank | Pain score (0–5) Value | Pain score (0–5) Rank |
|---------|------|------|------|------|
| 1 | 34 | 4 | 2 | 2.5 |
| 2 | 7 | 1 | 2 | 2.5 |
| 3 | 98 | 8 | 5 | 7.5 |
| 4 | 23 | 3 | 3 | 4 |
| 5 | 14 | 2 | 1 | 1 |
| 6 | 71 | 5 | 4 | 5.5 |
| 7 | 90 | 7 | 5 | 7.5 |
| 8 | 85 | 6 | 4 | 5.5 |

Rank values for serum C-reactive protein levels and pain score

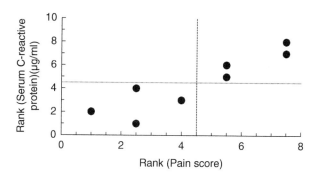

**Figure 19.6** Scatterplot of the rank values for the serum C-reactive protein levels and subjective pain scores taken from Table 19.9. The vertical dashed line indicates the mean rank of the pain scores (4.5), while the horizontal dotted line indicates the mean rank of the serum C-reactive protein levels (4.5).

## Spearman Rank Correlation analysis with tied ranks

The first point to notice about the scatterplot is that the data points include several **tied ranks** (at rank values of 2.5, 5.5 and 7.5). In such circumstances, the equations described above to perform correlation analysis of parametric data but applied to the rank values should be used (see Equations 19.1 to 19.3). [Please note; in the calculation Spearman's $r_s$, $x$ and $y$ now indicate the applied rank values for each observation, while $\bar{x}$ and $\bar{y}$ indicate the mean of the applied ranks and $s_x$ and $s_y$ indicate the respective standard deviations of the applied rank values.]. Where the ranked data **do not include tied ranks,** then the alternative equation described below should be used (see Example 19.5 and Equation 19.28).

Consequently, the next stage is to calculate the mean rank values for both variables together with the differences from the respective group means and the cross-product deviations for each ranked data pair, as shown in Table 19.10. The full correlation analysis, which uses the equations indicated earlier in this chapter even though this is the non-parametric procedure of correlation analysis, is summarised in Table 19.11.

**Table 19.10** Serum C-reactive protein and pain.

| Subject | C-reactive protein Rank | $(x-\bar{x})$ | Pain score Rank | $(y-\bar{y})$ | $(x-\bar{x})(y-\bar{y})$ |
|---|---|---|---|---|---|
| 1 | 4 | −0.5 | 2.5 | −2.0 | 1.0 |
| 2 | 1 | −3.5 | 2.5 | −2.0 | 7.0 |
| 3 | 8 | 3.5 | 7.5 | 3.0 | 10.5 |
| 4 | 3 | −1.5 | 4 | −0.5 | 0.75 |
| 5 | 2 | −2.5 | 1 | −3.5 | 8.75 |
| 6 | 5 | 0.5 | 5.5 | 1.0 | 0.5 |
| 7 | 7 | 2.5 | 7.5 | 3.0 | 7.5 |
| 8 | 6 | 1.5 | 5.5 | 1.0 | 1.5 |
| Mean | 4.50 | | 4.50 | | |
| St Dev | 2.449 | | 2.405 | | |
| $\sum$ | | | | | 37.5 |

For each set of data, the second column indicates the difference in the applied rank value for each observation from the respective group mean of the applied rank values indicated at the bottom of the previous column. The final column indicates the contribution of each paired data set to the covariance.

**Table 19.11** Correlation analysis of serum C-reactive protein and pain.

| Item | Value |
|---|---|
| Sum of cross-product deviations | 37.5 |
| Degrees of freedom $(N-1)$ | 7 |
| Covariance | 5.357 |
| Pooled standard deviation | 5.892 |
| Correlation coefficient, $r_s$ | 0.909 |

It should also be noticed that visual inspection of the resulting scatterplot of the ranked data values (Figure 19.6) suggests a *direct relationship* between the rank values of the two variables such that an increase in the *rank* of the serum levels of C-reactive protein may be associated with increase in the *rank* of the subjective joint pain score; i.e. the data points are limited to the bottom left and upper right sectors. This is supported by the positive value of the covariance (see data summarised in Table 19.11).

As in earlier examples, the value of the $t$-statistic may be directly calculated using the correlation coefficient, $r_s$, thus;

$$t_{r_s} = \frac{r_s\sqrt{N-2}}{\sqrt{1-r_s^2}} \tag{19.23}$$

$$t_{r_s} = \frac{0.909\sqrt{8-2}}{\sqrt{1-0.909^2}} = \frac{0.909 \times 2.449}{\sqrt{1-08263}} \tag{19.24}$$

$$t_{r_s} = \frac{2.226}{0.4168} = 5.341 \tag{19.25}$$

As we have already seen, the corresponding $p$ value may be determined by using the critical values of the $t$-distribution (Appendix C). The table shows that the critical value of $t$ with $N-2$ degrees of freedom (i.e. 6) for $p = 0.05$ is $t_{crit} = 2.447$, for $p = 0.01$, $t_{crit} = 3.707$, and for $p = 0.001$, $t_{crit} = 5.959$. Clearly, the probability of the calculated $t$-statistic with $N-2$ degrees of freedom lies between 0.001 and 0.01. Consequently, the probability of the Null Hypothesis being true may be summarised as follows,

$$t_{rs}(6) = 5.341, p < 0.01 \tag{19.26}$$

It therefore follows that the Spearman rank correlation analysis may be summarised as,

$$r_s = 0.909, p < 0.01 \tag{19.27}$$

## Example 19.5 Non-parametric rank correlation with no tied ranks

### Spearman Rank Correlation analysis with no tied ranks

An alternative method to perform Spearman's correlation analysis is to use the following equation for data sets that **do not include any applied tied ranks**.

$$r_s = 1 - \frac{6\sum d^2}{N(N^2-1)} \tag{19.28}$$

where $d$ is the difference between the corresponding rank values applied to each observation for both variables, and $N$ is the number of data pairs.

Consider the following data which compared the number of unfilled job vacancies for GPs in different districts to the number of working days lost in those districts through illness (Table 19.12).

**Table 19.12** Comparison of GP vacancies and lost working days.

| | Score | | Rank | | | |
|---|---|---|---|---|---|---|
| Area | GP vacancies | Working days lost | GP vacancies | Working days lost | $d$ | $d^2$ |
| 1 | 51 | 154 | 1 | 1 | 0 | 0 |
| 2 | 59 | 160 | 3 | 2 | 1 | 1 |
| 3 | 54 | 165 | 2 | 3 | −1 | 1 |
| 4 | 64 | 169 | 4 | 4 | 0 | 0 |
| 5 | 66 | 175 | 5 | 5 | 0 | 0 |
| 6 | 85 | 180 | 8 | 6 | 2 | 4 |
| 7 | 78 | 186 | 7 | 7 | 0 | 0 |
| 8 | 74 | 187 | 6 | 8 | −2 | 4 |
| | | | | | $\sum =$ | 10 |

Lost working days are per 10 000 workings days. $d$ and $d^2$ indicate difference between the assigned rank values and the squared difference, respectively.

The resulting scatterplot comparing the data for each variable is summarised in Figure 19.7, below.

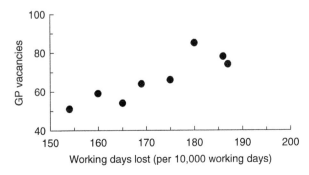

**Figure 19.7** **Scatterplot of GP vacancies against lost working days**. Working days lost are per 10 000 working days.

160

Experimental Design and Statistical Analysis for Pharmacology and the Biomedical S...

The arrangement of the data points suggests that there may be a relationship between the number of GP vacancies and the number of lost working days in the local population. However, parametric analysis is not appropriate here as the units of each variable are likely to violate the assumptions of data that is normally distributed. Consequently, it is appropriate to use the Spearman Rank correlation procedure. The first step is therefore to rank the data for both variables (see Table 19.12), the resulting scatterplot is summarised in Figure 19.8.

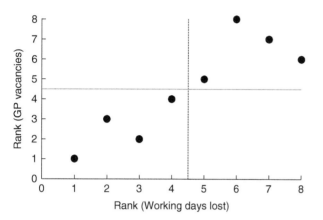

**Figure 19.8   Scatterplot of GP vacancies against lost working days**. Working days lost are per 10 000 working days. The vertical dashed line indicates the mean rank scores assigned to the number of lost working days (4.5), while the horizontal dotted line indicates the mean rank scores assigned to the number of GP vacancies (4.5).

Two important points to notice here.

**1** The arrangement of the data appears to suggest that there may be direct association between the number of GP vacancies and the number of lost working days in the local population. Note that the rank values of the data points are located in the bottom left and top right sectors of the scatterplot divided according to the mean values of the assigned rank values (Figure 19.8).

**2** Second, no tied ranks have been generated by assigning rank values to each data point (see Table 19.12 and Figure 19.8).

Since there are no tied ranks, the Spearman Rank Correlation coefficient may be calculated by the equation provided above (see Eq 19.28). Thus,

$$r_s = 1 - \frac{6 \sum d^2}{N(N^2 - 1)} = 1 - \frac{6 \times 10}{8(64 - 1)}$$
$$= 1 - \frac{60}{8(63)} \tag{19.29}$$

$$r_s = 1 - \frac{60}{504} = 1 - 0.119048 = 0.88095 \tag{19.30}$$

The probability of the Null Hypothesis being true (i.e. that $r_s$ is not different from 0) may be calculated by calculation of either the $t$-statistic (followed by inspection of the $t$-distribution with $N - 2$ degrees of freedom) or the $z$ score (followed by inspection of the standard normal distribution). Unfortunately, these estimations of $p$ are only recommended when $N \geq 10$ for the $t$-statistic and $N \geq 30$ for the $z$ score. However, tabulated *exact* critical values of Spearman's Rank Correlation coefficient, $r_s$, are available for $3 \leq N \leq 18$ and approximate values for $19 \leq N \leq 100$; see Appendix H, Table H.2.

Inspection of Appendix H, Table H.2, reveals that the critical value of $r_s$, with $N = 8$ pairs of data, for $p = 0.05$ is 0.738, for $p = 0.01$ is 0.881 and for $p = 0.001$ is 0.976. Since the calculated value of $r_s$ is greater than the critical value for $p = 0.05$, but lower (only just!) than $p = 0.01$, then we may reject the Null Hypothesis.

The Spearman Rank Correlation analysis may be summarised as

$$r_s = 0.88095, p < 0.05 \tag{19.31}$$

and we may conclude that there is a significant direct correlation between the number of working days lost and the number of GP vacancies in these districts.

## Example 19.6 Kendall's non-parametric rank correlation

Kendall's tau, $\tau$, is another method of non-parametric correlation that should be used with small data sets that have a large number of tied ranks where it provides a more accurate estimate of the correlation between two variables (it is more usual to call this version Kendall's tau-b, denoted by $\tau_b$).

Consider (again) the data provided in Table 19.9 which summarised the serum level of C-reactive protein and associated subjective pain reported by eight arthritic patients. Note that the usual procedure for tied ranks has been used. The first step is to order the rank values of one variable ($X$) in their natural order (i.e. 1, 2, 3, etc.) and then we will add the assigned rank values for the second variable ($Y$) immediately below as summarised in Table 19.13, where variable $X$ is the assigned rank values for the level of C-reactive protein and $Y$ is the assigned rank values for the subjective pain.

**Table 19.13**  Correspondence of assigned rank values for C-reaction protein and pain.

| Variable | \multicolumn{8}{c}{Assigned Ranks by Subject} | |
| | A | B | C | D | E | F | G | H | |
| --- | --- | --- | --- | --- | --- | --- | --- | --- | --- |
| X | 1 | 2 | 3 | 4 | 5 | 6 | 7 | 8 | |
| Y | 2.5 | 1 | 4 | 2.5 | 5.5 | 5.5 | 7.5 | 7.5 | Total |
| | 2.5→ | −1 | +1 | 0 | +1 | +1 | +1 | +1 | 4 |
| | | 1→ | +1 | +1 | +1 | +1 | +1 | +1 | 6 |
| | | | 4→ | −1 | +1 | +1 | +1 | +1 | 3 |
| | | | | 2.5→ | −1 | +1 | +1 | +1 | 4 |
| | | | | | 5.5→ | +1 | +1 | +1 | 2 |
| | | | | | | 5.5→ | +1 | +1 | 2 |
| | | | | | | | 7.5→ | 0 | 0 |
| | | | | | | | | 7.5→ | 0 |
| | | | | | | | Grand total | | 21 |

With the assigned rank values now listed in rows, we are now in a position to determine the degree of correspondence between the natural order of ranks for variable $X$ compared to the observed order of ranks for variable $Y$. Now, if we had a perfect set of data, then the increasing order of ranks for variable $Y$ would map exactly to the natural order of ranks for variable $X$, i.e. both sets of assigned ranks would follow 1, 2, 3, etc. However, this does not occur for variable $Y$, so we need to compare each rank for the $Y$ variable to the next rank in the order determined by variable $X$. Thus, the first rank for variable $Y$ is 2.5, but the next rank is 1. As the following rank is not in the natural order (i.e. it is not greater), then we score the correspondence as −1. We then compare the first rank for $Y$ against the third rank, i.e. 2.5 is compared to 4. This comparison does follow the natural order and so we score the correspondence as +1. The next comparison is between the first rank and the fourth rank for variable $Y$, i.e. 2.5 compared to 2.5. As these ranks are the same, we score the correspondence as 0. We then keep moving along row of data comparing the first rank against all the others until we complete the row. At this point, we subtract the negative scores from the total number of positive scores, i.e. +5 − 1, and put the total in the final column. We then move to the second assigned rank for variable $Y$ and assign the positive or negative correspondence scores as we move along the row. We keep repeating this until we have compared each assigned rank value for variable $Y$ against all the others. The total number of comparisons we have to make is,

$$\frac{N(N-1)}{2} = \frac{8(8-1)}{2} = \frac{56}{2} = 28 \tag{19.32}$$

Once we have completed the table (see Table 19.13), then we add up the scores to give a measure that indicates the total amount of agreement (i.e. where the assigned ranks follow the natural order) over and above the total amount of disagreement (i.e. where the assigned ranks do not follow the natural order) between the assigned ranks for the two variables; this is denoted by the symbol, $S$.

Kendall's Rank Coefficient is calculated by either of the following equations depending on whether there are tied ranks or not,

$$\text{No tied ranks}: \tau_b = \frac{\text{agreements} - \text{disagreements}}{N(N-1)} = \frac{2S}{N(N-1)} \tag{19.33}$$

$$\text{Tied ranks}: \tau_b = \frac{\text{agreements} - \text{disagreements}}{\sqrt{N(N-1)-T_X}.\sqrt{N(N-1)-T_Y}} = \frac{2S}{\sqrt{N(N-1)-T_X}.\sqrt{N(N-1)-T_Y}} \tag{19.34}$$

where $T_X$ indicates the number of tied ranks for variable $X$, while $T_Y$ indicates the number of tied ranks for variable $Y$. Notice that the only difference between these two equations is the calculation of the respective denominator.

For the C-reactive protein data, there are no tied ranks and thus $T_X = 0$. However, there a three pairs of pain values which have been assigned tied ranks, i.e. 2 at rank 2.5, 2 at rank 5.5 and 2 at rank 7.5. $T_Y$ is computed by,

$$T_Y = \sum t(t-1) \tag{19.35}$$

where $t$ indicates the number of ties at each tied rank value.

Thus,

$$T_Y = 2(2-1) + 2(2-1) + 2(2-1) = 6 \tag{19.36}$$

We now use the values of $T_X = 0$, $T_Y = 6$, $S = 21$, and $N = 8$ into the equation for $\tau_b$ for tied ranks indicated above. Thus,

$$\tau_b = \frac{2S}{\sqrt{N(N-1)-T_X}.\sqrt{N(N-1)-T_Y}}$$
$$= \frac{2 \times 21}{\sqrt{8(8-1)-0}.\sqrt{8(8-1)-6}} \tag{19.37}$$

$$\tau_b = \frac{2 \times 21}{\sqrt{8(8-1)-0}.\sqrt{8(8-1)-6}}$$
$$= \frac{42}{\sqrt{56-0}.\sqrt{56-6}} = \frac{42}{\sqrt{56}.\sqrt{50}} \tag{19.38}$$

$$\tau_b = \frac{42}{7.483 \times 7.071} = \frac{42}{52.912} = 0.794 \tag{19.39}$$

The critical values of Kendall's tau are provided in Appendix H, Table H.3. As in previous examples, if the value of the calculated statistic is greater than the critical value, then the Null Hypothesis may be rejected. Appendix H, Table H.3 indicates that for $N = 8$ pairs of observations, the critical value of $\tau_b$ for $p = 0.05$ is 0.643, while that for $p = 0.01$ is 0.786. Since the calculated value of $\tau_b$ exceeds the critical value for $p = 0.01$, then we may conclude that the probability of the Null Hypothesis (i.e. that there is no correspondence between the serum level of C-reactive protein and subjective pain) is <0.01, and so the Null Hypothesis may be rejected.

The Kendall Rank correlation analysis may therefore be summarised as

$$\tau_b = 0.794, p < 0.01 \tag{19.40}$$

i.e. there is a relationship or association between the serum levels of C-reactive protein and the reported intensity of subjective pain.

# Example output from statistical software

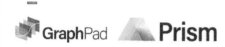

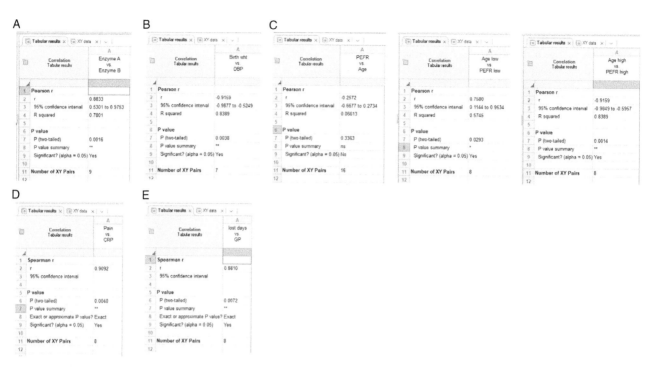

Summary statistical analysis from GraphPad Prism, v8. Panel A shows the summary of the correlation analysis of the enzyme data from Table 19.1. Panel B shows the correlation analysis of the birth weight and diastolic blood pressure data from Table 19.2. Panel C summarises the correlation analysis of the age and lung function data from Table 19.3, together with subsequent correlation analysis of the data divided into low and high age groups (see Tables 19.5 and 19.6, respectively). Panel D summarises the correlation analysis of the reported pain and serum CRP data from Table 19.8. Panel E summarises the correlation analysis of the lost working days and GP vacancies data from Table 19.12.

*Source*: GraphPad Software.

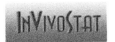

**A**

Table of results for the two-sided Pearson's product moment correlation coefficient

| Correlation | First variable | Second variable | n | Correlation Coefficient | Test statistic | p-value |
|---|---|---|---|---|---|---|
| 1 | Enzyme A | Enzyme B | 5 | 0.883 | 4.464 | 0.0016 |

Conclusion: The following pairwise correlations are statistically significant at the 5% level: Enzyme A vs. Enzyme B

**B**

Table of results for the two-sided Pearson's product moment correlation coefficient

| Correlation | First variable | Second variable | n | Correlation Coefficient | Test statistic | p-value |
|---|---|---|---|---|---|---|
| 1 | Birth wht | DBP | | -0.916 | -7.171 | 0.0035 |

Conclusion: The following pairwise correlations are statistically significant at the 5% level: Birth wht vs. DBP

**D**

Table of results for the two-sided Spearman's rho correlation coefficient

| Correlation | First variable | Second variable | n | Correlation Coefficient | Test statistic | p-value |
|---|---|---|---|---|---|---|
| 1 | Pain | CRP | | 0.909 | 6.24 | 0.0014 |

Conclusion: The following pairwise correlations are statistically significant at the 5% level: Pain vs. CRP

Table of results for the two-sided Kendall's tau correlation coefficient

| Correlation | First variable | Second variable | n | Correlation Coefficient | Test statistic | p-value |
|---|---|---|---|---|---|---|
| 1 | Pain | CRP | | 0.754 | 2.660 | 0.0078 |

Conclusion: The following pairwise correlations are statistically significant at the 5% level: Pain vs. CRP

**C**

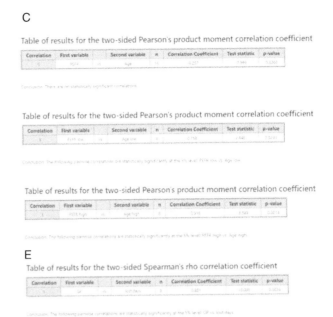

Table of results for the two-sided Pearson's product moment correlation coefficient

| Correlation | First variable | Second variable | n | Correlation Coefficient | Test statistic | p-value |
|---|---|---|---|---|---|---|
| 1 | PEFR | Age | | -0.257 | -0.946 | 0.3362 |

Conclusion: There are no statistically significant correlations.

Table of results for the two-sided Pearson's product moment correlation coefficient

| Correlation | First variable | Second variable | n | Correlation Coefficient | Test statistic | p-value |
|---|---|---|---|---|---|---|
| 1 | PEFR low | Age low | | 0.758 | 2.449 | 0.0291 |

Conclusion: The following pairwise correlations are statistically significant at the 5% level: PEFR low vs. Age low

Table of results for the two-sided Pearson's product moment correlation coefficient

| Correlation | First variable | Second variable | n | Correlation Coefficient | Test statistic | p-value |
|---|---|---|---|---|---|---|
| 1 | PEFR high | Age high | | -0.916 | -7.569 | 0.0010 |

Conclusion: The following pairwise correlations are statistically significant at the 5% level: PEFR high vs. Age high

**E**

Table of results for the two-sided Spearman's rho correlation coefficient

| Correlation | First variable | Second variable | n | Correlation Coefficient | Test statistic | p-value |
|---|---|---|---|---|---|---|
| 1 | GP | lost days | 5 | 0.881 | 0.001 | 0.0074 |

Conclusion: The following pairwise correlations are statistically significant at the 5% level: GP vs. lost days

Summary statistical analysis from InVivoStat, v4.0.2. Panel A shows the summary of the Pearson correlation analysis of the enzyme data from Table 19.1. Panel B shows the Pearson correlation analysis of the birth weight and diastolic blood pressure data from Table 19.2. Panel C summarises the Pearson correlation analysis of the age and lung function data from Table 19.3, together with, below, subsequent Pearson correlation analysis of the data divided into low and high age groups (see Tables 19.5 and 19.6, respectively). Panel D summarises the Spearman and Kendal tau (below) correlation analyses of the reported pain and serum CRP data from Table 19.8. Panel E summarises the Spearman correlation analysis of the lost working days and GP vacancies data from Table 19.12.

*Source*: InVivoStat.

## Minitab

**A** **Correlations**  **Covariances**

|  |  | Enz A | Enz B |
|---|---|---|---|
| Pearson correlation | 0.883 | Enz A | 0.0802694 | |
| P-value | 0.002 | Enz B | 0.0613319 | 0.0600694 |

**B** **Correlations**  **Covariances**

|  |  | Bdy Wht | DBP |
|---|---|---|---|
| Pearson correlation | -0.916 | Bdy Wht | 0.62952 | |
| P-value | 0.004 | DBP | -12.30714 | 286.80952 |

**C** **Correlation**  **Covariances**

|  |  | PEFR | Age |
|---|---|---|---|
| Pearson correlation | -0.257 | PEFR | 1.32917 | |
| P-value | 0.336 | Age | -5.37583 | 328.76250 |

**Correlation**  **Covariances**

|  |  | PEFR-L | Age-L |
|---|---|---|---|
| Pearson correlation | 0.758 | PEFR-L | 1.31411 | |
| P-value | 0.029 | Age-L | 2.85357 | 10.78571 |

**Correlations**  **Covariance**

|  |  | PEFR-H | Age-H |
|---|---|---|---|
| Pearson correlation | -0.916 | PEFR-H | 1.46411 | |
| P-value | 0.001 | Age-H | -19.54821 | 311.12500 |

**D** **Correlations**

| Spearman rho | 0.909 |
|---|---|
| P-value | 0.002 |

**E** **Correlations**

| Spearman rho | 0.881 |
|---|---|
| P-value | 0.004 |

Summary statistical analysis from MiniTab, v18. Panel A shows the summary of the Pearson correlation analysis of the enzyme data from Table 19.1. Panel B shows the Pearson correlation analysis of the birth weight and diastolic blood pressure data from Table 19.2. Panel C summarises the Pearson correlation analysis of the age and lung function data from Table 19.3, together with, below, subsequent Pearson correlation analysis of the data divided into low and high age groups (see Tables 19.5 and 19.6, respectively). Panel D summarises the Spearman and Kendal tau (below) correlation analyses of the reported pain and serum CRP data from Table 19.8. Panel E summarises the Spearman correlation analysis of the lost working days and GP vacancies data from Table 19.12.

*Source*: Minitab, LLC.

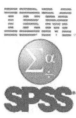

**A**

**Correlations**

| | | Enzyme_A | Enzyme_B |
|---|---|---|---|
| Enzyme_A | Pearson Correlation | 1 | .883** |
| | Sig. (2-tailed) | | .002 |
| | N | 9 | 9 |
| Enzyme_B | Pearson Correlation | .883** | 1 |
| | Sig. (2-tailed) | .002 | |
| | N | 9 | 9 |

**. Correlation is significant at the 0.01 level (2-tailed).

**B**

**Correlations**

| | | Birth_wht | DBP |
|---|---|---|---|
| Birth_wht | Pearson Correlation | 1 | -.916** |
| | Sig. (2-tailed) | | .004 |
| | N | 7 | 7 |
| DBP | Pearson Correlation | -.916** | 1 |
| | Sig. (2-tailed) | .004 | |
| | N | 7 | 7 |

**. Correlation is significant at the 0.01 level (2-tailed).

**C**

**Correlations**

| | | PEFR | Age |
|---|---|---|---|
| PEFR | Pearson Correlation | 1 | -.257 |
| | Sig. (2-tailed) | | .336 |
| | N | 16 | 16 |
| Age | Pearson Correlation | -.257 | 1 |
| | Sig. (2-tailed) | .336 | |
| | N | 16 | 16 |

**Correlations**

| | | PERF_Low | Age_Low |
|---|---|---|---|
| PERF_Low | Pearson Correlation | 1 | .758* |
| | Sig. (2-tailed) | | .029 |
| | N | 8 | 8 |
| Age_Low | Pearson Correlation | .758* | 1 |
| | Sig. (2-tailed) | .029 | |
| | N | 8 | 8 |

*. Correlation is significant at the 0.05 level (2-tailed).

**Correlations**

| | | PERF_High | Age_High |
|---|---|---|---|
| PERF_High | Pearson Correlation | 1 | -.916** |
| | Sig. (2-tailed) | | .001 |
| | N | 8 | 8 |
| Age_High | Pearson Correlation | -.916** | 1 |
| | Sig. (2-tailed) | .001 | |
| | N | 8 | 8 |

**. Correlation is significant at the 0.01 level (2-tailed).

**D**

**Nonparametric Correlations**

**Correlations**

| | | | Pain | CRP |
|---|---|---|---|---|
| Spearman's rho | Pain | Correlation Coefficient | 1.000 | .909** |
| | | Sig. (2-tailed) | . | .002 |
| | | N | 8 | 8 |
| | CRP | Correlation Coefficient | .909** | 1.000 |
| | | Sig. (2-tailed) | .002 | . |
| | | N | 8 | 8 |

**. Correlation is significant at the 0.01 level (2-tailed).

**E**

**Nonparametric Correlations**

**Correlations**

| | | | Lost_Days | GP |
|---|---|---|---|---|
| Spearman's rho | Lost_Days | Correlation Coefficient | 1.000 | .881** |
| | | Sig. (2-tailed) | . | .004 |
| | | N | 8 | 8 |
| | GP | Correlation Coefficient | .881** | 1.000 |
| | | Sig. (2-tailed) | .004 | . |
| | | N | 8 | 8 |

**. Correlation is significant at the 0.01 level (2-tailed).

Summary statistical analysis from SPSS, v27. Panel A shows the summary of the Pearson correlation analysis of the enzyme data from Table 19.1. Panel B shows the Pearson correlation analysis of the birth weight and diastolic blood pressure data from Table 19.2. Panel C summarises the Pearson correlation analysis of the age and lung function data from Table 19.3, together with subsequent Pearson correlation analysis of the data divided into low and high age groups (see Tables 19.5 and 19.6, respectively). Panel D summarises the Spearman correlation analysis of the reported pain and serum CRP data from Table 19.8. Panel E summarises the Spearman correlation analysis of the lost working days and GP vacancies data from Table 19.12.

*Source*: IBM Corporation.

**Write Your Own Notes**

# ⑳ Regression analysis

Like correlation analysis described in the previous chapter (see Chapter 19), **regression** analysis is also concerned with the relationship between variables. However, in regression analysis, we wish to describe the mathematical model of the relationship between the variables so that we can use the value of one variable to *predict* the value of the other corresponding variable. Consequently (and unlike correlation analysis), we must be able to control accurately the value of one variable (the **independent** variable, such as age, time, drug dose, or substrate concentration) and measure the resulting value of the corresponding **dependent** variable (also known as the *response variable*). Note that the value of the dependent variable is not only dependent on the value of the independent variable (which is chosen by the experimenter) but is also subject to experimental error.

For example, consider the situation where we wish to estimate the unknown concentration of a molecule in solution using an ultra-violet spectrometer. Our first step would be to prepare a range of solutions of known concentration of the molecule concerned and measure the absorbance at each concentration. We would then plot the data with the independent variable (concentration) on the horizontal $x$-axis and the dependent variable (absorbance) on the vertical $y$-axis to produce a scatterplot, which would act as our calibration data of the output from the spectrometer. Knowing how absorbance changed with concentration would allow us to determine a mathematical model (i.e. an **equation**) of the relationship between the two variables. Consequently, we would be able to measure the absorbance of any unknown concentration, substitute this value into the equation, and thereby predict the concentration of that solution. The mathematical technique to quantify the relationship between a dependent and independent variable is the basis of regression analysis and results in a mathematical model of the relationship. In linear regression, the result is the equation of a straight line.

It is vital to understand the difference between correlation and regression. In parametric correlation analysis, it is assumed that both variables are normally distributed; this is not the case in regression analysis where the independent variable is under the control of the experimenter and so the data are unlikely to follow a normal distribution. Furthermore, it is not justified to use a regression method where the independent variables is subject to considerable error of measurement, nor is it appropriate to only calculate a correlation coefficient and quote its probability (thereby excluding regression analysis) if regression is properly involved.

## Linear regression

As the name implies, linear regression assumes that the relationship between the independent and dependent variables is linear. However, we can only be certain that this applies over the range of the data we have from the experiment, and so it is always unwise to extrapolate to values *outside* the range. It is always advisable to plot the data as a scatterplot *before* performing regression analysis, since this allows a visual check of the relationship between the two variables and whether it is linear or non-linear (i.e. a curve). If the

scatter of the data suggests deviations from linearity, then it would be appropriate to consider transforming the data of one or both variables so that the relationship approximates to linearity or to apply a more complex non-linear model to the data – *but more about that later!*

Regression analysis also assumes a normal distribution for all values of the dependent variable ($y$) according to all values of the independent variable ($x$). Furthermore, the spread of the $y$ values (i.e. the variance of $y$) should be similar (homogeneity of variance) and independent for any given value of $x$, such that the scatter around a fitted line through the data points should not increase as $x$ increases; *take care here as this assumption is frequently violated!*

The assumptions of linear regression may be summarised as follows,

**1** The relationship between the independent ($x$) and dependent ($y$) variables is linear,
**2** The variability of errors for $y$ is constant for all values of $x$,
**3** The errors of y are independent of all values of x,
**4** The values and errors of y are normally distributed,
**5** The values of the independent variable are measured without error.

## Example 20.1 Linear regression without data transformation

Consider the following data from an experiment which examined the relationship between the level of a protein in the urine of expectant mothers throughout pregnancy (see Table 20.1).

**Table 20.1** Urinary protein levels throughout pregnancy.

| Subject | Time (wk) | Protein (mg/ml) |
|---|---|---|
| 1 | 11 | 0.38 |
| 2 | 13 | 0.51 |
| 3 | 17 | 0.58 |
| 4 | 19 | 0.84 |
| 5 | 22 | 0.78 |
| 6 | 27 | 0.65 |
| 7 | 29 | 0.83 |
| 8 | 31 | 0.84 |
| 9 | 34 | 0.92 |
| 10 | 36 | 0.92 |

The first step is to examine a scatterplot of the data to appreciate the possible relationship between the two variables, $x$ and $y$. In general terms, once a scatterplot has been drawn and the mathematical model of linear regression calculated and fitted to the data, then the observed data points will not necessarily lie on the fitted line (see Figure 20.1). The scatter about the straight line will depend on how good the mathematical model is. If we draw a vertical line from each observation to the fitted line, calculate the differences, square all the differences, and add them up then we obtain what is termed the **residual sum of squares** (for the sake of brevity, I have omitted some of the vertical lines from Figure 20.1 but you should get the general idea). We have come across this term repeatedly throughout previous chapters, especially when discussing analysis of variance (see Chapter 15); indeed, there is a lot of correspondence between ANOVA and linear regression which I shall discuss later.

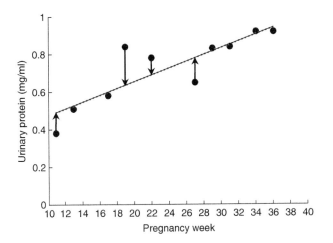

**Figure 20.1 Scatterplot of urinary protein levels and week of pregnancy.** Arrows indicate deviations of the observed protein level in the urine compared to the fitted line according to the mathematical model

We know that a straight line may be described by the equation:

$$y = a + bx \quad (20.1)$$

where $a$ = the intercept and $b$ = the gradient of the slope.

The gradient of the slope ($b$) may be calculated by dividing the sum of the cross-product deviations (a value which we used in correlation analysis, see Chapter 19) by total sum of squares for variable $x$. Thus,

$$b = \frac{\sum(x - \bar{x})(y - \bar{y})}{\sum(x - \bar{x})^2} \quad (20.2)$$

while the intercept may be calculated by simple re-arrangement of the equation to describe the straight line. Thus,

$$a = \bar{y} - b\bar{x} \quad (20.3)$$

The straight line fitted through the data points according to the mathematical model involves finding estimates of the slope and intercept that results in a straight line that best fits the data, a process that minimises the residual sum of squares. Consequently, this process is called the **least squares** method.

So, let's extend Table 20.1 to allow calculation of the mathematical model for linear regression.

Sum of squares values are calculated by squaring the difference of each observation for $x$ and $y$ from the respective group means, $\bar{x}$ and $\bar{y}$, and adding the respective values together for each variable (see Table 20.2).

As indicated above, the slope of the straight line fitted through the data may be calculated by dividing the **sum of the cross-product deviations** (see final column in Table 20.2) by the **total sum of squares for the independent variable, $x$.**

**Table 20.2** Regression analysis of urinary protein levels throughout pregnancy.

| Subject | Time (wk) | Protein (mg/ml) | $(x - \bar{x})$ | $(y - \bar{y})$ | $(x - \bar{x})(y - \bar{y})$ |
|---|---|---|---|---|---|
| 1 | 11 | 0.38 | −12.9 | −0.345 | 4.4505 |
| 2 | 13 | 0.51 | −10.9 | −0.215 | 2.3435 |
| 3 | 17 | 0.58 | −6.9 | −0.145 | 1.0005 |
| 4 | 19 | 0.84 | −4.9 | 0.115 | −0.5635 |
| 5 | 22 | 0.78 | −1.9 | 0.055 | −0.1045 |
| 6 | 27 | 0.65 | 3.1 | −0.075 | −0.2325 |
| 7 | 29 | 0.83 | 5.1 | 0.105 | 0.5355 |
| 8 | 31 | 0.84 | 7.1 | 0.115 | 0.8165 |
| 9 | 34 | 0.92 | 10.1 | 0.195 | 1.9695 |
| 10 | 36 | 0.92 | 12.1 | 0.195 | 2.3595 |
| Sum | 239 | 7.25 | | | 12.575 |
| Mean | 23.9 | 0.725 | | | |
| Sum of squares | | | 694.9 | 0.30845 | |

The total sum of squares for $x$,

$$ssqx = \sum(x - \bar{x})^2 = 694.9 \quad (20.4)$$

Therefore,

$$b = \frac{12.575}{694.9} = 0.0181 \quad (20.5)$$

The slope is equal to the number of units of the $y$ variable that change per unit of the $x$ variable; in the example used here this reflects the mg/ml change per unit time (i.e. per week).

The re-arranged equation for the fitted straight line allows calculation of the constant, $a$, for any appropriate values of $x$ and $y$. So now we can complete the re-arranged equation by simply using the mean values of the two variables.

Thus,

$$a = \bar{y} - b\bar{x} = 0.725 - 0.0181 \times 23.9 = 0.2924 \quad (20.6)$$

We can now express the equation in terms of $y$:

$$y = a + bx = 0.2924 + 0.0181.x \quad (20.7)$$

where $y$ is expressed as mg/ml and $x$ in weeks of pregnancy.

Therefore, an increase of one week in pregnancy is associated with an average increase in urinary protein level of 0.0181 mg/ml. Conversely, the current length of pregnancy may be estimated by measuring the urinary protein level and re-arranging the equation in terms of $x$.

Regression analysis further allows us to examine whether the mathematical model may explain a proportion of the total variation in the dependent variable, $y$. This is best calculated by partitioning the sum of squares of $y$ into two parts:

**1** The part explained by the model, i.e. **the regression sum of squares**
**2** The part not explained by the model, i.e. **the residual variation** about the line

These sums of squares values may then be arranged in an analysis of variance table, and an F-test between the residual and regression variances will reveal whether the fitted model accounts for a significant variation in the dependent variable.

The first stage is to calculate the **total sum of squares for the dependent variable, $y$** (see Table 20.2). So, for the current example,

$$\text{ssqy} = \sum (y - \bar{y})^2 = 0.30845,$$
$$\text{with } n-1 \text{ degrees of freedom} \tag{20.8}$$

The **regression sum of squares (regssq)** is calculated by dividing **the square of the sum of the cross-products** by the **total sum of squares for the independent variable, $x$.** Therefore,

$$\text{regssq} = \frac{12.575^2}{694.9} = \frac{158.13}{694.9} = 0.22756,$$
$$\text{with } 1 \text{ degree of freedom} \tag{20.9}$$

The **residual sum of squares (residssq)** is simply the difference between the total sum of squares for y and the regression sum of squares. Thus,

$$\text{residssq} = \text{ssqy} - \text{regssq} =$$
$$0.30845 - 0.22756 = 0.08089 \tag{20.10}$$
$$\text{with } n-2 \text{ degrees of freedom}$$

These values are then summarised in an ANOVA table (see Table 20.3). Thus,

Table 20.3  Linear regression ANOVA.

| Source | Sum of squares | df | Variance (mean square) | F ratio | p |
|---|---|---|---|---|---|
| Regression | 0.22756 | 1 | 0.22756 | 22.508 | <0.01 |
| Residual error | 0.08089 | 8 | 0.01011 | | |
| Total | 0.30845 | 9 | | | |

If the independent variable, $x$, had no impact on the observed changes in the dependent variable, $y$, then it would be expected that the regression variance and the residual variance to be estimates of the same quantity, and consequently the value of $F$ would approach unity, i.e. $F = 1$. Inspection of the critical values of $F$ (with 1 and 8 degrees of freedom) summarised in Appendix E indicate that for $p = 0.05$, 0.01, and 0.001, the critical values of $F(1,8)$ are 5.32, 11.26, and 25.42, respectively. Clearly, the calculated value of $F$ (1,8) indicates that the probability to support the Null Hypothesis (i.e. that there is no difference between the regression and residual variation in protein levels) lies between 0.01 and 0.001. We may therefore reject the Null Hypothesis and conclude that a significant proportion of the variance in urinary protein levels may be explained by the time of pregnancy.

The regression ANOVA is summarised as:

$$F(1,8) = 22.51, p < 0.01 \tag{20.11}$$

In addition, the regression sum of squares may be expressed as a percentage of the total sum of squares for $y$; this is known as the **coefficient of determination**. Thus,

$$\left(\frac{0.22756}{0.30845}\right) \times 100 = 73.8 \tag{20.12}$$

Therefore, almost 74% of the sum of squares of the urinary protein levels may be accounted for by fitting the mathematical model.

Interestingly, the coefficient of determination may also be determined by squaring the correlation coefficient between the independent and dependent variables. As described in Chapter 19, the correlation coefficient is calculated as follows:

$$r = \frac{\sum(x - \bar{x})(y - \bar{y})}{(N-1).s_x.s_y} = \frac{12.575}{9 \times 8.78699 \times 0.18513} \tag{20.13}$$
$$= 0.8589$$

The coefficient of determination may therefore be determined as:

$$r^2 = 0.8589^2 = 0.738 \tag{20.14}$$

As discussed in Chapter 19, the probability of the Null Hypothesis for the correlation coefficient may be obtained by calculating the $t$-statistic with $N-2$ degrees of freedom. Thus,

$$t_r = \frac{r\sqrt{N-2}}{\sqrt{1-r^2}} = \frac{0.8589\sqrt{8}}{\sqrt{1-0.738}} = \frac{0.8589 \times 2.8284}{\sqrt{0.262}} \tag{20.15}$$

$$t_r = \frac{2.4293}{0.51186} = 4.746 \tag{20.16}$$

The corresponding $p$-value may be determined by using the critical values of the $t$-distribution summarised in Appendix C. The table shows that for $p = 0.05$ then $t_{\text{crit}}(8) = 2.306$, for $p = 0.01$, $t_{\text{crit}}(8) = 3.355$ and for $p = 0.001$, $t_{\text{crit}}(8) = 5.041$. As the calculated value of $t_r$ lies between the $t_{\text{crit}}$ values of 3.355 and 5.041, we may conclude that the probability of the Null Hypothesis being true is <0.01. Consequently, we may reject the Null Hypothesis in favour of the alternate hypothesis and conclude that the correlation is significant.

The correlation analysis may therefore be summarised as:

$$r = 0.8589, p < 0.01 \tag{20.17}$$

A final point to note regarding regression analysis is that when summarising the data, it is important to report both the regression (i.e. the ANOVA analysis) and the correlation (i.e. the coefficient values with the $t$-statistic and probability) results.

## Example 20.2 Linear regression with single variable transformation

In the introduction to linear regression, I indicated that transformation of the data for one or both variables is permissible if the scatterplot of the original data shows deviation from linearity.

As an example, consider the following data which summarise the degradation of an aqueous solution of atropine sulphate over time (see Table 20.4).

Table 20.4  Degradation of atropine sulphate solution.

| Observation | Time (h) | % Atropine sulphate remaining |
|---|---|---|
| 1 | 0 | 100 |
| 2 | 12 | 73 |
| 3 | 24 | 53 |
| 4 | 36 | 38 |
| 5 | 48 | 27 |
| 6 | 72 | 15 |
| 7 | 96 | 7.2 |

The resulting scatterplot of the data clearly suggests exponential decay of the atropine sulphate solution and demonstrates deviation from linearity (Figure 20.2).

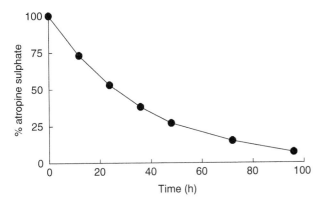

**Figure 20.2** Degradation of aqueous atropine sulphate: original data.

However, if we transform the dependent variable by calculating the $Log_{10}$ of the percentage atropine sulphate remaining values and replot the data, then the following scatterplot is produced (see Figure 20.3).

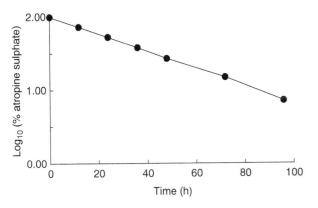

**Figure 20.3** Degradation of aqueous atropine sulphate: transformed data.

Transforming the values of the dependent variable results in a scatterplot that approximates to linearity, thereby allowing the application of the linear regression model to the transformed data.

Clearly, the data now approximate to linearity across the range of time values. Consequently, we may now apply linear regression analysis to the data using the values summarised in Table 20.5.

Thus,

$$b = \frac{\sum(x-\bar{x})(y-\bar{y})}{\sum(x-\bar{x})^2} = \frac{-81.13628}{6870.85714} \tag{20.18}$$

$$= -0.011809$$

where $y$ and $\bar{y}$ are the $Log_{10}$ values and the mean of the $Log_{10}$ values for the dependent variable as summarised in Table 20.5, and

$$a = \bar{y} - b\bar{x} = 1.5189 - (-0.011809 \times 41.1429)$$
$$= 1.5189 - (-0.48586) \tag{20.19}$$
$$a = 2.00476$$

where $\bar{y}$ is the mean of the $Log_{10}$ values (i.e. the geometric mean of the original non-transformed data) for the dependent variable as summarised in Table 20.5.

We can now express the regression equation in terms of $y$:

$$y = a + bx = 2.00476 + (-0.011809.x) \tag{20.20}$$

where $y$ is expressed as $Log_{10}$ of the atropine sulphate concentration and may be predicted by the value of $x$ expressed in hours.

As in the previous example, if we now calculate the total sum of squares for y, and the regression sum of squares then we can produce the linear regression ANOVA table (see Table 20.6) to examine whether the fitted model may account for any significant variation in the dependent variable.

Thus,

**1** Total sum of squares for y (see Table 20.5),

$$ssqy = \sum(y-\bar{y})^2 = 0.95885, \tag{20.21}$$
$$\text{with } n-1 \text{ degrees of freedom}$$

**2** Regression sum of squares,

$$regssq = \frac{-80.13628^2}{6870.85714} = \frac{6583.09593}{6870.85714} = 0.95812, \tag{20.22}$$
$$\text{with 1 degree of freedom}$$

**3** Residual sum of squares,

$$residssq = ssqy - regssq$$
$$= 0.95885 - 0.95812 = 0.00073 \tag{20.23}$$
$$\text{with } n-2 \text{ degrees of freedom}$$

**Table 20.5** Degradation of atropine sulphate solution: transformed data.

| Subject | Time (h) | $Log_{10}$ [atropine] | $(x-\bar{x})$ | $(y-\bar{y})$ | $(x-\bar{x})(y-\bar{y})$ |
|---|---|---|---|---|---|
| 1 | 0 | 2.00 | −41.14 | 0.4811 | −19.79385 |
| 2 | 12 | 1.86 | −29.14 | 0.3444 | −10.03681 |
| 3 | 24 | 1.72 | −17.14 | 0.2054 | −3.52115 |
| 4 | 36 | 1.58 | −5.14 | 0.0609 | −0.31320 |
| 5 | 48 | 1.43 | 6.86 | −0.0875 | −0.60000 |
| 6 | 72 | 1.18 | 30.86 | −0.3428 | −10.57781 |
| 7 | 96 | 0.86 | 54.86 | −0.6616 | −36.29346 |
| | | | | | −81.13628 |
| Sum | 288 | 10.63 | | | |
| Mean | 41.1429 | 1.5189 | | | |
| StDev | 33.84 | 0.39975 | | | |
| Sum of squares | | | 6870.85714 | 0.95885 | |

170

Experimental Design and Statistical Analysis for Pharmacology and the Biomedical Sc...

**Table 20.6** Linear regression ANOVA; atropine degradation.

| Source | Sum of squares | df | Variance (mean square) | F ratio | p |
|---|---|---|---|---|---|
| Regression | 0.95812 | 1 | 0.95812 | 6562.46575 | <0.001 |
| Residual error | 0.00073 | 5 | 0.000146 | | |
| Total | 0.95885 | 6 | | | |

Inspection of the critical values of $F$, with 1 and 5 degrees of freedom, summarised in Appendix E, indicate that for $p = 0.001 F_{crit}(1, 5) = 47.18$. Since the calculated F value exceeds the critical value for $p = 0.001$, then we may reject the Null Hypothesis and conclude that a significant proportion of the variance in the dependent variable may be explained by the time at which the percentage atropine concentration remaining was measured.

The regression ANOVA is summarised as:

$$F(1,5) = 6562.46575, p < 0.001 \qquad (20.24)$$

Furthermore, the correlation coefficient is calculated as follows (see Table 20.5 for standard deviations for $x$ and $y$):

$$r = \frac{\sum(x-\bar{x})(y-\bar{y})}{(N-1).s_x.s_y} = \frac{-80.13628}{6 \times 33.84 \times 0.39975} \qquad (20.25)$$
$$= -0.99964$$

and the probability of the Null Hypothesis for the correlation coefficient may be obtained by calculating the $t$-statistic with $N-2$ degrees of freedom. Thus,

$$t_r = \frac{r\sqrt{N-2}}{\sqrt{1-r^2}} = \frac{-0.99964\sqrt{5}}{\sqrt{1-0.99928}}$$
$$= \frac{-0.99964 \times 2.2361}{\sqrt{0.00072}} \qquad (20.26)$$

$$t_r = \frac{-2.235295}{0.026833} = -83.304 \qquad (20.27)$$

The corresponding $p$-value may be determined by using the critical values of the $t$-distribution summarised in Appendix C. The table shows that for $p = 0.001$, then $t_{crit}(5) = 6.869$. As the calculated value of $t_r$ exceeds the $t_{crit}$ values of 6.869, we may conclude that the probability of the Null Hypothesis being true is <0.001. Consequently, we may reject the Null Hypothesis in favour of the alternate hypothesis and conclude that the correlation is significant.

The correlation analysis may therefore be summarised as:

$$r = -0.99964, p < 0.001 \qquad (20.28)$$

Finally, the coefficient of determination, $r^2 = 0.988$ reveals that nearly 99% of the sum of squares of the atropine values may be accounted for by fitting the mathematical model.

The important point about this example is that it demonstrates how transformation of one of the variables, in this case $Log_{10}$ transformation the dependent variable, results in a scatterplot where the fitted line approximates to linearity, thereby allowing linear regression analysis. In other examples, the data may require transformation of the independent variable, rather than the dependent variable, in order to reveal a linear relationship between the pairs of observations. Consider Figure 1.3 which summarises the relationship between the magnitude of contraction of the isolated rat anococcygeus muscle and the concentration of the $\alpha_1$-adrenoreceptor agonist,

phenylephrine, to which the tissue has been exposed. Notice that the independent variable, the molar concentration of phenylephrine, has been subjected to $Log_{10}$ transformation. The reason for this is that if the response was plotted against the molar concentration of phenylephrine, then the resulting scatterplot would have the shape of a rectangular hyperbola, but data plotted in this way are very difficult to work with! Pharmacologists therefore plot their concentration–effect data with the response plotted against the $Log_{10}$ of the agonist concentration. This produces a classic shape of the scatterplot known as a sigmoid curve, the advantage of which is that the area of the curve between 25 and 75% of maximum approximates to a straight line and may therefore be subjected to linear regression analysis.

## Example 20.3 Linear regression with dual variable transformation

However, consider the following experiment where the unknown concentration of methylene blue was estimated by colorimetric assay. Here students were instructed to prepare a range of six serial 1 in 4 dilutions (with distilled water) of methylene blue, 800 μM. 200 μl of each solution was then pipetted in *triplicate* into a 96-well microtitre plate. The students were then provided with four solutions of methylene blue of unknown concentration from which 200 μl were pipetted in triplicate into the plate. Finally, 200 μl of distilled water were pipetted into three wells to provide a blank measurement in triplicate. Absorbance at 650 nm was measured using a spectrophotometer and the absorbance data summarised in the table below (Table 20.7).

**Table 20.7** Colorimetric assay of methylene blue.

| Concentration (M) | Absorbance (650 nm) Triplicate values | | | | Average – |
|---|---|---|---|---|---|
| | 1 | 2 | 3 | Average | Blank |
| Blank (H₂O) | 0.054 | 0.051 | 0.058 | 0.0543 | |
| $1.95 \times 10^{-7}$ | 0.064 | 0.066 | 0.062 | 0.0640 | 0.0097 |
| $7.81 \times 10^{-7}$ | 0.074 | 0.076 | 0.072 | 0.0740 | 0.0197 |
| $3.125 \times 10^{-6}$ | 0.106 | 0.110 | 0.102 | 0.1060 | 0.0517 |
| $1.25 \times 10^{-5}$ | 0.218 | 0.214 | 0.222 | 0.2180 | 0.1637 |
| $5.0 \times 10^{-5}$ | 0.734 | 0.732 | 0.736 | 0.7340 | 0.6797 |
| $2.0 \times 10^{-4}$ | 3.046 | 3.035 | 3.057 | 3.0460 | 2.9917 |
| $8.0 \times 10^{-4}$ | 4.100 | 4.112 | 4.020 | 4.0773 | 4.0230 |
| Unknown A | 0.060 | 0.065 | 0.058 | 0.0610 | 0.0067 |
| Unknown B | 0.110 | 0.114 | 0.106 | 0.1100 | 0.0557 |
| Unknown C | 0.230 | 0.235 | 0.225 | 0.2300 | 0.1757 |
| Unknown D | 1.190 | 1.120 | 1.260 | 1.1900 | 1.1357 |

The objective of assays of this type is to obtain the most accurate measurement possible of each solution used in the experiment. However, spectrophotometers and similar pieces of equipment are renowned for reporting variability in the readings even though the same solution may be assayed on numerous occasions. Consequently, it is usual for each solution to be assayed numerous times. So, the first thing to notice about the summary of data (Table 20.7) is that the absorbance of each solution of methylene blue was measured in triplicate (although in other experiments duplicate, quadruplicate, or even more reading may be taken) and the average of the readings calculated. Notice that the *average* reading is based on repeated absorbance measurements of the *same* solution and thus reflects a *single* reading (i.e. $n = 1$) and not multiple readings (i.e. $n = 3$). The reason for this is that we are interested in the best estimate of the reading for each concentration to be used in further analysis (and multiple readings improve the accuracy of the assay – see also discussion on accuracy and precision in Chapter 3) and **not** primarily in the consistency of the equipment used; if we were interested in the latter, then we would report the mean of the readings together an index of the variability (i.e. spread) of the readings obtained (most likely the standard deviation). Second, the medium used to dilute methylene blue (i.e. distilled water) has its own absorbance value, so the next step is to subtract the absorbance value of the water (i.e. the blank) away from all the other values used in the assay so that the absorbance values used in further analysis relate to the amount methylene blue in each solution only and *not* the methylene blue plus the distilled water; the final column in Table 20.7 summarises these values.

As in previous examples, the next step is to examine the scatterplot of the data to ensure approximate linearity before performing linear regression analysis. Figure 20.4 summarises the data where the concentration of methylene blue (the independent variable, $x$) is plotted against the corresponding average absorbance value (the dependent variable, $y$). Although the lower concentrations suggest possible linearity, it is difficult to be absolutely certain since the lowest four data points ($1.25 \times 10^{-5}$ M and below) are all clustered together, and clearly the relationship deviates from linearity above $5 \times 10^{-5}$ M. Consequently, some form of transformation of one or both of the variables may be justified.

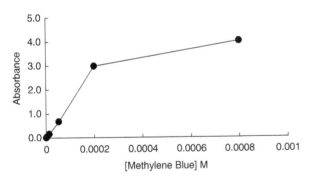

**Figure 20.4  Spectrophotometer absorbance measurements of methylene blue.** Solid circles indicate the absorbance values for various standard concentrations of methylene blue. Some lower values have been omitted for brevity.

A suitable transformation that may resolve the problem would be to try and spread the lower concentrations apart while squeezing the higher concentrations closer together; such a transformation may be achieved by using the logarithm$_{10}$ of the concentration values of the methylene blue solutions. A similar Log$_{10}$ transformation of the absorbance values may also be applied if necessary. Table 20.8 summarises the concentrations of methylene blue and the corresponding absorbance values (taken from Table 20.7) together with the Log$_{10}$ transformed values of both variables.

**Table 20.8** Log$_{10}$ transformation of methylene blue absorbance data.

| Concentration (M) | Log$_{10}$ (M) | Absorbance | Log$_{10}$ absorbance |
|---|---|---|---|
| $1.95 \times 10^{-7}$ | −6.7100 | 0.0097 | −2.0147 |
| $7.81 \times 10^{-7}$ | −6.1073 | 0.0197 | −1.7063 |
| $3.125 \times 10^{-6}$ | −5.5051 | 0.0517 | −1.2868 |
| $1.25 \times 10^{-5}$ | −4.9031 | 0.1637 | −0.7860 |
| $5.0 \times 10^{-5}$ | −4.3010 | 0.6797 | −0.1677 |
| $2.0 \times 10^{-4}$ | −3.6990 | 2.9917 | 0.4759 |
| $8.0 \times 10^{-4}$ | −3.0969 | 4.0230 | 0.6046 |
| Unknown A | | 0.0067 | −2.1761 |
| Unknown B | | 0.0557 | −1.2544 |
| Unknown C | | 0.1757 | −0.7553 |
| Unknown D | | 1.1357 | 0.0553 |

Figure 20.5 summarises the data where the Log$_{10}$ transformed concentration values of methylene blue are plotted against the corresponding average absorbance value. The resulting scatterplot shows that the data points are now more evenly spread across the range of values for the independent variable ($x$-axis); however, the data still exhibit deviation from linearity.

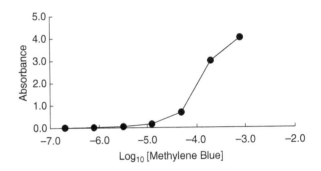

**Figure 20.5  Spectrophotometer absorbance measurements of methylene blue: Log$_{10}$ transformation of methylene blue concentration.**

The next step is to examine whether the additional Log$_{10}$ transformation of the dependent variable values (i.e. the corresponding absorbance values) allows the relationship between the data points to approximate to linearity. Figure 20.6 summarises the resulting scatterplot following Log$_{10}$ transformation of both the independent and dependent variables (i.e. of both the molarity concentrations of the methylene blue solutions and the corresponding absorbance values); clearly, the scatterplot now suggests a near-linear relationship between the data points.

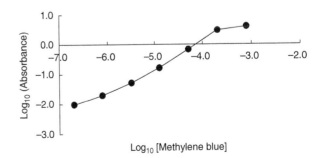

**Figure 20.6  Spectrophotometer absorbance measurements of methylene blue: Log$_{10}$ transformation of methylene blue concentration and corresponding absorbance values.**

With a near-linear relationship between the two variables, we are now in a position to perform a linear regression analysis but notice this must use the $Log_{10}$ transformed data points of both variables only; see values summarised in Table 20.9.

Table 20.9 Methylene blue absorbance data: transformed data.

| | $Log_{10}$ (M) | $Log_{10}$ absorbance | $(x-\bar{x})$ | $(y-\bar{y})$ | $(x-\bar{x})(y-\bar{y})$ |
|---|---|---|---|---|---|
| 1 | −6.7100 | −2.0147 | −1.8068 | −1.3174 | 2.3803 |
| 2 | −6.1073 | −1.7063 | −1.2041 | −1.0090 | 1.2149 |
| 3 | −5.5051 | −1.2868 | −0.6019 | −0.5895 | 0.3548 |
| 4 | −4.9031 | −0.7860 | 0.0001 | −0.0887 | 0.0000 |
| 5 | −4.3010 | −0.1677 | 0.6022 | 0.5296 | 0.3189 |
| 6 | −3.6990 | 0.4759 | 1.2042 | 1.1732 | 1.4128 |
| 7 | −3.0969 | 0.6046 | 1.8063 | 1.3019 | 2.3516 |
| | | | | | |
| Sum | −34.3224 | −4.8810 | | | 8.0333 |
| Mean | −4.9032 | −0.6973 | | | |
| StDev | 1.3008 | 1.0377 | | | |
| Sum of Squares | | | 10.1521 | 6.4608 | |

Thus,

$$b = \frac{\sum(x-\bar{x})(y-\bar{y})}{\sum(x-\bar{x})^2} = \frac{8.0333}{10.1521} = 0.7913 \quad (20.29)$$

and

$$a = \bar{y} - b\bar{x} = -0.6973 - (0.7913 \times -4.9032) \quad (20.30)$$

$$a = -0.6973 - (-3.8799) \quad (20.31)$$

$$a = 3.1826 \quad (20.32)$$

We can now express the regression equation in terms of $x$:

$$x = \frac{y-a}{b} = \frac{y-3.1826}{0.7913} \quad (20.33)$$

where $x$ is expressed as $Log_{10}$ of the methylene blue concentration and may be predicted by the value of $y$ expressed in $Log_{10}$ of the absorbance value. We are now in a position to calculate the concentrations of the four unknown solutions of methylene blue from their respective absorbance values determined in the experiment. However, before that we should complete the regression analysis by calculating the linear regression ANOVA table (see Table 20.10) to examine whether the fitted model may account for any significant variation in the dependent variable.

Thus,

**1** Total sum of squares for $y$ (see Table 20.9),

$$ssqy = \sum(y-\bar{y})^2 = 6.4608, \quad (20.34)$$

with $n-1$ degrees of freedom

**2** Regression sum of squares,

$$regssq = \frac{8.0333^2}{10.1521} = \frac{64.5339}{10.1521} = 6.3567, \quad (20.35)$$

with 1 degree of freedom

**3** Residual sum of squares,

$$residssq = ssqy - regssq = 6.4608 - 6.3567 = 0.1041 \quad (20.36)$$

with $n-2$ degrees of freedom

Table 20.10 Linear regression ANOVA; methylene blue absorbance

| Source | Sum of Squares | df | Variance (mean square) | F ratio | p |
|---|---|---|---|---|---|
| Regression | 6.3567 | 1 | 6.3567 | 305.317 | <0.001 |
| Residual error | 0.1041 | 5 | 0.02082 | | |
| | | | | | |
| Total | 6.4608 | 6 | | | |

Inspection of the critical values of $F$, with 1 and 5 degrees of freedom, summarised in Appendix E, indicate that for $p = 0.001$ then $F_{crit}(1, 5) = 47.18$.

Since the calculated F value exceeds the critical value for $p = 0.001$, then we may reject the Null Hypothesis and conclude that a significant proportion of the variance in the dependent variable may be explained by the time at which the percentage atropine concentration remaining was measured.

The regression ANOVA is summarised as:

$$F(1,5) = 305.317, p < 0.001 \quad (20.37)$$

Furthermore, the correlation coefficient is calculated as follows (see Table 20.9 for standard deviations for $x$ and $y$):

$$r = \frac{\sum(x-\bar{x})(y-\bar{y})}{(N-1).s_x.s_y} = \frac{8.0333}{6 \times 1.3008 \times 1.0377} = 0.9919 \quad (20.38)$$

and the probability of the Null Hypothesis for the correlation coefficient may be obtained by calculating the $t$-statistic with $N-2$ degrees of freedom. Thus,

$$t_r = \frac{r\sqrt{N-2}}{\sqrt{1-r^2}} = \frac{0.9919\sqrt{5}}{\sqrt{1-0.9839}} = \frac{0.9919 \times 2.236}{\sqrt{0.017}} \quad (20.39)$$

$$t_r = \frac{2.2179}{0.1304} = 17.008 \quad (20.40)$$

The corresponding $p$-value may be determined by using the critical values of the $t$-distribution summarised in Appendix C. The table shows that for $p = 0.001$, then $t_{crit}(5) = 6.869$. As the calculated value of $t_r$ exceeds the $t_{crit}$ values of 6.869, we may conclude that the probability of the Null Hypothesis being true is <0.001. Consequently, we may reject the Null Hypothesis in favour of the alternate hypothesis and conclude that the correlation is significant.

The correlation analysis may therefore be summarised as:

$$r = 0.9914, p < 0.001 \quad (20.41)$$

Finally, the coefficient of determination $r^2 = 0.9839$ reveals that over 98% of the sum of squares of the absorbance values may be accounted for by fitting the mathematical model.

The important point about this example is that it demonstrates how transformation of both independent and dependent variables, in both cases a $Log_{10}$ transformation, results in a scatterplot where the fitted line approximates to linearity, thereby allowing linear regression analysis.

Finally (!), we can now use the linear regression equation expressed in terms of $x$, the independent variable, to determine the four unknown concentrations of methylene blue.

Thus,

$$x = \frac{y-a}{b} = \frac{y-3.1826}{0.7913} \quad (20.42)$$

We need to remember that the various values of absorbance we substitute into this equation (i.e. $y$) must be the $Log_{10}$ values of the respective average absorbance for each concentration (see Table 20.8), and the calculated value of $x$ will be the $Log_{10}$ value of the respective concentration of methylene blue. Consequently, the actual molar concentrations of the unknown solutions of methylene blue will be the $antilog_{10}$ of the calculated values of the independent variable, $x$. These values are summarised in Table 20.11.

Table 20.11 Summary of calculated unknown concentrations of methylene blue.

| Solution | $Log_{10}$ y | $Log_{10}$ x | [Unknown] M |
|---|---|---|---|
| A | −2.1761 | −6.7720 | $1.690 \times 10^{-7}$ |
| B | −1.2544 | −5.6072 | $2.471 \times 10^{-6}$ |
| C | −0.7553 | −4.9965 | $1.056 \times 10^{-5}$ |
| D | 0.0553 | −3.9521 | $1.117 \times 10^{-4}$ |

The examples provided in this chapter demonstrate how linear regression may be used to analyse the relationship between quite complex series of data, although as you will appreciate by now, sometimes it is necessary to transform the values of one or both variables in order to tease out the relationship so that the mathematical model may be used as a predictor of unknown values.

# Example output from statistical software

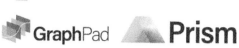

**A**

| Simple linear regression Tabular results | A<br>Protein | |
|---|---|---|
| 1 **Best-fit values** | | |
| 2 Slope | 0.01810 | |
| 3 Y-intercept | 0.2925 | |
| 4 X-intercept | -16.16 | |
| 5 1/slope | 55.26 | |
| 6 | | |
| 7 **Std. Error** | | |
| 8 Slope | 0.003815 | |
| 9 Y-intercept | 0.09655 | |
| 10 | | |
| 11 **95% Confidence Intervals** | | |
| 12 Slope | 0.009300 to 0.02689 | |
| 13 Y-intercept | 0.06985 to 0.5152 | |
| 14 X-intercept | -54.48 to -2.641 | |
| 15 | | |
| 16 **Goodness of Fit** | | |
| 17 R squared | 0.7377 | |
| 18 Sy.x | 0.1006 | |
| 19 | | |
| 20 **Is slope significantly non-zero?** | | |
| 21 F | 22.51 | |
| 22 DFn, DFd | 1, 8 | |
| 23 P value | 0.0015 | |
| 24 Deviation from zero? | Significant | |
| 25 | | |
| 26 **Equation** | Y = 0.01810*X + 0.2925 | |

**B**

| Simple linear regression Tabular results | A<br>Log [Atropine] | B |
|---|---|---|
| 1 **Best-fit values** | | |
| 2 Slope | -0.01174 | |
| 3 Y-intercept | 2.000 | |
| 4 X-intercept | 170.4 | |
| 5 1/slope | -85.19 | |
| 6 | | |
| 7 **Std. Error** | | |
| 8 Slope | 0.0001625 | |
| 9 Y-intercept | 0.008402 | |
| 10 | | |
| 11 **95% Confidence Intervals** | | |
| 12 Slope | -0.01216 to -0.01132 | |
| 13 Y-intercept | 1.979 to 2.022 | |
| 14 X-intercept | 165.8 to 175.3 | |
| 15 | | |
| 16 **Goodness of Fit** | | |
| 17 R squared | 0.9990 | |
| 18 Sy.x | 0.01347 | |
| 19 | | |
| 20 **Is slope significantly non-zero?** | | |
| 21 F | 5220 | |
| 22 DFn, DFd | 1, 5 | |
| 23 P value | <0.0001 | |
| 24 Deviation from zero? | Significant | |
| 25 | | |
| 26 **Equation** | Y = -0.01174*X + 2.000 | |

**C**

| Simple linear regression Tabular results | A<br>Log Absorb | |
|---|---|---|
| 1 **Best-fit values** | | |
| 2 Slope | 0.7913 | |
| 3 Y-intercept | 3.183 | |
| 4 X-intercept | -4.022 | |
| 5 1/slope | 1.264 | |
| 6 | | |
| 7 **Std. Error** | | |
| 8 Slope | 0.04528 | |
| 9 Y-intercept | 0.2286 | |
| 10 | | |
| 11 **95% Confidence Intervals** | | |
| 12 Slope | 0.6749 to 0.9077 | |
| 13 Y-intercept | 2.595 to 3.770 | |
| 14 X-intercept | -4.225 to -3.780 | |
| 15 | | |
| 16 **Goodness of Fit** | | |
| 17 R squared | 0.9839 | |
| 18 Sy.x | 0.1443 | |
| 19 | | |
| 20 **Is slope significantly non-zero?** | | |
| 21 F | 305.4 | |
| 22 DFn, DFd | 1, 5 | |
| 23 P value | <0.0001 | |
| 24 Deviation from zero? | Significant | |
| 25 | | |
| 26 **Equation** | Y = 0.7913*X + 3.183 | |

Summary statistical analysis from GraphPad Prism, v8. Panels A, B, and C show the summary linear regression analysis of the urinary protein levels (Table 20.1), the transformed atropine data (Table 20.5), and the transformed methylene blue data (Table 20.9), respectively.

*Source*: GraphPad Software.

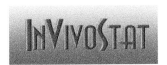

A

### Table of model coefficients

| | Estimate | Lower 95% CI | Upper 95% CI |
|---|---|---|---|
| (Intercept) | 0.2925 | 0.0698 | 0.5152 |
| Weeks | 0.0181 | 0.0093 | 0.0269 |

### Estimates of the coefficients of the best-fit regression line

| Categorisation Factor levels | Intercept estimate | Slope estimate |
|---|---|---|
| Overall regression line | 0.2925 | 0.0181 |

### R-squared and Adjusted R-squared statistics

| | R-squared | Adjusted R-sq |
|---|---|---|
| Estimate | 0.7377 | 0.7050 |

### Analysis of variance (ANOVA) table

| Effect | Sums of squares | Degrees of freedom | Mean square | F-value | p-value |
|---|---|---|---|---|---|
| Weeks | 0.23 | 1 | 0.229 | 22.51 | 0.0015 |
| Residual | 0.08 | 8 | 0.010 | | |

B

### Table of model coefficients

| | Estimate | Lower 95% CI | Upper 95% CI |
|---|---|---|---|
| (Intercept) | 2.000 | 1.979 | 2.022 |
| Hrs | -0.012 | -0.012 | -0.011 |

### Estimates of the coefficients of the best-fit regression line

| Categorisation Factor levels | Intercept estimate | Slope estimate |
|---|---|---|
| Overall regression line | 2.0001 | -0.0117 |

### R-squared and Adjusted R-squared statistics

| | R-squared | Adjusted R-sq |
|---|---|---|
| Estimate | 0.9990 | 0.9989 |

### Analysis of variance (ANOVA) table

| Effect | Sums of squares | Degrees of freedom | Mean square | F-value | p-value |
|---|---|---|---|---|---|
| Hrs | 0.95 | 1 | 0.947 | 3220.28 | < 0.0001 |
| Residual | 0.00 | 3 | 0.000 | | |

C

### Table of model coefficients

| | Estimate | Lower 95% CI | Upper 95% CI |
|---|---|---|---|
| (Intercept) | 3.16 | 2.56 | 3.77 |
| Log Methylu | 0.79 | 0.67 | 0.91 |

### Estimates of the coefficients of the best-fit regression line

| Categorisation Factor levels | Intercept estimate | Slope estimate |
|---|---|---|
| Overall regression line | 1.1626 | 0.7912 |

### R-squared and Adjusted R-squared statistics

| | R-squared | Adjusted R-sq |
|---|---|---|
| Estimate | 0.9839 | 0.9807 |

### Analysis of variance (ANOVA) table

| Effect | Sums of squares | Degrees of freedom | Mean square | F-value | p-value |
|---|---|---|---|---|---|
| Log Methylu | 6.35 | 1 | 6.357 | 305.41 | < 0.0001 |
| Residual | 0.10 | 5 | 0.021 | | |

Summary statistical analysis from InVivoStat, v4.0.2. Panels A, B, and C show the summary linear regression analysis of the urinary protein levels (Table 20.1), the transformed atropine data (Table 20.5), and the transformed methylene blue data (Table 20.9), respectively.

*Source*: InVivoStat.

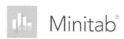

## A

### Coefficients

| Term | Coef | SE Coef | T-value | P-value | VIF |
|------|------|---------|---------|---------|-----|
| Constant | 0.2925 | 0.0966 | 3.03 | 0.016 | |
| Weeks | 0.01810 | 0.00381 | 4.74 | 0.001 | 1.00 |

### Analysis of variance

| Source | DF | Adj SS | Adj MS | F-Value | P-Value |
|--------|----|--------|--------|---------|---------|
| Regression | 1 | 0.22756 | 0.22756 | 22.51 | 0.001 |
| Weeks | 1 | 0.22756 | 0.22756 | 22.51 | 0.001 |
| Error | 8 | 0.08089 | 0.01011 | | |
| Total | 9 | 0.30845 | | | |

### Model summary

| S | R-sq | R-sq(adj) | R-sq(pred) |
|---|------|-----------|------------|
| 0.100555 | 73.77% | 70.50% | 61.45% |

### Regression equation

Protein = 0.2925 + 0.01810 Weeks

## B

### Coefficients

| Term | Coef | SE Coef | T-Value | P-Value | VIF |
|------|------|---------|---------|---------|-----|
| Constant | 2.00472 | 0.00754 | 266.02 | 0.000 | |
| Hours | −0.011809 | 0.000146 | −81.03 | 0.000 | 1.00 |

### Analysis of variance

| Source | DF | Adj SS | Adj MS | F-Value | P-Value |
|--------|----|--------|--------|---------|---------|
| Regression | 1 | 0.958093 | 0.958093 | 6566.49 | 0.000 |
| Hours | 1 | 0.958093 | 0.958093 | 6566.49 | 0.000 |
| Error | 5 | 0.000730 | 0.000146 | | |
| Total | 6 | 0.958822 | | | |

### Model summary

| S | R-sq | R-sq(adj) | R-sq(pred) |
|---|------|-----------|------------|
| 0.0120792 | 99.92% | 99.91% | 99.78% |

### Regression equation

Log At = 2.00472 − 0.011809 Hours

## C

### Coefficients

| Term | Coef | SE Coef | T-Value | P-Value | VIF |
|------|------|---------|---------|---------|-----|
| Constant | 3.183 | 0.229 | 13.92 | 0.000 | |
| Log Conc | 0.7913 | 0.0453 | 17.48 | 0.000 | 1.00 |

### Analysis of variance

| Source | DF | Adj SS | Adj MS | F-Value | P-Value |
|--------|----|--------|--------|---------|---------|
| Regression | 1 | 6.3567 | 6.35666 | 305.45 | 0.000 |
| Log Conc | 1 | 6.3567 | 6.35666 | 305.45 | 0.000 |
| Error | 5 | 0.1041 | 0.02081 | | |
| Total | 6 | 6.4607 | | | |

### Model summary

| S | R-sq | R-sq(adj) | R-sq(pred) |
|---|------|-----------|------------|
| 0.144259 | 98.39% | 98.07% | 96.35% |

### Regression equation

Log Abs = 3.183 + 0.7913 Log Conc

Summary statistical analysis from MiniTab, v18. Panels A, B, and C show the summary linear regression analysis of the urinary protein levels (Table 20.1), the transformed atropine data (Table 20.5), and the transformed methylene blue data (Table 20.9), respectively.

*Source*: Minitab, LLC.

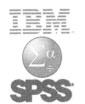

**A**

**Model Summary**

| Model | R | R Square | Adjusted R Square | Std. Error of the Estimate | R Square Change | F Change | df1 | df2 | Sig. F Change |
|---|---|---|---|---|---|---|---|---|---|
| 1 | .859[a] | .738 | .705 | .10056 | .738 | 22.505 | 1 | 8 | .001 |

a. Predictors: (Constant), Weeks

**Coefficients[a]**

| Model | | Unstandardized Coefficients B | Std. Error | Standardized Coefficients Beta | t | Sig. | 95.0% Confidence Interval for B Lower Bound | Upper Bound |
|---|---|---|---|---|---|---|---|---|
| 1 | (Constant) | .293 | .097 | | 3.029 | .016 | .070 | .515 |
| | Weeks | .018 | .004 | .859 | 4.744 | .001 | .009 | .027 |

a. Dependent Variable: Protein

**ANOVA[a]**

| Model | | Sum of Squares | df | Mean Square | F | Sig. |
|---|---|---|---|---|---|---|
| 1 | Regression | .228 | 1 | .228 | 22.505 | .001[b] |
| | Residual | .081 | 8 | .010 | | |
| | Total | .308 | 9 | | | |

a. Dependent Variable: Protein
b. Predictors: (Constant), Weeks

**B**

**Model Summary**

| Model | R | R Square | Adjusted R Square | Std. Error of the Estimate | R Square Change | F Change | df1 | df2 | Sig. F Change |
|---|---|---|---|---|---|---|---|---|---|
| 1 | 1.000[a] | .999 | .999 | .01347 | .999 | 5220.258 | 1 | 5 | .000 |

a. Predictors: (Constant), Hours

**Coefficients[a]**

| Model | | Unstandardized Coefficients B | Std. Error | Standardized Coefficients Beta | t | Sig. | 95.0% Confidence Interval for B Lower Bound | Upper Bound |
|---|---|---|---|---|---|---|---|---|
| 1 | (Constant) | 2.000 | .008 | | 238.049 | .000 | 1.979 | 2.022 |
| | Hours | -.012 | .000 | -1.000 | -72.251 | .000 | -.012 | -.011 |

a. Dependent Variable: Log_atropine

**ANOVA[a]**

| Model | | Sum of Squares | df | Mean Square | F | Sig. |
|---|---|---|---|---|---|---|
| 1 | Regression | .947 | 1 | .947 | 5220.258 | .000[b] |
| | Residual | .001 | 5 | .000 | | |
| | Total | .948 | 6 | | | |

a. Dependent Variable: Log_atropine
b. Predictors: (Constant), Hours

**C**

**Model Summary**

| Model | R | R Square | Adjusted R Square | Std. Error of the Estimate | R Square Change | F Change | df1 | df2 | Sig. F Change |
|---|---|---|---|---|---|---|---|---|---|
| 1 | .992[a] | .984 | .981 | .14427 | .984 | 305.415 | 1 | 5 | .000 |

a. Predictors: (Constant), Log_MethBlue

**Coefficients[a]**

| Model | | Unstandardized Coefficients B | Std. Error | Standardized Coefficients Beta | t | Sig. | 95.0% Confidence Interval for B Lower Bound | Upper Bound |
|---|---|---|---|---|---|---|---|---|
| 1 | (Constant) | 3.183 | .229 | | 13.922 | .000 | 2.595 | 3.770 |
| | Log_MethBlue | .791 | .045 | .992 | 17.476 | .000 | .675 | .908 |

a. Dependent Variable: Log_Absorp

**ANOVA[a]**

| Model | | Sum of Squares | df | Mean Square | F | Sig. |
|---|---|---|---|---|---|---|
| 1 | Regression | 6.357 | 1 | 6.357 | 305.415 | .000[b] |
| | Residual | .104 | 5 | .021 | | |
| | Total | 6.461 | 6 | | | |

a. Dependent Variable: Log_Absorp
b. Predictors: (Constant), Log_MethBlue

Summary statistical analysis from SPSS, v27. Panels A, B, and C show the summary linear regression analysis of the urinary protein levels (Table 20.1), the transformed atropine data (Table 20.5), and the transformed methylene blue data (Table 20.9), respectively.

*Source*: IBM Corporation.

# 21 Chi-square analysis

As I said way back in Chapter 4, in general terms, there are three types of data (nominal, ordinal, and measurement), but for both descriptive and inferential statistics I have concentrated on topics related solely to ordinal and measurement data. It is now time to examine how nominal data sets may be analysed.

Nominal data are where numerals are applied to attributes or **categories**. Imagine the situation where you are quietly going about your business on a weekend, doing your weekly shopping, for example, and you're approached by a Gandalf lookalike who asks if you could spare a few minutes to answer some questions. *[This happened to me a month or so ago when shopping at Waitrose (now you know this scenario is fictitious – like I can afford to shop at Waitrose!)].* It quickly becomes obvious that this is a marketing exercise and the subsequent questions are focused on your personal preference and product placement, etc. So, the questioner simply works his/her way through the series of questions noting your responses as a series of ticks on their questionnaire. Clearly this is a survey, but the data produced are very different from that which we have encountered so far in our journey through the vagaries of statistical analysis. All of the *individual* responses you provided to the questions asked become mixed up with all the answers (similar or otherwise) provided by other independent responders, and at the end of the survey the questioner has a series of values associated with each of the possible outcomes for each question; essentially, you have lost your individuality and are just grouped into a category with the rest of the hoi polloi!

Such data are generally summarised in a table where the series of columns and rows reflect various options within the column variable and the row variable. These tables are known as contingency tables and the data analysed by a technique known as chi-square analysis ($\chi^2$ analysis).

## Assumptions of chi-square analysis

The basic assumption of chi-square analysis is that all of the observations are independent from each other. This means that first, an individual's response would have no effect on another individual's response and second, any individual's response may be recorded in one cell *only* within the contingency table. Consequently, chi-square analysis may not be used to analyse data from a repeated measures design experiment.

Another assumption relates to inclusivity. Imagine the situation where subjects respond either positively or negatively to a question by the interviewer. It is unacceptable to analyse just the positive responses to the question because this would fail to account for all the negative responses (known in the statistical literature as *non-occurrences*) to the question. Failure to take account of non-occurrences will invalidate the chi-square analysis (it will also reduce the value of the test statistic, $\chi^2$, making you more likely to accept the Null Hypothesis). One way around this is to double-check that the total number in the contingency table equals the number of subjects in the study.

The utility of contingency tables relies on making the correct calculation of the expected frequency for each cell within the table. For $2 \times 2$ contingency tables, no expected frequency should be less than 5 (this is addressed in Example 21.2 below). For larger tables, the general rule is that all expected counts should be larger than 1 with no more than 20% of the expected counts less than 5. If the assumption of expected frequencies is violated, there is a large reduction in power of the test which will risk making a Type 2 error.

For most contingency tables, the method described below to calculate the expected frequencies will apply. However, in some cases, we may already be aware of the expected frequencies from the type of experiment concerned. Consider a genetic experiment examining Mendel's *Law of Segregation* to explain how genes are inherited. In genetic terminology, if two *Yy* hybrids cross-fertilise, then at fertilisation ¼ of the progeny will be *YY*, ¼ *Yy*, ¼ *yY*, and ¼ *yy*. As far as the progeny are concerned, then *Yy* is equivalent to *yY*. Phenotypically, 75% of the progeny will have the same dominant trait and 25% will have the same recessive trait. However, the dominant phenotype will consist of 33.3% of pure *YY* and 66.7% of the heterozygous *Yy* hybrid. Quite clearly, therefore, genetics allows us to accurately *predict* the expected frequency of each phenotype and genotype in the offspring. However, as we shall see in the subsequent examples described below, prior knowledge of expected frequencies in general populations for most applications of chi-square analysis of contingency tables is not a luxury we can usually enjoy. Consequently, the expected frequencies have to be estimated as part of the statistical procedure.

## Example 21.1 3 × 3 contingency table and $\chi^2$

As an example, consider the following task which we set a small group of final year pharmacy students a few years ago. The students were asked to go into the local town and ask people at random a series of questions related to their preference for medication (type of formulation, colour, taste, etc.). From the resulting data, we were really only interested in whether there was a relationship between the age of the interviewee and their colour preference for tablets. The contingency table below summarises the resulting data (see Table 21.1), and each number represents the number or frequency of people which fell into each cell.

Table 21.1 Summary of age and colour preference.

| Age group (yr) | Colour preference | | |
| --- | --- | --- | --- |
| | Pink | Orange | White |
| 18–35 | 26 | 40 | 32 |
| 36–60 | 14 | 57 | 49 |
| Over 60 | 9 | 28 | 35 |

Summary of observed frequencies.

On the basis of these data, can we conclude that there is a link or relationship between age and colour preference in the population as a whole? Our **Null Hypothesis** for experiments of this type would be that there is **no association between the two classes of category (i.e. the variables age and colour preference).**

The problem with data sets of this type is that each value represents the *frequency* of responders according to each cell within the table rather than a single observation from clearly defined individual subjects. So how do we analyse such data that are based on categories? To answer this question, we use a statistic calculated by **Pearson's chi-square ($\chi^2$)** test, which measures the degree of association between two categorical variables. The basis of chi-squared analysis, in simple terms, is that the test assumes the patterning of the cells in each row is similar across all the columns, and likewise the patterning down each column is similar across all the rows. I realise this is somewhat difficult to imagine so I'll return to this argument once I've discussed the test and how to interpret the result of the analysis (see Example 21.4).

So, let's return to our example data and see how chi-squared analysis may help us draw appropriate conclusions about the results of the students' survey. The first stage is to calculate all the row and column totals of the table (see Table 21.2).

Table 21.2  Summary of age and colour preference: column and row totals.

| Age group (yr) | Colour preference | | | Total |
| | Pink | Orange | White | |
|---|---|---|---|---|
| 18–35 | 26 | 40 | 32 | 98 |
| 36–60 | 14 | 57 | 49 | 120 |
| Over 60 | 9 | 28 | 35 | 72 |
| Total | 49 | 125 | 116 | 290 |

Summary of observed frequencies including column and row totals.

First, consider the 49 subjects who preferred pink tablets and how these should be distributed between the 3 age groups under the Null Hypothesis (we need to do this because the number of interviewees in each age group is different). The total number of interviewees is 290 and so the proportion of all interviewees in row one (18–35 years age group) is 98/290. The total number of interviewees in column one (pink preference) is 49 and so this coupled with the 98/290 in the youngest age range would lead us to *expect* $49 \times 98/290 = 16.6$ individuals in the 18–35 years age range who preferred pink tablets. Consequently, we can now calculate the *expected frequency* for each cell within the contingency table, according to the formula:

$$\text{Expected frequency} = \frac{\text{column total} \times \text{row total}}{\text{grand total}} \quad (21.1)$$

Note that the actual values substituted into the equation will differ for each cell within the table; Table 21.3 summarises the categorical data including the expected frequencies for each cell.

Table 21.3  Summary of age and colour preference: expected frequencies.

| Age group (yr) | | Colour preference | | | Total |
| | | Pink | Orange | White | |
|---|---|---|---|---|---|
| 18–35 | Obs | 26 | 40 | 32 | 98 |
| | Expt | 16.6 | 42.2 | 39.2 | |
| 36–60 | Obs | 14 | 57 | 49 | 120 |
| | Expt | 20.3 | 51.7 | 48.0 | |
| Over 60 | Obs | 9 | 28 | 35 | 72 |
| | Expt | 12.2 | 31.0 | 28.8 | |
| Total | | 49 | 125 | 116 | 290 |

Obs indicates the observed counts for each cell. Expt indicates the expected frequency for each cell.

The point to notice here is that if the patterning across the columns and down the rows were consistent in line with the Null Hypothesis, then the expected frequencies should be similar to the observed data. Inspection of Table 21.3 shows that in some cases this is true (see orange preference for the youngest age group, white preference for the middle age group, and the pink and orange preferences for the oldest age group), but not for all cells in the table (see pink preference for the youngest age group). Also, in some cases, the expected frequencies are larger than the observed values in some cells, but smaller than the observed frequencies in other cells. Notice also that the sum of the expected frequencies is equal to the sum of the observed frequencies.

The next step is to determine the importance of any differences between the observed and expected frequencies. This is achieved by calculating the contribution of each cell to the overall level of chi-square according to the following formula:

$$\chi^2 = \sum \frac{(\text{Obs} - \text{Expt})^2}{\text{Expt}} \quad (21.2)$$

If you look closely, the equation uses the technique of squaring differences between values to get rid of negative values (we met this previously in all the sum of squares calculation we've performed to calculate variances and standard deviations, correlation, and regression analysis). Table 21.4 summarises the categorical data with the addition of the cell contributions to chi-square.

Table 21.4  Summary of age and colour preference: expected frequencies.

| Age group (yr) | | Colour preference | | | Total |
| | | Pink | Orange | White | |
|---|---|---|---|---|---|
| 18–35 | Obs | 26 | 40 | 32 | 98 |
| | Expt | 16.6 | 42.2 | 39.2 | |
| | $\chi^2$ | 5.323 | 0.115 | 1.322 | |
| 36–60 | Obs | 14 | 57 | 49 | 120 |
| | Expt | 20.3 | 51.7 | 48.0 | |
| | $\chi^2$ | 1.955 | 0.543 | 0.021 | |
| Over 60 | Obs | 9 | 28 | 35 | 72 |
| | Expt | 12.2 | 31.0 | 28.8 | |
| | $\chi^2$ | 0.839 | 0.290 | 1.335 | |
| Total | | 49 | 125 | 116 | 290 |

Obs indicates the observed counts for each cell. Expt indicates the expected frequency for each cell. $\chi^2$ indicates cell contribution to chi-square.

The individual cell contributions to chi-square are then added together to produce the total chi-square for the contingency table; thus $\chi^2 = 11.74$. We now need to determine the probability of obtaining such a chi-square value. To do so, we consult the critical values of the chi-square distribution which are summarised in the table found in Appendix F. However, in order to find the probability associated with critical values of chi-square, we need to determine the degrees of freedom for the contingency table. For any contingency table, the number of degrees of freedom is the product of ($n$ rows -1) and ($n$ columns -1). In the table used here, there are three rows and three columns and therefore there are $(3-1) \times (3-1)$ degrees of freedom = 4. Consulting Appendix F reveals that with four degrees of freedom, $\chi^2_{crit}$ for $p = 0.05$, $p = 0.01$, and $p = 0.001$ equals 9.49, 13.28, and 18.47, respectively. Consequently, the probability of the Null Hypothesis being true (i.e. that there is *no* association between the two variables, age and colour preference) is less than 0.05 but greater than 0.01. We may therefore reject the Null Hypothesis. The chi-square analysis may therefore be summarised as:

$$\chi^2(4) = 11.74, p < 0.05 \qquad (21.3)$$

and we may conclude that therefore there is an association between age and tablet colour preference.

At this point we hit a problem! If you think back to the discussion on analysis of variance (see Chapters 15–18), then a common theme throughout was that while an ANOVA model may indicate significant variation between the various groups in the experiment, it doesn't indicate exactly which groups differ from each other – to answer that question we need to use the tests of pairwise comparisons. A similar issue arises here with chi-square analysis. The analysis may indicate that one variable may influence the other, but the test fails to indicate immediately whether each observed frequency is similar or different from the corresponding expected frequency. One method to look at the relation between the observed and expected frequencies more closely is to calculate the **standardised residuals**.

I've not used this term much so far, but any residual is the difference between the experimental observation and the value predicted by the statistical model. So, the residual may be the difference between the observation of a single subject and the subject's group mean (I used the term *deviation* in discussing correlation and regression, Chapters 19 and 20 but this is really the same as the term *residual*). Or, as here in chi-square analysis, the difference between the observed and expected frequency for any particular cell in the contingency table. This may be summarised as the equation:

$$\text{Residual} = \text{observation} - \text{statistical model} \qquad (21.4)$$

Of course, for chi-square analysis, the totals of the various columns and rows are different according to each cell and so we need to *standardise* the residual, and we achieve this by dividing the difference between the observed and expected frequency by the square root of the expected frequency. Thus, for chi-square analysis,

$$\text{Standardised residual} = \frac{\text{Obs} - \text{Expt}}{\sqrt{\text{Expt}}} \qquad (21.5)$$

Table 21.5 summarises the survey data with the addition of the standardised residual for each cell.

Table 21.5 Summary of age and colour preference: standardised residuals.

| Age group (yr) | | Colour preference | | | Total |
|---|---|---|---|---|---|
| | | Pink | Orange | White | |
| 18–35 | Obs | 26 | 40 | 32 | 98 |
| | Expt | 16.6 | 42.2 | 39.2 | |
| | $\chi^2$ | 5.323 | 0.115 | 1.322 | |
| | StRes | 2.307 | −0.339 | −1.150 | |
| 36–60 | Obs | 14 | 57 | 49 | 120 |
| | Expt | 20.3 | 51.7 | 48.0 | |
| | $\chi^2$ | 1.955 | 0.543 | 0.021 | |
| | StRes | −1.398 | 0.737 | 0.144 | |
| Over 60 | Obs | 9 | 28 | 35 | 72 |
| | Expt | 12.2 | 31.0 | 28.8 | |
| | $\chi^2$ | 0.839 | 0.290 | 1.335 | |
| | StRes | −0.916 | −0.539 | 1.155 | |
| Total | | 49 | 125 | 116 | 290 |

Obs indicates the observed counts for each cell. Expt indicates the expected frequency for each cell. $\chi^2$ indicates cell contribution to chi-square. StRes indicates the standardised residual.

There are three important points to note about the standardised residuals:

• First, because the standardised residual is dependent on the difference between the observed and expected frequencies then there is a direct relationship to the cell's contribution to the overall chi-square statistic.
• Second, the positive or negative nature of the standardised residual provides useful information as to whether the observed frequency is larger or smaller than the expected frequency predicted by the statistical model.
• Third, each standardised residual is a *z*-score and thus has a direct relationship to the probability distribution of a standard normal distribution curve.

If you examine the table in Appendix B (standard normal probabilities), then for $z = -1.96$ the probability remaining in the left tail of the distribution curve is 0.0250, for $z = -2.58$ the probability in the left tail is 0.0049 and for $z = -3.29$ the probability is 0.0005. Of course, we need to consider the area of the curve in *both* tails (for a two-tailed test) and so the *total* probability for a standardised residual value that lies outside ±1.96 is significant at <0.05, if the value lies outside ±2.58 then $p < 0.01$ and if it lies outside ±3.29 then $p < 0.001$.

If we now refer back to Table 21.5, then the only standardised residual that is larger than ±1.96 is that for the youngest age group that preferred pink tablets (i.e. $p < 0.05$). We would therefore reject the Null Hypothesis (which would state that there is *no* difference between the observed and expected frequencies) for this cell *only* and conclude that the observed frequency of 18–35 years old participants who preferred pink tablets was significantly greater than the expected frequency predicted by the statistical model.

### Care!

At this point we must be very careful not to overemphasise any conclusions based on significant standardised residual values since they simply relate to the observed and expected frequencies in a single cell, and not to the whole contingency table. If you look at the colour preference data across the row for 18–35 years olds in Table 21.5, then the greatest preference was for orange tablets (40/98 = 40.8%), followed by a preference for white (32/98 = 32.7%) and then pink (26/98 = 26.5%), it is just that the analysis revealed a larger preference for pink tablets than we expected!

## Example 21.2 $\chi^2$ and expected frequencies

Consider the following chi-square analysis (Table 21.6) of data obtained to determine whether there was a gender bias in arthritic disease.

Table 21.6 Gender bias, rheumatoid, and osteoarthritis.

| Gender | | Patient status | | | Total |
| --- | --- | --- | --- | --- | --- |
| | | Healthy | Rheumatoid | Osteo | |
| Male | Obs | 143 | 13 | 4 | 160 |
| | Expt | 135.38 | 15.04 | 9.57 | |
| Female | Obs | 55 | 9 | 10 | 74 |
| | Expt | 62.62 | 6.96 | 4.43 | |
| Total | | 198 | 22 | 14 | 234 |

Obs indicates the observed counts for each cell. Expt indicates the expected frequency for each cell. Osteo indicates osteoarthritis.

In the previous example, we used the observed and expected frequencies to estimate the chi-square statistic and then used the summary table of critical values of the chi-square statistic to determine the probability that the Null Hypothesis was true. In fact, the calculated chi-square statistic has a sampling distribution that is only *approximately* a chi-square distribution, and in general terms the approximation becomes better as the sample size increases. Consequently, in small sample sizes, the approximation is not good enough such that the calculated chi-square statistic is inaccurate. Indeed, when the expected frequencies are greater than 5, then the sampling distribution of the calculated $\chi^2$ test statistic is sufficiently close enough to the chi-square distribution for us not to be too concerned about any difference. However, when the expected frequency is *less* than 5, then the calculated chi-square statistic is unlikely to be accurate. This is especially a problem when analysing $2 \times 2$ contingency tables (see below).

Table 21.6 summarises the observed and expected counts from the study examining gender bias in arthritic disease. Note especially the expected frequency for female subjects suffering from osteoarthritis, here the expected frequency equals 4.43. As explained above, this raises a confidence issue in the calculated test statistic.

So, what can we do in this situation? Well, we have three clear choices:

**1** Do nothing and accept the loss of power in the analysis, but this will risk making a Type 1 error in the affected cell.
**2** Collect more data so that the expected frequency of the affected cell is greater than 5.
**3** Collapse data across one of the variables.

I've argued throughout this book that as experimental scientists the last thing we want to do is risk making a Type 1 or Type 2 error in drawing conclusions from our experimental data, so I am always loath to choose option 1. In a number of experimental situations increasing the sample size may not be an option (see option 2), so let's collapse data across one of the variables and examine whether that provides any meaningful statistical data.

In this example, we can't collapse across gender because we only have two subgroups to start with; collapsing would only produce one group in the gender variable with consequently zero degrees of freedom – so this is not an option! The best choice here would be to collapse across the two arthritic subgroups in the patient status variable – at least this way we'll still be able to examine whether there is a gender bias in arthritic disease, we just will not have sufficient data to see if any gender bias resides in the rheumatoid or osteoarthritic conditions. The modified sample data together with the complete chi-square analysis (including calculation of the standard residuals) is summarised below (Table 21.7).

Table 21.7 Gender bias and arthritic disease.

| Gender | | Patient status | | Total |
| --- | --- | --- | --- | --- |
| | | Healthy | Arthritis | |
| Male | Obs | 143 | 17 | 160 |
| | Expt | 135.38 | 24.62 | |
| | $\chi^2$ | 0.428 | 2.356 | |
| | StRes | 0.654 | −1.535 | |
| Female | Obs | 55 | 19 | 74 |
| | Expt | 62.62 | 11.38 | |
| | $\chi^2$ | 0.926 | 5.094 | |
| | StRes | −0.962 | 2.257 | |
| Total | | 198 | 22 | 234 |

Obs indicates the observed counts for each cell. Expt indicates the expected frequency for each cell. $\chi^2$ indicates cell contribution to chi-square. StRes indicates the standardised residual.

The first point to notice about the revised data set is that all four cells in the contingency table now have expected frequencies greater than 5. We now need to calculate the sum of the individual cell contributions to the overall level of chi-square, which may be summarised thus,

$$\chi^2(1) = 8.804, p < 0.01 \qquad (21.6)$$

with one degree of freedom and where $p$ may be determined by consulting the critical values of chi-square summarised in Appendix F. The probability of the Null Hypothesis being true (i.e. no relationship between gender and arthritic disease) is <0.01 and may therefore be rejected. However, we have to inspect the standardised residuals to determine the relationship between the observed and expected frequencies in each of the four cells. We saw in the earlier example that for $p = 0.05$, the standardised residual is ±1.96, while for $p = 0.01$, the standardised residual is ±2.58. Consequently, for the female + arthritic cell only (bottom right in Table 21.7), the standardised residual indicates that there is a significant difference between the observed and expected frequencies, $p < 0.05$.

So, from these data, we may conclude that the observed frequency of female patients suffering arthritis is significantly greater than the number expected. Furthermore, we may also conclude that the observed frequencies of the other three patient groups were not significantly different from the expected frequencies.

### Fisher's Exact test

The problem associated with situations with cells where the expected frequency is less than 5 was resolved by Fisher who developed a method to compute the exact probability of the chi-square statistic for small sample sizes. The method is usually only used in situations with two variables each with two subgroups (i.e. $2 \times 2$ contingency tables); there is little advantage in using it on larger tables with large sample sizes where the sampling distribution approximates to the chi-square distribution. For example of Fisher's Exact test see screenshots from software packages at the end of this chapter.

## Example 21.3 2 × 2 contingency tables

Consider data where the death rates 10 years after standard drug therapy alone or coronary bypass surgery were examined in patients suffering from heart disease; Table 21.8 summarises the chi-square analysis including calculation of the standardised residuals.

**Table 21.8** Heart disease and treatment.

| Gender | | Dead | Alive | Total |
|--------|------|------|-------|-------|
| | | **Patient status** | | |
| **Drug** | **Obs** | 440 | 921 | **1361** |
| | **Expt** | 400.44 | 960.56 | |
| | $\chi^2$ | 3.908 | 1.629 | |
| | **StRes** | 1.977 | −1.276 | |
| **Surgery** | **Obs** | 350 | 974 | **1324** |
| | **Expt** | 389.56 | 934.44 | |
| | $\chi^2$ | 4.017 | 1.675 | |
| | **StRes** | −2.004 | 1.2941 | |
| **Total** | | **790** | **1895** | **2685** |

Obs indicates the observed counts for each cell. Expt indicates the expected frequency for each cell. $\chi^2$ indicates cell contribution to chi-square. StRes indicates the standardised residual.

In summary,

$$\chi^2(1) = 11.229, p < 0.001 \qquad (21.7)$$

where the p-value was determined by consulting the table in Appendix F. Consequently, we may conclude that there is a relationship between treatment type and patient status 10 years later. Furthermore, inspection of the standardised residuals suggests that for patients still alive after treatment, there was no difference between the observed and expected frequencies regardless of whether the patients had been treated with drug or cardiac surgery; the standardised residuals were both *within* the range of ±1.96, and therefore p > 0.05 in both cases. In contrast, the standardised residuals of patients who had died were both *outside* the range of ±1.96 indicating significant differences between the observed and expected frequencies. For patients who received drug treatment, the observed frequency was significantly <u>greater</u> than the expected frequency, while for patients who had had surgery the observed frequency was significantly <u>less</u> than the expected frequency.

### Yate's correction

One of the problems with a 2 × 2 contingency table is that the difference between the observed and expected frequencies is overemphasised leading to greater contributions of each cell to the overall chi-square test statistic. The result of this is to produce a Type 1 error where the probability in support of the Null Hypothesis is too small. The **Yate's correction** (more correctly called **Yate's continuity correction**) slightly reduces the difference between the observed and expected frequencies used in calculating each cell's contribution to chi-square, thereby lowering the overall chi-square test statistic and reducing the chance of making a Type 1 error. However, the adjustment is somewhat arbitrary and has been criticised for overcorrecting the chi square values and making them

too small. Consequently, while you may come across Yate's correction in many software packages, *it is best left ignored.*

## Risk, relative risk, and odds ratio

Data sets presented in contingency tables derived from clinical trials may be used in different ways to give an indication of the likelihood that a particular event may occur.

The **risk** is a measure of the likelihood of an event occurring in a population. Using the data from Table 21.8, we can calculate the risk of death associated with each treatment protocol.

The equation is simply

$$\text{Risk} = \frac{\text{Observed frequency}}{\text{Variable total frequency}} \qquad (21.8)$$

Therefore,

$$\text{Risk with drug treatment} = \frac{440}{1361} = 0.323 \qquad (21.9)$$

$$\text{Risk with surgery} = \frac{350}{1324} = 0.264 \qquad (21.10)$$

We can now determine the **relative risk** (also known as the **risk ratio**) which reflects the likelihood of the variable (in this example death) occurring in an individual suffering from heart disease exposed to event 1 (i.e. drug treatment) compared to those exposed to event 2 (i.e. surgery). Thus,

$$\text{Relative Risk} = \frac{\text{Risk of event 1}}{\text{Risk of event 2}} = \frac{0.323}{0.264} = 1.223 \qquad (21.11)$$

Consequently, there is a 1.223 increase in the risk of death following drug treatment compared to surgery.

The **odds** of an event is the probability of an event occurring divided by the probability of that event not occurring. From the data in Table 21.8, we can therefore determine the odds of death occurring following drug treatment or surgery:

$$\text{Odds with drug treatment} = \frac{440}{921} = 0.4777 \qquad (21.12)$$

$$\text{Odds with surgery} = \frac{350}{974} = 0.3593 \qquad (21.13)$$

We can now determine the **odds ratio** of these two odds. Thus,

$$\text{Odds ratio} = \frac{0.4777}{0.3593} = 1.3295 \qquad (21.14)$$

The odds ratio is a useful statistic, especially for 2 × 2 contingency tables, since it is unaffected by sample size and identifies the degree to which one variable may influence the other.

## Example 21.4 Patterning across contingency tables and $\chi^2$

Consider the following *hypothetical* 3 × 3 contingency table summarised in Table 21.9. If you look very closely at each row of data in Table 21.9, then you'll quickly appreciate that the proportional changes in the observed frequencies from cell to cell across the columns are the same, and likewise down each column across the rows. This consistency in patterning across the whole contingency table is important with respect to both the Null Hypothesis associated with chi-square analysis and the expected frequencies for each cell. The Null Hypothesis states that there is no relationship or association between the column and row variables. This means that the row variable should have no effect on the column variable, and *vice versa*.

**Table 21.9** 3 × 3 contingency table, observed frequencies.

|       | 1   | 2   | 3  | Total |
|-------|-----|-----|----|-------|
| A     | 90  | 60  | 30 | 180   |
| B     | 60  | 40  | 20 | 120   |
| C     | 30  | 20  | 10 | 60    |
| Total | 180 | 120 | 60 | 360   |

Summary of the hypothetical observed counts for each cell.

Consequently, if the patterning of change in the observed frequencies across the rows is the same as that down the columns, then we can safely predict that the expected frequency should be the same as the observed frequency in each cell! If we now calculate the expected frequencies then, as predicted, they are the same as the observed frequencies (see Table 21.10), and consequently, each cell's contribution to chi-square is zero – I've not included the individual $\chi^2$ values in Table 21.10 but if you're not sure why each cell's contribution to chi-square is zero then refer back to the equation provided in Example 21.1.

**Table 21.10** 3 × 3 contingency table, observed and expected frequencies.

|       |      | 1   | 2   | 3  | Total |
|-------|------|-----|-----|----|-------|
| A     | Obs  | 90  | 60  | 30 | 180   |
|       | Expt | 90  | 60  | 30 |       |
| B     | Obs  | 60  | 40  | 20 | 120   |
|       | Expt | 60  | 40  | 20 |       |
| C     | Obs  | 30  | 20  | 10 | 60    |
|       | Expt | 30  | 20  | 10 |       |
| Total |      | 180 | 120 | 60 | 360   |

Obs indicates the observed counts for each cell. Expt indicates the expected frequency for each cell.

Now consider what happens to the expected frequencies for each cell if we disrupt the constant patterning across the contingency table simply by making a sizeable change to the observed frequency of just one cell, in this case by increasing the value of the top left cell from 90 to 135; see Table 21.11. As you can see, by just

**Table 21.11** 3 × 3 contingency table, observed and expected frequencies.

|       |      | 1    | 2    | 3    | Total |
|-------|------|------|------|------|-------|
| A     | Obs  | 135  | 60   | 30   | 225   |
|       | Expt | 125  | 66.7 | 33.3 |       |
| B     | Obs  | 60   | 40   | 20   | 120   |
|       | Expt | 66.7 | 35.5 | 17.8 |       |
| C     | Obs  | 30   | 20   | 10   | 60    |
|       | Expt | 33.3 | 17.8 | 8.9  |       |
| Total |      | 225  | 120  | 60   | 405   |

Obs indicates the observed counts for each cell. Expt indicates the expected frequency for each cell.

changing the value of one observed frequency, we now start to see differences between the observed and the calculated expected frequency for each cell.

Furthermore, now that if there are differences between all the observed and expected frequencies within the contingency table, then each cell will contribute to the overall chi-square value, as summarised in Table 21.12.

For the hypothetical data in Table 21.12, the overall chi-square analysis, with four degrees of freedom, may be summarised as:

$$\chi^2(4) = 4.047, p > 0.05 \tag{21.15}$$

[The critical value of $\chi^2$ with four degrees of freedom for $p = 0.05$ is 9.49; see table in Appendix F].

**Table 21.12** 3 × 3 contingency table, contributions to $\chi^2$.

|       |          | 1     | 2     | 3     | Total |
|-------|----------|-------|-------|-------|-------|
| A     | Obs      | 135   | 60    | 30    | 225   |
|       | Expt     | 125   | 66.67 | 33.33 |       |
|       | $\chi^2$ | 0.800 | 0.667 | 0.333 |       |
| B     | Obs      | 60    | 40    | 20    | 120   |
|       | Expt     | 66.67 | 35.56 | 17.78 |       |
|       | $\chi^2$ | 0.667 | 0.554 | 0.277 |       |
| C     | Obs      | 30    | 20    | 10    | 60    |
|       | Expt     | 33.33 | 17.78 | 8.89  |       |
|       | $\chi^2$ | 0.333 | 0.277 | 0.139 |       |
| Total |          | 225   | 120   | 60    | 405   |

Obs indicates the observed counts for each cell. Expt indicates the expected frequency for each cell. $\chi^2$ indicates cell contribution to chi-square.

For this set of data at least, chi-square analysis reveals no significant relationship or association between the row and column variables. However, what would happen if we were to make an even larger change to the value of that top left cell, by increasing the observed frequency to 180? The summary data for chi-square analysis is summarised in Table 21.13.

**Table 21.13** 3 × 3 contingency table, contributions to $\chi^2$.

|       |          | 1     | 2     | 3     | Total |
|-------|----------|-------|-------|-------|-------|
| A     | Obs      | 180   | 60    | 30    | 270   |
|       | Expt     | 162   | 72    | 36    |       |
|       | $\chi^2$ | 2.0   | 2.0   | 1.0   |       |
|       | StRes    | 1.414 | 1.414 | 1.0   |       |
| B     | Obs      | 60    | 40    | 20    | 120   |
|       | Expt     | 72    | 32    | 16    |       |
|       | $\chi^2$ | 2.0   | 2.0   | 1.0   |       |
|       | StRes    | 1.414 | 1.414 | 1.0   |       |
| C     | Obs      | 30    | 20    | 10    | 60    |
|       | Expt     | 36    | 16    | 8     |       |
|       | $\chi^2$ | 1.0   | 1.0   | 0.5   |       |
|       | StRes    | 1.0   | 1.0   | 0.707 |       |
| Total |          | 270   | 120   | 60    | 450   |

Obs indicates the observed counts for each cell. Expt indicates the expected frequency for each cell. $\chi^2$ indicates cell contribution to chi-square. StRes indicates the standardised residual.

Clearly, there are now larger differences between the observed and expected frequencies resulting in greater individual cell contributions to the overall chi-square.

For Table 21.13, the overall chi-square analysis, with four degrees of freedom, may be summarised as:

$$\chi^2(4) = 12.5, p < 0.05 \qquad (21.16)$$

[The critical value of $\chi^2$ with four degrees of freedom for $p = 0.05$ is 9.49; see table in Appendix F].

So, the overall chi-square analysis indicates that the probability of the Null Hypothesis being true (i.e. that there is no association between the column and row totals) is less than 0.05. Consequently, the Null Hypothesis may be rejected, and we may conclude that the one of the two variables has an influence over the other. Interestingly, for this set of hypothetical data, calculation of the standardised residuals fails to identify a significant difference between the observed and expected frequencies for any of the cells in the contingency table, and so no further conclusions about the observed frequencies may be drawn.

The interesting point about this hypothetical contingency table is that we started with a table where the patterning of the values was constant across all the columns and rows, resulting in no difference between the observed and expected frequencies. However, as the patterning became increasingly disrupted so differences between the observed and expected frequencies started to appear, and the greater the disruption, the larger the differences until the resulting overall chi-square value was sufficiently large to allow the rejection of the Null Hypothesis. I would predict that even further disruption of the patterning of the data would start to produce sufficiently large standardised residuals such that significant differences between the observed and expected frequencies for individual cells would also start to appear. This hypothetical example shows how and why chi-square analysis works – for such a simple analysis it is rather elegant!

# Example output from statistical software

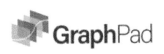 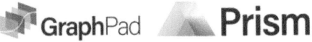

**A**

| | Contingency | A |
|---|---|---|
| 1 | **Table Analyzed** | Complete data set for stats analysis |
| 2 | | |
| 3 | **P value and statistical significance** | |
| 4 | Test | Chi-square |
| 5 | Chi-square, df | 11.78, 4 |
| 6 | P value | 0.0191 |
| 7 | P value summary | * |
| 8 | One- or two-sided | NA |
| 9 | Statistically significant (P < 0.05)? | Yes |
| 10 | | |
| 11 | **Data analyzed** | |
| 12 | Number of rows | 3 |
| 13 | Number of columns | 3 |

**B**

| | Contingency | A |
|---|---|---|
| 1 | **Table Analyzed** | Complete data set for stats analysis |
| 2 | | |
| 3 | **P value and statistical significance** | |
| 4 | Test | Chi-square |
| 5 | Chi-square, df | 12.49, 2 |
| 6 | P value | 0.0019 |
| 7 | P value summary | ** |
| 8 | One- or two-sided | NA |
| 9 | Statistically significant (P < 0.05)? | Yes |
| 10 | | |
| 11 | **Data analyzed** | |
| 12 | Number of rows | 2 |
| 13 | Number of columns | 3 |

| | Contingency | A |
|---|---|---|
| 1 | **Table Analyzed** | Complete data set for stats analysis |
| 2 | | |
| 3 | **P value and statistical significance** | |
| 4 | Test | Chi-square |
| 5 | Chi-square, df | 8.805, 1 |
| 6 | z | 2.967 |
| 7 | P value | 0.0030 |
| 8 | P value summary | ** |
| 9 | One- or two-sided | Two-sided |
| 10 | Statistically significant (P < 0.05)? | Yes |

**C**

| | Contingency | A |
|---|---|---|
| 1 | **Table Analyzed** | Complete data set for stats analysis |
| 2 | | |
| 3 | **P value and statistical significance** | |
| 4 | Test | Chi-square |
| 5 | Chi-square, df | 11.23, 1 |
| 6 | z | 3.351 |
| 7 | P value | 0.0008 |
| 8 | P value summary | *** |
| 9 | One- or two-sided | Two-sided |
| 10 | Statistically significant (P < 0.05)? | Yes |

| | Contingency | A | B |
|---|---|---|---|
| 1 | **Table Analyzed** | Complete data set for stats analysis | |
| 2 | | | |
| 3 | **P value and statistical significance** | | |
| 4 | Test | Fisher's exact test | |
| 5 | P value | 0.0008 | |
| 6 | P value summary | *** | |
| 7 | One- or two-sided | Two-sided | |
| 8 | Statistically significant (P < 0.05)? | Yes | |
| 9 | | | |
| 10 | **Effect size** | Value | 95% CI |
| 11 | Relative Risk | 1.223 | 1.087 to 1.377 |
| 12 | Reciprocal of relative risk | 0.8177 | 0.7263 to 0.9201 |
| 13 | | | |
| 14 | Odds ratio | 1.329 | 1.126 to 1.572 |
| 15 | Reciprocal of odds ratio | 0.7522 | 0.6362 to 0.8879 |

Summary statistical analysis from GraphPad Prism, v8. Panel A summarises the chi-square analysis of the tablet colour preference data from Table 21.3. Panel B summarises the chi-square analysis of the rheumatoid and osteoarthritis data from Table 21.6 together with the analysis after collapsing the data across the two arthritis columns from Table 21.7 (see text for details). Panel C summarises the chi-square analysis of the heart disease data from Table 21.8, together with analysis by Fisher's exact test (including relative risk and odds ratio analysis), respectively.

*Source*: GraphPad Software.

**InVivoStat**

**A**

### Contingency table of counts

|  | Orange | Pink | White |
|---|---|---|---|
| >60 | 28 | 9 | 35 |
| 70-75 | 40 | 26 | 32 |
| 36-60 | 57 | 14 | 49 |

The values in this table are the sum of the individual entries in the imported dataset.

### Table of expected results (under the null hypothesis of no association)

|  | Orange | Pink | White | Column totals |
|---|---|---|---|---|
| >65 | 31.03 | 12.17 | 28.80 | 72 |
| 18-35 | 42.24 | 16.56 | 39.20 | 98 |
| 36-60 | 51.72 | 20.28 | 48.00 | 120 |
| Row totals | 128 | 49 | 116 | 290 |

The values in this table are the expected results, given the row and column totals, under the assumption of no association between the grouping factor and the response categories.

### Chi-squared test

|  | Test statistic | Degrees of freedom | p-value |
|---|---|---|---|
| Result | 11.78 | 4 | 0.0191 |

The chi-squared test is significant at the 5% level of significance as the p-value is less than 0.05.

**B**

### Contingency table of counts

|  | Healthy | Osteo | Rheumatoid |
|---|---|---|---|
| Female | 55 | 10 | 9 |
| Male | 141 | 4 | 18 |

The values in this table are the sum of the individual entries in the imported dataset.

### Table of expected results (under the null hypothesis of no association)

|  | Healthy | Osteo | Rheumatoid | Column totals |
|---|---|---|---|---|
| Female | 62.62 | 4.43 | 6.96 | 74 |
| Male | 135.38 | 9.57 | 15.04 | 160 |
| Row totals | 196 | 14 | 27 | 234 |

The values in this table are the expected results, given the row and column totals, under the assumption of no association between the grouping factor and the response categories.

### Chi-squared test

|  | Test statistic | Degrees of freedom | p-value |
|---|---|---|---|
| Result | 12.48 | 2 | 0.0019 |

The chi-squared test is significant at the 5% level of significance as the p-value is less than 0.05.

### Contingency table of counts

|  | Arthritic | Healthy |
|---|---|---|
| Female | 19 | 55 |
| Male | 17 | 143 |

The values in this table are the sum of the individual entries in the imported dataset.

### Table of expected results (under the null hypothesis of no association)

|  | Arthritic | Healthy | Column totals |
|---|---|---|---|
| Female | 11.38 | 62.62 | 74 |
| Male | 24.62 | 135.38 | 160 |
| Row totals | 36 | 198 | 234 |

The values in this table are the expected results, given the row and column totals, under the assumption of no association between the grouping factor and the response categories.

### Chi-squared test

|  | Test statistic | Degrees of freedom | p-value |
|---|---|---|---|
| Result | 7.69 | 1 | 0.0056 |

Note: For the 2 × 2 case, the chi-squared test is calculated with Yates' continuity correction.

The chi-squared test is significant at the 5% level of significance as the p-value is less than 0.05.

**C**

### Contingency table of counts

|  | Alive | Dead |
|---|---|---|
| Drug | 921 | 440 |
| Surgery | 974 | 350 |

The values in this table are the sum of the individual entries in the imported dataset.

### Table of expected results (under the null hypothesis of no association)

|  | Alive | Dead | Column totals |
|---|---|---|---|
| Drug | 960.56 | 400.44 | 1361 |
| Surgery | 934.44 | 389.56 | 1324 |
| Row totals | 1895 | 790 | 2685 |

The values in this table are the expected results, given the row and column totals, under the assumption of no association between the grouping factor and the response categories.

### Chi-squared test

|  | Test statistic | Degrees of freedom | p-value |
|---|---|---|---|
| Result | 10.95 | 1 | 0.0009 |

Note: For the 2 × 2 case, the chi-squared test is calculated with Yates' continuity correction.

The chi-squared test is significant at the 5% level of significance as the p-value is less than 0.05.

### Fisher's exact test

|  | p-value |
|---|---|
| Result | 0.0009 |

The Fisher's exact test is significant at the 5% level of significance as the p-value is less than 0.05.

Summary statistical analysis from InVivoStat, v4.0.2. Panel A summarises the chi-square analysis of the tablet colour preference data from Table 21.3. Panel B summarises the chi-square analysis of the rheumatoid and osteoarthritis data from Table 21.6 together with the analysis after collapsing the data across the two arthritis columns (see Table 21.7 and text for details). Panel C summarises the chi-square analysis of the heart disease data from Table 21.8 together with analysis by Fisher's exact test, respectively.

*Source*: InVivoStat.

## Minitab

**A**

| | Pink | Orange | White | All |
|---|---|---|---|---|
| 1 | 26 | 40 | 32 | 98 |
| | 16.56 | 42.24 | 39.20 | |
| | 2.3202 | −0.3449 | −1.1500 | |
| | 5.3833 | 0.1189 | 1.3224 | |
| 2 | 14 | 57 | 49 | 120 |
| | 20.28 | 51.72 | 48.00 | |
| | −1.3937 | 0.7336 | 0.1443 | |
| | 1.9425 | 0.5381 | 0.0208 | |
| 3 | 9 | 28 | 35 | 72 |
| | 12.17 | 31.03 | 28.80 | |
| | −0.9076 | −0.5447 | 1.1553 | |
| | 0.8237 | 0.2967 | 1.3347 | |
| All | 49 | 125 | 116 | 290 |

### Chi-square test

| | Chi-square | DF | P-value |
|---|---|---|---|
| Pearson | 11.781 | 4 | 0.019 |
| Likelihood ratio | 11.296 | 4 | 0.023 |

Cell Contents
  Count
  Expected count
  Standardized residual
  Contribution to Chi-square

**B**

| | Healthy | Rheumatoid | Osteo | All |
|---|---|---|---|---|
| 1 | 143 | 13 | 4 | 160 |
| | 135.38 | 15.04 | 9.57 | |
| | 0.6545 | −0.5267 | −1.8011 | |
| | 0.4284 | 0.2774 | 3.2441 | |
| 2 | 55 | 9 | 10 | 74 |
| | 62.62 | 6.96 | 4.43 | |
| | −0.9624 | 0.7744 | 2.6484 | |
| | 0.9262 | 0.5998 | 7.0142 | |
| All | 198 | 22 | 14 | 234 |

### Chi-square test

| | Chi-square | DF | P-value |
|---|---|---|---|
| Pearson | 12.490 | 2 | 0.002 |
| Likelihood Ratio | 11.541 | 2 | 0.003 |

1 cell(s) with expected counts less than 5.

Cell Contents
  Count
  Expected count
  Standardized residual
  Contribution to Chi-square

| | Healthy | Arthritic | All |
|---|---|---|---|
| 1 | 143 | 17 | 160 |
| | 135.38 | 24.62 | |
| | 0.6545 | −1.5349 | |
| | 0.4284 | 2.3560 | |
| 2 | 55 | 19 | 74 |
| | 62.62 | 11.38 | |
| | −0.9624 | 2.2570 | |
| | 0.9262 | 5.0941 | |
| All | 198 | 36 | 234 |

### Chi-square test

| | Chi-square | DF | P-value |
|---|---|---|---|
| Pearson | 8.805 | 1 | 0.003 |
| Likelihood Ratio | 8.264 | 1 | 0.004 |

Cell Contents
  Count
  Expected count
  Standardized residual
  Contribution to Chi-square

**C**

| | Dead | Alive | All |
|---|---|---|---|
| 1 | 440 | 921 | 1361 |
| | 400.4 | 960.6 | |
| | 1.977 | −1.276 | |
| | 3.908 | 1.629 | |
| 2 | 350 | 974 | 1324 |
| | 389.6 | 934.4 | |
| | −2.004 | 1.294 | |
| | 4.017 | 1.675 | |
| All | 790 | 1895 | 2685 |

### Chi-square test

| | Chi-square | DF | P-value |
|---|---|---|---|
| Pearson | 11.228 | 1 | 0.001 |
| Likelihood Ratio | 11.248 | 1 | 0.001 |

### Fisher's exact test

| P-value |
|---|
| 0.0008210 |

Cell Contents
  Count
  Expected count
  Standardized residual
  Contribution to Chi-square

Summary statistical analysis from MiniTab, v18. Panel A summarises the chi-square analysis of the tablet colour preference data from Table 21.3. Panel B summarises the chi-square analysis of the rheumatoid and osteoarthritis data from Table 21.6 together with the analysis after collapsing the data across the two arthritis columns (see Table 21.7 and text for details). Panel C summarises the chi-square analysis of the heart disease data from Table 21.8 including analysis by Fisher's exact test.

*Source*: Minitab, LLC.

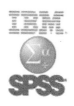

**A**

**Tablet_Age \* Tablet_Colour Crosstabulation**

| | | | Tablet_Colour | | | |
| --- | --- | --- | --- | --- | --- | --- |
| | | | Orange | Pink | White | Total |
| Tablet_Age | 18-35 | Count | 40a | 26a | 32a | 98 |
| | | Expected Count | 42.2 | 16.6 | 39.2 | 98.0 |
| | | Standardized Residual | -.3449 | 2.3202 | -1.1590 | |
| | 36-60 | Count | 57a | 14a | 49a | 120 |
| | | Expected Count | 51.7 | 20.3 | 48.0 | 120.0 |
| | | Standardized Residual | .7336 | -1.3937 | .1443 | |
| | 60-90 | Count | 28a | 9a | 35a | 72 |
| | | Expected Count | 31.0 | 12.2 | 28.8 | 72.0 |
| | | Standardized Residual | -.5447 | -.9076 | 1.1553 | |
| Total | | Count | 125 | 49 | 116 | 290 |
| | | Expected Count | 125.0 | 49.0 | 116.0 | 290.0 |

Each subscript letter denotes a subset of Tablet_Colour categories whose column proportions do not differ significantly from each other at the .05 level.

**Chi-Square Tests**

| | Value | df | Asymptotic Significance (2-sided) |
| --- | --- | --- | --- |
| Pearson Chi-Square | 11.781a | 4 | .019 |
| Likelihood Ratio | 11.296 | 4 | .023 |
| N of Valid Cases | 290 | | |

a. 0 cells (0.0%) have expected count less than 5. The minimum expected count is 12.17.

**B**

**Status \* Gender Crosstabulation**

| | | | Gender | | |
| --- | --- | --- | --- | --- | --- |
| | | | Female | Male | Total |
| Status | Healthy | Count | 55a | 143b | 198 |
| | | Expected Count | 62.6 | 135.4 | 198.0 |
| | | Standardized Residual | -1.0 | .7 | |
| | Osteo | Count | 10a | 4b | 14 |
| | | Expected Count | 4.4 | 9.6 | 14.0 |
| | | Standardized Residual | 2.6 | -1.8 | |
| | Rheumat. | Count | 9a | 13a | 22 |
| | | Expected Count | 7.0 | 15.0 | 22.0 |
| | | Standardized Residual | .8 | -.5 | |
| Total | | Count | 74 | 160 | 234 |
| | | Expected Count | 74.0 | 160.0 | 234.0 |

Each subscript letter denotes a subset of Gender categories whose column proportions do not differ significantly from each other at the .05 level.

**Chi-Square Tests**

| | Value | df | Asymptotic Significance (2-sided) |
| --- | --- | --- | --- |
| Pearson Chi-Square | 12.490a | 2 | .002 |
| Likelihood Ratio | 11.541 | 2 | .003 |
| N of Valid Cases | 234 | | |

a. 1 cells (16.7%) have expected count less than 5. The minimum expected count is 4.43.

**Status2 \* Gender_2 Crosstabulation**

| | | | Gender_2 | | |
| --- | --- | --- | --- | --- | --- |
| | | | Female | Male | Total |
| Status2 | Arthrit | Count | 19a | 17b | 36 |
| | | Expected Count | 11.4 | 24.6 | 36.0 |
| | | Standardized Residual | 2.3 | -1.5 | |
| | Healthy | Count | 55a | 143b | 198 |
| | | Expected Count | 62.6 | 135.4 | 198.0 |
| | | Standardized Residual | -1.0 | .7 | |
| Total | | Count | 74 | 160 | 234 |
| | | Expected Count | 74.0 | 160.0 | 234.0 |

Each subscript letter denotes a subset of Gender_2 categories whose column proportions do not differ significantly from each other at the .05 level.

**Chi-Square Tests**

| | Value | df | Asymptotic Significance (2-sided) | Exact Sig. (2-sided) | Exact Sig. (1-sided) |
| --- | --- | --- | --- | --- | --- |
| Pearson Chi-Square | 8.905a | 1 | .003 | | |
| Continuity Correction b | 7.686 | 1 | .006 | | |
| Likelihood Ratio | 8.264 | 1 | .004 | | |
| Fisher's Exact Test | | | | .006 | .003 |
| N of Valid Cases | 234 | | | | |

a. 0 cells (0.0%) have expected count less than 5. The minimum expected count is 11.38.
b. Computed only for a 2x2 table

**C**

**Treatment \* DorA Crosstabulation**

| | | | DorA | | |
| --- | --- | --- | --- | --- | --- |
| | | | Alive | Dead | Total |
| Treatment | Drug | Count | 921a | 440a | 1361 |
| | | Expected Count | 960.6 | 400.4 | 1361.0 |
| | | Standardized Residual | -1.3 | 2.0 | |
| | Surgery | Count | 974a | 350a | 1324 |
| | | Expected Count | 934.4 | 389.6 | 1324.0 |
| | | Standardized Residual | 1.3 | -2.0 | |
| Total | | Count | 1895 | 790 | 2685 |
| | | Expected Count | 1895.0 | 790.0 | 2685.0 |

Each subscript letter denotes a subset of DorA categories whose column proportions do not differ significantly from each other at the .05 level.

**Chi-Square Tests**

| | Value | df | Asymptotic Significance (2-sided) | Exact Sig. (2-sided) | Exact Sig. (1-sided) |
| --- | --- | --- | --- | --- | --- |
| Pearson Chi-Square | 11.228a | 1 | .001 | | |
| Continuity Correction b | 10.946 | 1 | .001 | | |
| Likelihood Ratio | 11.248 | 1 | .001 | | |
| Fisher's Exact Test | | | | .001 | .000 |
| N of Valid Cases | 2685 | | | | |

a. 0 cells (0.0%) have expected count less than 5. The minimum expected count is 389.56.
b. Computed only for a 2x2 table

Summary statistical analysis from SPSS, v27. Panel A summarises the chi-square analysis of the tablet colour preference data from Table 21.3. Panel B summarises the chi-square analysis of the rheumatoid and osteoarthritis data from Table 21.6 together with the analysis after collapsing the data across the two arthritis columns (see Table 21.7 and text for details). Panel C summarises the chi-square analysis of the heart disease data from Table 21.8 including analysis by Fisher's exact test.

*Source*: IBM Corporation.

# Decision Flowchart 3: Inferential Statistics – Tests of Association

| Test type and data distribution | Test of Association | Group type | | Inferential test |
|---|---|---|---|---|
| Parametric (Normal distribution) | Correlation | Independent | ⬆ | Pearson's product-moment correlation test (Chapter 19) |
| | Regression | Independent and dependent | ⬆ | Linear regression (Chapter 20) |

| | | | | |
|---|---|---|---|---|
| Non-parametric (Non-normal or distribution unknown) | Correlation | Independent | ⬆ | Spearman's test (tied ranks) Spearman's test (no tied ranks) Kendall's test (Chapter 19) |
| | Categorical | Independent | ⬆ | Chi-square test (Chapter 21) |

# 22 Confidence intervals

Throughout this book, I have described different inferential statistical tests whereby 2 or more groups of data may be compared, either to determine the *probability* that the groups were similar (or not!) or whether there was any level of *association* or *relationship* between them. One of the problems with the tests described so far lies in the random nature of the experimental samples obtained, each of which are assumed to represent the population from which those samples were taken (see discussion in Chapter 4). Consequently, results from a single sample set will include statistical uncertainty which we try to overcome by increasing the sample size. However, this doesn't change the fact that samples will always provide imprecise estimates of the population. Furthermore, the focus of the inferential statistical tests described in this book concentrate on hypothesis testing (see Chapter 10) where data sets are compared to each other in relation to a statistical Null Hypothesis. It should be recognised that the results of statistical hypothesis testing rely on the arbitrary use of the 5% level of probability to define the two possible outcomes, i.e. either accept or reject the Null Hypothesis, to conclude a significant difference, or not, between two or more groups. In fact, the *p* value determined by inferential statistical tests fails to convey anything about the *size* of the differences between experimental groups. For example, statistical significance may be attributed to the small, inconsequential, differences between groups with large sample sizes, while large, important, differences between groups may be non-significant due to the small sample sizes used.

## Overview

In contrast to a single value estimate such as the sample mean, a **confidence interval** is an estimate that proposes a range of values for a parameter where there is a specified probability in which the true value of the parameter lies within. The rationale for using confidence intervals, therefore, is that they allow the reporting of experimental details on the original measurement scale with information on the imprecise variability due to sampling. The confidence interval thereby indicates the boundary, in the appropriate experimental units, within which the population will be contained.

There is a strong argument that confidence intervals are relevant whenever sampled data are used to infer the relationship of experimental results to the whole world. The calculated confidence interval provides a range of values within which we will have confidence, at a level of *our* choosing, that it will contain the value of the population. So, while the sample estimate of the population will be imprecise, the degree of imprecision will be indicated by the width of the confidence interval which depends on three factors,

**1** Variability – the less variable the data (see Precision and Accuracy in Chapter 2), the more precise the sample estimate and the narrower the confidence interval.
**2** Sample size – the larger the sample size, the more precise the estimate and consequently the narrower the confidence interval.

**3** Required degree of confidence – the level of confidence is directly related to the size of the confidence interval; the greater the confidence (e.g. 99% compared to 95%), the wider the confidence interval.

In Chapter 5, I introduced the branch of statistical analysis where various values derived from our data may be used to describe our data, i.e. Descriptive Statistics. For data that follows a normal distribution, we usually use the mean value together with either the Standard Deviation or Standard Error of the Mean. It is worth reminding ourselves at this point exactly what we mean by these terms.

- *Mean*: this is the average of the data set. But remember, there are three different mean values (arithmetic, geometric, and harmonic) so it may de important to define which mean value you use in your reports.
- *Standard Deviation*: this value reflects the spread of the data and is, in turn, derived from the Sum of Squares and variance of the data set. Consequently, the larger the Standard Deviation, then the greater the spread of data around the sample mean.
- *Standard Error of the Mean*: this value reflects the level of confidence in the position of the sample mean. Consequently, the larger the Standard Error of the Mean, the greater the uncertainty in the value of the *sample* mean as truly representing the *population* mean.

It is important to remember that the Standard Error of the Mean depends on the Standard Deviation and the sample size (and hence also on the Sum of Square and variance) and, consequently, we should accept that it is unlikely to determine the exact value of the population mean. The Standard Error of the Mean is therefore a measure of imprecision in the value of the sample mean! As such the Standard Error of the Mean is of little importance and is really only favoured in summary data (either in text or plotted on figures in published manuscripts, experimental reports etc.) because the size of the error bars is shorter than those that represent the Standard Deviation, thereby conveying the highly questionable impression that the data are precise, accurate, and of high quality. However, the Standard Error of the Mean is useful in that it is used to calculate the confidence interval.

Previously, at the beginning of Chapter 4, we met the *Central Limit Theorem*, and to refresh your memory, this states that as the number of samples taken from a population increases so the mean of those sampled values approximates the true population mean. Furthermore, if the number of samples is large (usually taken to be *greater* than $n = 30$), then the sampling distribution has a normal distribution with a sample mean equal to the population mean. However, when the sample size is relatively small (i.e. $n < 30$), then the sampling distribution is not normal and instead has a different shape known as the *t*-distribution. Furthermore, as the degrees of freedom of the *t*-distribution increase, so the shape of the resulting sampling distribution approximates towards the normal distribution (see Figure 4.9). This has, as we shall see below, important consequences for calculating the confidence intervals of sampled data.

## Example 22.1 Calculating confidence intervals for large sample sizes ($n \geq 30$).

To calculate the confidence interval of a given set of data, we first need to decide the limits within which a percentage of the sample means will fall. Typically, we use limits such as 95 or 99% (although sometimes 99.9% may be required). As described above, we know that the sampling distribution of means for large samples will be normal. We also know that the *Standard Normal Distribution* has a mean of 0 and a standard deviation of 1 (see Chapter 7) and this information is extremely useful since it allows us to compute either the probability of a particular score occurring or the limits within which a particular percentage of scores will fall. For example, for a standard normal distribution with mean of 0 and a standard deviation of 1, we know that 95% of the area under the curve lies between −1.96 and +1.96 z-scores either side of the mean (see Figure 10.1), while 99% lies between *z-scores* of −2.58 to +2.58 (see also Appendix B). It is very rare that our experimental data will result in a mean of 0 and a standard deviation of 1, but we can convert our values to z scores by the following equation;

$$z = \frac{x - \bar{x}}{s} \tag{22.1}$$

where $\bar{x}$ is the mean and $s$ is the standard deviation.

If we replace the value of $z$ in the equation above by the appropriate *z-scores* for our desired percentage interval, i.e. −1.96 and +1.96 for the 95% interval, then we get two equations, as follows,

$$\text{Lower value}: -1.96 = \frac{x - \bar{x}}{s}$$
$$\text{Upper value}: +1.96 = \frac{x - \bar{x}}{s} \tag{22.2}$$

Re-arranging in terms of $x$,

$$-1.96 \times s = x - \bar{x} \qquad +1.96 \times s = x - \bar{x} \tag{22.3}$$

$$(-1.96 \times s) + \bar{x} = x \qquad (+1.96 \times s) + \bar{x} = x \tag{22.4}$$

So, once we know the standard deviation, $s$, and the mean, $\bar{x}$, of the set of data, then we can calculate the value of the upper and lower limits of the 95% confidence interval for the *individual observations* in the set of data.

However, in this discussion, we are more interested in the confidence limits due to the variability of the sample means and so we use the standard error of the mean rather than the standard deviation of the data set. The standard error of the mean is simply the standard deviation divided by the square root of the number of observations. Thus,

$$\text{Standard error of the mean (SEM)} = \frac{s}{\sqrt{n}} \tag{22.5}$$

The lower value of the 95% confidence interval is now defined as the mean minus 1.96 times the standard error of the mean, whereas the upper boundary is the mean plus 1.96 times the standard error of the mean, thus

$$\text{Lower boundary value}: \quad \bar{x} - (1.96 \times \text{SEM}) \tag{22.6}$$

$$\text{Upper boundary value}: \quad \bar{x} + (1.96 \times \text{SEM}) \tag{22.7}$$

Of course, as a consequence, the mean value is always at the centre of the confidence interval. Furthermore, if the interval is very small, then the sample mean must be very close to the true population mean, but if the confidence interval is large, then there may be a large difference between the sample mean and the true population mean.

If we wished to calculate the 99% confidence interval for our data, then we simply substitute the *z-score* value of 2.58 into equations 22.6 and 22.7, above.

As an example, look back at Chapter 5, Tables 5.1, and 5.2, which summarised the individual heights of 40 female and 33 male undergraduate students, respectively (notice that $n > 30$ for both groups). Later, I summarised the descriptive statistical data derived from these two sets of data (see Table 5.5).

Thus, the respective mean ± standard error of the mean values are as follows,

$$\text{Female}: \qquad 1.651 \pm 0.01105 \text{ m} \tag{22.8}$$

$$\text{Male}: \qquad 1.808 \pm 0.01016 \text{ m} \tag{22.9}$$

In contrast, the mean ± 95% confidence intervals are,
Female:

$$\text{Lower 95\% limit}; \quad 1.651 - (1.96 \times 0.01105) = 1.6293 \tag{22.10}$$

$$\text{Upper 95\% limit}; \quad 1.651 + (1.96 \times 0.01105) = 1.6727 \tag{22.11}$$

Male:

$$\text{Lower 95\% limit}; \quad 1.808 - (1.96 \times 0.01016) = 1.7881 \tag{22.12}$$

$$\text{Upper 95\% limit}; \quad 1.808 + (1.96 \times 0.01016) = 1.8999 \tag{22.13}$$

When confidence intervals are reported, the normal format is to quote the actual values of the lower and upper limits in parenthesis immediately following the mean value.

$$\text{General format}: \qquad \text{mean (lower limit, upper limit)} \tag{22.14}$$

$$\text{Female}: \qquad 1.651 \,(1.6293, 1.6727) \text{ m} \tag{22.15}$$

$$\text{Male}: \qquad 1.808 \,(1.7881, 1.8999) \text{ m} \tag{22.16}$$

Notice that there is no crossover in the range of the limits for the two sets of height data. From this, we can infer that the respective mean values for the height data from male and female students are from different populations.

## Example 22.2 Calculating confidence intervals for small sample sizes ($n < 30$).

The method described above to calculate the confidence intervals for large data sets is fine since the central limit theorem indicates that the sampling distribution of the mean values is normal. However, when $n$ is small, then the sampling distribution is not normal, and instead follows that of a *t*-distribution. Consequently, for small data sets, we use the appropriate value of $t$ (which depends on the degrees of freedom) to calculate the confidence interval rather than using the *z*-score.

Thus, the respective equations for small sample sizes may be summarised as,

Lower boundary value : $\qquad \bar{x} - (t_{n-1} \times \text{SEM})$ (22.17)

Upper boundary value : $\qquad \bar{x} + (t_{n-1} \times \text{SEM})$ (22.18)

where $n - 1$ is the degrees of freedom. For the 95% confidence intervals, we use the value of $t$ for a two-tailed test and a probability of 0.05 (see the critical values of the $t$-distribution provided in Appendix C).

As an example, look at Table 11.1 which summarised the locomotor activity of eight rats treated with Drug A compared to a control group, whereas Table 11.2 summarised the descriptive statistics of these data sets. The mean ± standard error of the mean locomotor activity of the treatment groups may be summarised as,

Control : $\qquad 603.0 \pm 25.60$ (22.19)

Drug A : $\qquad 368.5 \pm 25.42$ (22.20)

In contrast, the mean ± 95% confidence intervals are,
Control:

Lower 95% limit; $\qquad 603.0 - (2.365 \times 25.60) = 542.456$ (22.21)

Upper 95% limit; $\qquad 603.0 + (2.365 \times 25.60) = 663.544$ (22.22)

Drug A:

Lower 95% limit; $\qquad 368.5 - (2.365 \times 25.42) = 308.3817$ (22.23)

Upper 95% limit; $\qquad 368.5 + (2.365 \times 25.42) = 428.6183$ (22.24)

where the critical value of $t$ (with 7 degrees of freedom at $p = 0.05$) is equal to 2.365.

These values may be further summarised as,

Control : $\qquad 603.0\ (542.456, 663.544)$ (22.25)

Drug A : $\qquad 368.5\ (308.382, 428.618)$ (22.26)

As we saw with the previous example, you should note the lack of crossover between the respective range of the confidence intervals, and similarly we can infer that the respective mean values for the locomotor activity exhibited by the two groups of rats are from different populations.

## Statistical significance of confidence intervals

Of course, the last statement begs the question '*How significantly different are these two sets of data?*'. The general assumption is that if the 95% confidence intervals do not overlap, then the respective means come from different populations and are therefore significantly different at the *assumed* level of $p < 0.05$. In fact, the following general guidelines apply;

**1** If there is a *moderate* overlap of the 95% confidence limits, then you may conclude that the probability of the Null Hypothesis is true is $p < 0.05$! A moderate overlap is defined as half the length of the average *margin of error* (MOE). The MOE is the difference between the mean value and the length of the confidence interval in

one direction. So, if we take the *average* of the MOEs for each set of data, we wish to compare and half that value then that is the maximum amount of overlap we would accept for $p = 0.05$. For example, for the locomotor activity data above, the MOE for the control confidence interval is 60.5440 (i.e. $2.365 \times 25.60$; see equations above), while that for the Drug A data is 60.1183 (i.e. $2.365 \times 25.42$), resulting in an average MOE equal to 60.33115. Consequently, if the maximum amount of overlap is half this value, i.e. a maximum of 30.166, then we would accept $p < 0.05$.
**2** If the confidence intervals just meet, then the $p$ value of the Null Hypothesis (i.e. probability of no difference between the mean values) is approximately 0.01.
**3** If there is a gap between the upper end of one confidence limit and the lower end of the other, then $p < 0.01$.

## Example 22.3 Confidence interval of differences between two independent groups

A similar method to those described above may be applied to the difference in the sample mean values from two groups. The first step is to calculate the *pooled estimate* of the standard deviation according to the formula (see also Chapter 11).

$$s_p = \sqrt{\frac{(n_1 - 1)s_1^2 + (n_2 - 1)s_2^2}{n_1 + n_2 - 2}}$$ (22.27)

where $s_1^2$ and $s_2^2$ are the variance values for the two groups, respectively, and $n_1$ and $n_2$ are the respective sample sizes.

This allows calculation of the standard error for the difference between the two mean values,

$$\text{SEM}(d) = s_p \times \sqrt{\frac{1}{n_1} + \frac{1}{n_2}}$$ (22.28)

where $d$ is the difference between the mean values, $\bar{x}_1 - \bar{x}_2$.

The confidence interval for the difference in the two sets of data is given by

Lower boundary value : $\qquad d - (t \times \text{SEM}(d))$ (22.29)

Upper boundary value : $\qquad d + (t \times \text{SEM}(d))$ (22.30)

where $t$ is the critical value of the $t$-distribution for $n_1 + n_2 - 2$ degrees of freedom for a two-tailed test the appropriate value of probability (e.g. 0.05).

Using data from Table 11.2 to examine the difference between the mean values of locomotor activity expressed by control and Drug A-treated rats (i.e. $603.0 - 368.5 = 234.5$), then the pooled standard deviation equals

$$s_p = \sqrt{\frac{7 \times 5244 + 7 \times 5170.57}{8 + 8 - 2}}$$ (22.31)

$$s_p = \sqrt{\frac{72901.99}{14}} = \sqrt{5207.285} = 72.1615$$ (22.32)

while the standard error of the mean equals

$$\text{SEM}(d) = 72.1615 \times \sqrt{\frac{1}{8} + \frac{1}{8}}$$ (22.33)

$$\text{SEM}(d) = 72.1615 \times \sqrt{0.25} = 36.08$$ (22.34)

Consequently,

Lower boundary value :     $234.5 - (2.145 \times 36.08) = 157.11$

$$(22.35)$$

Upper boundary value :     $234.5 + (2.145 \times 36.08) = 311.89$

$$(22.36)$$

So, the 95% confidence interval of the difference between the two mean values is from 157.11 to 311.89.

## Example 22.4 Confidence interval of differences between two paired groups

Previously, I discussed how the paired $t$-test may be used to compare two sets of observations from the same experimental subjects. The example experiment looked at the effect of coffee on the resting heart rate of eight young adult males. We can also compute the confidence interval of the change in scores arising from paired data. Table 12.1 summarises the measurements in heart rate of the eight volunteers (see Chapter 12). To calculate the confidence interval of the change in heart rate scores, we use the formula for the single sample case described (see locomotor activity example above), where $\bar{x}$ and $s$ are the mean and standard deviation of the *differences* between the two sets of heart rate observations. From the data in Table 12.1,

Mean change in heart rate;    +4.125 beats per minute (bpm)
Standard deviation;    4.5806 bpm
Standard error    1.6195 bpm

The critical value of $t$ for the 95% confidence interval with 7 degrees of freedom (i.e. $n - 1$ pairs of observations) = 2.365. Therefore, the 95% confidence interval for the population value of the mean increase in heart rate after coffee is given by,

$$4.125 - (2.365 \times 1.6195) \text{ to } 4.125 + (2.365 \times 1.6195) \quad (22.37)$$

$$4.125 - 3.830 \text{ to } 4.125 + 3.830 \quad (22.38)$$

$$0.295 \text{ to } 7.955 \quad (22.39)$$

The mean increase in heart rate with 95% confidence limits may therefore be summarised as,

$$4.125 \, (0.295, 7.955) \text{ bpm} \quad (22.40)$$

## Example 22.5 Confidence intervals and correlation

In chapter 19, I discussed a number of methods of performing correlation analysis to examine the relationship or association between two variables, and in Example 19.1, I described two procedures to determine the probability of the Null Hypothesis. The second of these uses $z$-scores derived from the Pearson correlation coefficient, $r$ (see Chapter 19), according to the formula;

$$z_r = \frac{1}{2} \log_e \left( \frac{1+r}{1-r} \right) \quad (22.41)$$

with a standard error;

$$SE_{z_r} = \frac{1}{\sqrt{N-3}} \quad (22.42)$$

With these values, we can now compute the 95% confidence intervals; thus,

$$\text{Lower boundary} = z_r - (1.96 \times SE_{z_r}) \quad (22.43)$$

$$\text{Upper boundary} = z_r + (1.96 \times SE_{z_r}) \quad (22.44)$$

For the data given in Example 19.1 and Table 19.1,

$$z_r = 1.391 \quad (22.45)$$

and

$$SE_{z_r} = 0.408 \quad (22.46)$$

Therefore,

$$\text{Lower boundary} = 1.391 - (1.96 \times 0.408) = 0.59132 \quad (22.47)$$

$$\text{Upper boundary} = 1.391 + (1.96 \times 0.408) = 2.19068 \quad (22.48)$$

We must now convert these upper and lower boundary values from the $z_r$ metric back to a correlation coefficient;

$$\text{Lower boundary} = \frac{e^{2 \times z_r} - 1}{e^{2 \times z_r} + 1} = \frac{e^{2 \times 0.59132} - 1}{e^{2 \times 0.59132} + 1} \quad (22.49)$$

$$\frac{e^{1.18264} - 1}{e^{1.18264} + 1} = \frac{2.263}{4.263} = 0.531 \quad (22.50)$$

$$\text{Upper boundary} = \frac{e^{2 \times z_r} - 1}{e^{2 \times z_r} + 1} = \frac{e^{2 \times 2.19068} - 1}{e^{2 \times 2.19068} + 1} \quad (22.51)$$

$$\frac{e^{4.38136} - 1}{e^{4.38136} + 1} = \frac{78.947}{80.947} = 0.975 \quad (22.52)$$

Consequently, the Pearson correlation coefficient for Example 19.1 with 95% confidence limits may be expressed as;

$$r = 0.8835 \, (0.531, 0.975) \quad (22.53)$$

# 23 Permutation test of exact inference

The Permutation Test (sometimes referred to as the *Randomisation Test*) provides a further alternative method to the established inferential statistical tests to examine whether two or more groups of data are similar (where upon the Null Hypothesis is accepted) or dissimilar to such an extent that the Null Hypothesis is rejected in favour of the Alternate Hypothesis.

## Rationale

If we randomly divide a series of samples from a population into two groups and calculate the respective group means, then the Null Hypothesis is that there is no difference between the means of those two groups and we can test this hypothesis by applying the independent *t*-test (see Chapter 11). As a consequence of the Null Hypothesis and that all observations were taken at random from the same population, then all the observations in the two groups are interchangeable and the Null Hypothesis will *always* be true. Furthermore, by examining all the possible permutations of dividing the samples into two groups, we are able to calculate the exact probability of each permutation.

## Example 23.1 A simple hypothetical data set

To demonstrate this, let's consider a simple example. Consider the following hypothetical set of data where the first three subjects are the control group and the second three subjects are our test group (see Table 23.1).

Table 23.1 Hypothetical control and test data.

| Group | Hypothetical data | | | | | |
|---|---|---|---|---|---|---|
| | Control | | | Test | | |
| Subject | A | B | C | D | E | F |
| Score | 1 | 2 | 2 | 4 | 5 | 5 |

We could, of course, compare these groups in a number of ways; by calculating the sum of scores in each group, by comparing the mean, median, or sum of the values in each group, or even by comparing the groups by either an independent *t*-test or a Mann–Whitney *U*-test, as summarised in Table 23.2.

Table 23.2 Summary of hypothetical control and test data.

| | Control | Test |
|---|---|---|
| Mean | 1.667 | 4.667 |
| Median | 2 | 5 |
| Sum | 5 | 14 |
| *t*-test | $t(4) = -6.364, p = 0.003$ | |
| MW *U*-test | $U = 0.000, p = 0.043$ | |

Independent *t*-test and Mann–Whitney *U*-test by SPSS, v26.

However, permutation theory provides an alternative way of looking at the data. For example, let us consider the *sum* of the values in the control and test groups from Table 23.1. Here the data values for the control are labelled as A, B, and C, while the test group data are labelled as D, E, and F, and the sum of the data in each group are 5 and 14, respectively. In the permutation test, the experimental groups from which the observations are taken are ignored and all possible permutations of the values in the complete data set are examined which allows us to determine the probability of how often an observed sum value will occur. Table 23.3 lists all the possible permutations of the six observations divided into two equal groups of three observations per group (note that the first arrangement is the grouping of our hypothetical observations into the control and test groups); for clarity the two groups are now labelled as Group 1 and Group 2, respectively.

Table 23.3 All possible permutations of hypothetical control and test data.

| Permutation | Group 1 observations | Sum | Group 2 observations | Sum | Difference (Gp2–Gp1) |
|---|---|---|---|---|---|
| 1 | ABC | 5 | DEF | 14 | 9 |
| 2 | ABD | 7 | CEF | 12 | 5 |
| 3 | ABE | 8 | CDF | 11 | 3 |
| 4 | ABF | 8 | CDE | 11 | 3 |
| 5 | ACD | 7 | BEF | 12 | 5 |
| 6 | ACE | 8 | BDF | 11 | 3 |
| 7 | ACF | 8 | BDE | 11 | 3 |
| 8 | ADE | 10 | BEF | 9 | −1 |
| 9 | ADF | 10 | BCE | 9 | −1 |
| 10 | AEF | 11 | BCD | 8 | −3 |
| 11 | BCD | 8 | AEF | 11 | 3 |
| 12 | BCE | 9 | ADF | 10 | 1 |
| 13 | BCF | 9 | ADE | 10 | 1 |
| 14 | BDE | 11 | ACF | 8 | −3 |
| 15 | BDF | 11 | ACE | 8 | −3 |
| 16 | BEF | 12 | ACD | 7 | −5 |
| 17 | CDE | 11 | ABF | 8 | −3 |
| 18 | CDF | 11 | ABE | 8 | −3 |
| 19 | CEF | 12 | ABD | 7 | −5 |
| 20 | DEF | 14 | ABC | 5 | −9 |

The first point to notice is that there are only (!) 20 possible permutations of dividing the 6 observations into 2 groups of 3 observations per group without repetition. The total number of permutations is calculated according to the formula:

$$\text{Number of permutations} = \frac{N!}{(n_1)!(n_2)!} \quad (23.1)$$

where $N$ indicates the total number of observations, and $n_1$ and $n_2$ indicate the number of observations in each group (i.e. $N = n_1 + n_2$).

*Experimental Design and Statistical Analysis for Pharmacology and the Biomedical Sciences*, First Edition. Paul J. Mitchell.

Note that these are factorial numbers as indicated by the ! sign. Therefore,

$$\text{Number of permutations} = \frac{6!}{(3)!(3)!} = \frac{720}{6 \times 6} = \frac{720}{36} = 20$$

$$(23.2)$$

Since there are only 20 different permutations, the probability of each permutation occurring is $1/20 = 5\%$ (i.e. $p = 0.05$). However, if we consider the various differences between the sum of the values, then the probability for each difference value may be summarised as follows (see Table 23.4).

Table 23.4 All possible permutations of hypothetical control and test data.

| Difference | Permutation numbers | Total probability |
|---|---|---|
| 9 | 1 | 0.05 |
| 5 | 2, 5 | 0.10 |
| 3 | 3, 4, 6, 7, 11 | 0.25 |
| 1 | 12, 13 | 0.10 |
| −1 | 8, 9 | 0.10 |
| −3 | 10, 14, 15, 17, 18 | 0.25 |
| −5 | 16, 19 | 0.10 |
| −9 | 20 | 0.05 |

Difference values are the differences between the sum values for each group according to the permutation numbers listed in Table 23.3.

If we now refer back to Table 23.1, where our control data comprised of samples A, B, and C (sum = 5), while the test data samples were D, E, and F (sum = 14), then the *exact* probability of this arrangement occurring is $1/20 = 0.05$ (see Table 23.3, permutation 1). Likewise, the probability of a difference between the sum of the two groups of +9 (where the test group is 9 units *greater* than the control group, i.e. permutation 1) is also 0.05, while the probability of the test group being *at least* five units greater than the control group is 0.15 (see Table 23.4, permutations 1, 2, and 5). Consequently, the result of the permutation test agrees with the pairwise comparisons using the independent *t*-test or Mann–Whitney *U*-test (see Table 23.2). It is important to note, however, that while the *t*-test generally assumes random sampling of our individual subjects which are then randomly assigned to the treatment groups, such assumptions do not apply to the permutation test because all possible permutations are included. This is a very simple example, but it does demonstrate the important aspect of the permutation test in that if all possible permutations of the data are examined then it enables the determination of the *exact* probability of how often the observed value is likely to occur.

*But therein lies the problem.*

The total number of permutations depends on the respective factorial values (for example see Table 23.5) of the total number of subjects in the experiment, the number of different groups, and the number of subjects/observations in each group and may be calculated according to the general equation:

$$\text{Number of permutations} = \frac{N!}{n_1! n_2! n_3! \ldots n_k!} \quad (23.3)$$

where $N$ is the total number of subjects or observations for $k$ groups where there are $n_i$ observations in group $i$ (and $i = 1, 2, 3 \ldots$ to $k$).

Table 23.6 summarises the total number of permutations, without repetition, according to different experimental designs each with different numbers of groups and numbers of subjects per

Table 23.5 Example factorial values.

| N | Factorial N (i.e. N!) |
|---|---|
| 1 | 1 |
| 2 | 2 |
| 3 | 6 |
| 4 | 24 |
| 5 | 120 |
| 6 | 720 |
| 7 | 5040 |
| 8 | 40 320 |
| 9 | 362 880 |
| 10 | 3 628 800 |
| 15 | 1 307 674 368 000 |
| 20 | 2 432 902 008 177 000 000 |

Table 23.6 Example total permutations, without repetition.

| Number of groups | Subjects per group | $\dfrac{N!}{n_1! n_2! n_3! \ldots n_k!}$ |
|---|---|---|
| 2 | 4 | $\dfrac{8!}{4!4!} = \dfrac{40\ 320}{24^2} = \dfrac{40\ 320}{576} = 70$ |
| 2 | 6 | $\dfrac{12!}{6!6!} = \dfrac{479\ 001\ 600}{720^2} = 924$ |
| 2 | 8 | $\dfrac{16!}{8!8!} = \dfrac{20\ 922\ 789\ 888\ 000}{40\ 320^2} = 1\ 625\ 702\ 400$ |
| 3 | 6 | $\dfrac{18!}{6!6!6!} = \dfrac{6\ 402\ 373\ 705\ 728\ 000}{720^3}$ <br> $= 17\ 153\ 136$ |
| 4 | 6 | $\dfrac{24!}{6!6!6!6!} = \dfrac{6.204484 \times 10^{23}}{2.6873856 \times 10^{11}}$ <br> $= 2.308743493 \times 10^{12}$ |
| 5 | 6 | $\dfrac{30!}{6!6!6!6!6!} = \dfrac{2.6525286 \times 10^{32}}{1.934917362 \times 10^{14}}$ <br> $= 1.3708742 \times 10^{18}$ |

group that are typically used in pharmacological experiments (I have used equal number of subjects in each case to demonstrate good experimental design!).

It is clear from Table 23.6 with increasing total number of subjects and increasing number of groups, the total number of possible permutations becomes unwieldly. Consequently, the permutation test, even with reasonable group and subject numbers, is only practical with access to high-speed and high-power computers due to the high number of permutations involved, where even a simple experiment involving three groups of six subjects per group would involve over 17 million permutations to compute. In practice, if it is not possible to compute all the possible permutations without repetition, then a random selection of 1000–2000 of the possible permutations is usually sufficient to obtain a reasonable approximation of the *p*-value (this process is sometimes referred to as the *Monte Carlo* version of the permutation test).

The advantage of the permutation test is that it is a very elegant method to calculate the *exact* probability of obtaining two (or more) sets of data where the differences in the respective values are equal to or greater than the desired difference between the groups.

I have yet to come across a generally available statistical package that includes the permutation test to analyse experimental data; however, there are various websites that enable data to be analysed by this method.

# 24 General Linear Model

**O**K, it's admission time!

If you've managed to read this book all the way through to this final chapter (or perhaps you just dipped in whenever you felt the need – and that's equally OK), then you probably have the impression that I have spent a lifetime immersed in statistical theory and application.

Oh, my poor misguided reader, you couldn't be further from the truth!

In fact, I've never had any formal training in statistics! Everything I know about this subject is based on learning statistical analysis 'on-the-hoof' in order to apply the correct statistical method to the analysis of experimental data. To me, as it is for most experimental pharmacologists, statistics is simply a *tool* to understand what my experimental data are able to tell me about drug effects on whatever experimental output I am measuring (from changes in the tension in an isolated tissue preparation, changes in cardiovascular or respiratory function in anaesthetised whole animal preparations through to changes in social, agonistic, or consummatory behaviour in conscious animals) and also, *most importantly*, to stop me making a complete idiot of myself by drawing erroneous conclusions about the drugs I am studying.

Consequently, my knowledge of statistical analysis is really based on a need-to-know basis, and the style and structure of this book reflects that. Indeed, this approach is very 'traditional' where the nature of the data (continuous, rank, or categorical data, number of groups, paired or independent) determines the appropriate statistic which is then used to test the Null Hypothesis (look back at the three aims of this book outlined at the end of the Foreword). Interestingly, however, the teaching of statistical method has become very polarised between the traditional method I use and an alternative approach based on linear regression; to my mind, both approaches have merit (a position not accepted by all statisticians, some of whom have a very blinkered and biased view and consequently favour one approach to the exclusion of the other).

Throughout this book, I have tried to present ways by which the use of descriptive and inferential statistics may be used to examine experimental data so that we may gain a greater understanding of the real world; does a change in the value of an **independent variable** (which may be viewed as a *predictor*) cause a change in the **dependent variable** (the experimental output, which is our observation, and may be viewed as the *outcome*)? In all cases, regardless of whether we calculated the mean, variance, standard deviation, or standard error of the mean, or compared two or more groups by *t*-test, ANOVA, correlation, or regression, we essentially used or developed a statistical model that enabled us to predict an outcome. In its most simple form, any statistical model may be described mathematically by the following equation which infers that any data we observe may be predicted by the model plus some degree of error;

$$\text{outcome} = (\text{model}) + \text{error} \qquad (24.1)$$

Here, the (model) relates to the design of your experiment, the type of data produced by the experiment, the objective of your model (e.g. comparison, similarity, association, etc.), and its complexity.

In general terms, statistical models are composed of *variables* and *parameters*. As we have seen throughout this book, variables are measured constructs whose values vary, e.g. dependent and independent variables (denoted by the symbols $Y$ and $X$, respectively), while parameters are constants (e.g. measures of central tendency like the mean or median or measures of association or the relationship between two variables like the correlation or regression coefficients), usually denoted by $b$.

So, we could re-write the equation above as

$$\text{outcome} = (b) + \text{error} \qquad (24.2)$$

if we wish to predict an outcome from a single parameter (e.g. the mean).

If, however, we want to predict the outcome from a variable (denoted by $X$) then we simply expand the equation which then becomes:

$$\text{outcome}_i = (b_0 + b_1 X_i) + \text{error} \qquad (24.3)$$

where the outcome is dependent not only on the parameter alone ($b_0$) but also from the predictor variable ($X$) whose value is modified by another parameter ($b_1$).

Now, let's just stop a minute (or longer if you're still trying to keep up!) and think back to Chapter 20 on regression analysis. In that chapter, the first equation I introduced was that which described the linear relationship between the variable $x$ and $y$; thus,

$$y = a + bx \qquad (24.4)$$

In this latter equation, we are able to predict the outcome ($y$) based on the value of a constant ($a$) and the value of a predictor ($x$) multiplied by another constant ($b$). If we assume zero error, then the *outcome*$_i$ equation given above (Equation 24.3) is exactly the same as the linear regression equation (Equation 24.4) used to predict values of $y$ (the **dependent** variable) based on measured values of $x$ (the **independent** variable), where $a$ is the intercept (or offset) along the x-axis and $b$ is the gradient of the slope (i.e. another constant that determines the relationship between $x$ and $y$). This is the basis of the **General Linear Model** (GLM) in statistics where $b_0$ and $b_1$ are the equivalents of $a$ and $b$, respectively.

In fact, we can keep adding predictor variables (with their associated parameters) to the general equation:

$$\text{outcome}_i = (b_0 + b_1 X_i + b_2 X_{2i} \ldots\ldots + b_n X_{ni}) + \text{error} \qquad (24.5)$$

## The General Linear Model and Descriptive Statistics

Let's return to the first equation and consider its relationship to a simple parameter, the mean. In fact, the mean is a hypothetical value in that it is calculated from the experimental observations we make. Indeed, it is not beyond the realms of possibility that in a given set of data, we do not make an observation that has

*Experimental Design and Statistical Analysis for Pharmacology and the Biomedical Sciences*, First Edition. Paul J. Mitchell.

the exact value of the mean. Consequently, all of the individual observations in the data set will contain a certain amount of error (i.e. difference) from the calculated mean value. Indeed, we could express equation 24.1 in terms of the error component; thus,

$$error_i = outcome_i - (model_i) \qquad (24.6)$$

Indeed, look back at Table 5.4 in Chapter 5 (surprise, surprise!), and you will see a list of *error* values between the calculated mean height of a group of 40 female undergraduate students and their individual height values (see column headed $\bar{x} - x$). So, our trusted mean value, which we use whenever we can as a measure of central tendency of our data, is purely hypothetical in that it is simply a statistical model we use to summarise our experimental data, and it contains an *error*!

In Chapter 5, I used the female height data not only to calculate the mean height value but also to calculate the sum of the differences from the mean, the sum of the squared values, and the variance, the equations for each of which may be expressed in terms of the error according to the statistical model and each observation; thus,

- the sum of the differences of the mean from each observation equals the sum of the individual errors;

$$\sum(x - \bar{x}) = \sum(outcome_i - model_i) \qquad (24.7)$$

- the sum of the square of the differences of the mean from each observation equals the sum of the squared errors;

$$\sum(x - \bar{x})^2 = \sum(outcome_i - model_i)^2 \qquad (24.8)$$

- the variance equals the mean squared error;

$$s^2 = \frac{\sum(x - \bar{x})^2}{n - 1} = \frac{\sum(outcome_i - model_i)^2}{n - 1} \qquad (24.9)$$

So, we can see how the General Linear Model relates to Descriptive Statistics, but how does this approach apply to Inferential Statistics when we wish to compare two or more sets of data?

## The General Linear Model and Inferential Statistics

When we wish to compare the differences between the mean values of two groups, we are essentially predicting an *outcome* that is dependent on membership of one group or the other. Remember that an Independent *t*-test (see Chapter 11) really examines whether the model (i.e. the difference between the two mean values) equals zero or not, and the value of *t* is determined by the general equation,

$$t = \frac{\bar{x}_1 - \bar{x}_2}{\text{estimate of the standard error of the difference between two sample means}} \qquad (24.10)$$

So how does the equation to calculate *t* relate to the general equation for the General Linear Model?

We have already seen that the general equation of

$$outcome_i = (b_0 + b_1 X_i) + error \qquad (24.11)$$

may be expressed as

$$Y_i = (b_0 + b_1 X_{1i}) + error_i \qquad (24.12)$$

where $b_0$ indicates the value of the outcome ($Y_i$) when the predictor variable ($X_{1i}$) is zero, and $b_1$ is the quantifiable relationship (a constant multiplier) between $X_{1i}$ and $Y_i$.

Let's apply this latter equation (Equation 24.12) to the rodent locomotor activity data summarised in Table 11.1, which examined the effect of Drug A on exploratory locomotor activity expressed by a group of eight rats compared to a Control group. In terms of the experiment, the equation may be expressed as

$$Locomotion = (b_0 + b_1\,Drug\,A) + error_i \qquad (24.13)$$

First, let's consider the Control group that were *not* treated with Drug A. Here the best estimate or prediction of the level of locomotor activity would be the group mean of the Control group (*i.e.* $\bar{X}_{Control}$) because this is the summary statistic that has the least squared error for the Control-treated rats. Consequently, the value of $Y_i$ in the equation above (Equation 24.12) would be $\bar{X}_{Control} = 603.0$ (see Table 11.2), and the value of $X_{1i}$ (i.e. Drug A) would be zero (i.e. no drug!). Consequently, Equation 24.12 becomes,

$$\bar{X}_{Control} = (b_0 + b_1\,Drug\,A) + error_i \qquad (24.14)$$

which, if we ignore the error term and Drug A = 0, in turn becomes,

$$\bar{X}_{Control} = b_0 + (b_1 \times 0) \qquad (24.15)$$

Thus,

$$\bar{X}_{Control} = b_0 = 603 \qquad (24.16)$$

We saw earlier that $b_0$ is the equivalent of $a$ in the linear regression equation (see Equation 24.4 and compare to Equation 24.3). Consequently, the intercept of the linear model (i.e. $b_0$) is equal to the mean of the Control group. We can now use this value to predict the level of locomotor activity expressed by rats treated with Drug A.

Thus, substituting the new values into Equation 24.14 where the predicted outcome is the group mean for the locomotor activity of rats treated with Drug A (i.e. $\bar{X}_{Drug\,A}$, again because this is the summary statistic for Drug A-treated rats with the least squared error value) and the value of Drug A equals 1 (i.e. drug present!), then Equation 24.14 becomes

$$\bar{X}_{Drug\,A} = (b_0 + b_1\,Drug\,A) \qquad (24.17)$$

$$\bar{X}_{Drug\,A} = b_0 + (b_1 \times 1) \qquad (24.18)$$

$$\bar{X}_{Drug\,A} = b_0 + b_1 \qquad (24.19)$$

We already know that $b_0$ equals $\bar{X}_{Control}$ (see above), so,

$$\bar{X}_{Drug\,A} = \bar{X}_{Control} + b_1 \qquad (24.20)$$

If we re-arrange in terms of $b_1$

$$b_1 = \bar{X}_{Drug\,A} - \bar{X}_{Control} \qquad (24.21)$$

Consequently, $b_1$ is the *difference* between the two group means; thus,

$$b_1 = 368.5 - 603 = -234.5 \qquad (24.22)$$

This is really important because it demonstrates that in a statistical model with two predictors, then $b_0$ is the mean value of one group (usually the control group), and $b_1$ is the *difference* between the two group means. Remember that in the context of the *t*-test, then the resulting *t*-statistic would examine whether the difference between the two group means is equal to zero. In GLM terms, therefore, the *t*-statistic examines whether $b_1 = 0$ or $b_1 \neq 0$!

We can extend this argument to apply to experimental situations where we have more than two groups. In Chapter 15, I described the one-way ANOVA model (where we have 1 Between-Group Factor). Table 15.11 summarised the effect of three different drugs administered to different groups of rats compared to a control group on systolic blood pressure.

In this situation, the General Linear Model may be summarised as

$$\text{outcome}_i = (b_0 + b_1X_i + b_2X_i + b_3X_i) + \text{error} \qquad (24.23)$$

First, we'll ignore the error term so that our equation becomes

$$\text{outcome}_i = (b_0 + b_1X_i + b_2X_i + b_3X_i) \qquad (24.24)$$

In terms of the outcome for each group (i.e. the respective group mean values since these are the respective summary descriptive statistics with the least squared error values), then each outcome may be expressed as follows (group mean values taken from Table 15.11);

Control:

$$\overline{X}_{\text{Control}} = b_0 + (b_1 \times 0) + (b_2 \times 0) + (b_3 \times 0) = b_0 = 1.000 \qquad (24.25)$$

Drug A:

$$\overline{X}_{\text{Drug A}} = b_0 + (b_1 \times 1) + (b_2 \times 0) + (b_3 \times 0) = b_0 + b_1 = -2.833 \qquad (24.26)$$

Therefore,

$$b_1 = \overline{X}_{\text{Drug A}} - \overline{X}_{\text{Control}} = -2.833 - 1.000 = -3.833 \qquad (24.27)$$

Drug B:

$$\overline{X}_{\text{Drug B}} = b_0 + (b_1 \times 0) + (b_2 \times 1) + (b_3 \times 0) = b_0 + b_2 = 7.500 \qquad (24.28)$$

Therefore,

$$b_2 = \overline{X}_{\text{Drug B}} - \overline{X}_{\text{Control}} = 7.500 - 1.000 = 6.500 \qquad (24.29)$$

Drug C:

$$\overline{X}_{\text{Drug C}} = b_0 + (b_1 \times 0) + (b_2 \times 0) + (b_3 \times 1) = b_0 + b_3 = 2.167 \qquad (24.30)$$

Therefore,

$$b_3 = \overline{X}_{\text{Drug C}} - \overline{X}_{\text{Control}} = 2.167 - 1.000 = 1.167 \qquad (24.31)$$

In any ANOVA test, it is important to remember that the $F$-statistic doesn't identify differences between the different group mean values. However, as can be seen above, the $b_0$ value is the group mean of the control group (or base category if there is no clear control group), while the remaining $b$ values ($b_1$, $b_2$, $b_3$) are the *differences* between the respective group mean values remaining groups and that of the control (or base) group.

There are many textbooks describing the General Linear Model approach to statistical analysis to which I refer you if this chapter has piqued your interest. As an introduction to this approach to statistics, I have now said all I need to say. The important point to realise from this chapter is that the General Linear Model may be applied to both Descriptive and Inferential statistics.

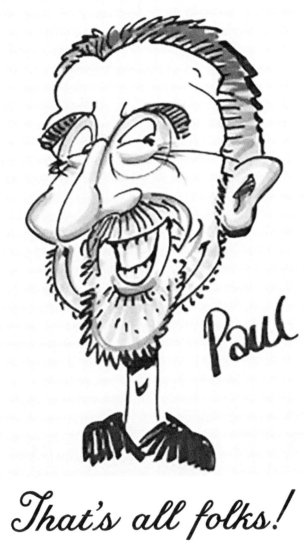

Paul

*That's all folks!*

# Appendix A: Data distribution: probability mass function and probability density functions

## A.1 Binomial distribution (Chapter 4.iii, Figure 4.4): Probability mass function

The binomial distribution with $n$ independent experiments, each with a success-failure result or question (where the respective probabilities are $p$ (for success) and $1 - p$ (for failure)) is the discrete probability distribution of the number of successes in a sequence of trials. The probability of obtaining a specific number of successes, $k$, in $n$ trials is given by the **probability mass function**, according to the formula;

$$\mathrm{Pr} = \binom{n}{k} p^k (1-p)^{n-k}$$

Where;

Pr = probability of success,

$$\binom{n}{k} = \frac{n!}{k!(n-k)!}$$

which is known as the **binomial coefficient,**

$p^k$ = probability of success ($p$) to the power of $k$ successes,

$(1-p)^{n-k}$ = probability of failure ($1 - p$) to the power of $n - k$ failures.

In the example provided in Chapter 4 (see Figure4.4), students were asked to count the number of heads (success) from 10 tosses ($n$) of a coin. Consequently, there could be $k = 0, 1, 2, 3,....10$ successful tosses of the coin (i.e. heads), with a corresponding $n-k = 10$, 9, 8, .....0 unsuccessful tosses of the coin (i.e. tails).

The first stage is to calculate the corresponding binomial coefficients for each number of possible successes. Thus,

| $k$ success | Factorial equations | | Binomial Coefficient |
|---|---|---|---|
| 0 | $\dfrac{10!}{0!10!}$ | $\dfrac{3\,628\,800}{1 \times 3\,628\,800}$ | 1 |
| 1 | $\dfrac{10!}{1!9!}$ | $\dfrac{3\,628\,800}{1 \times 362\,880}$ | 10 |
| 2 | $\dfrac{10!}{2!8!}$ | $\dfrac{3\,628\,800}{2 \times 40\,320}$ | 45 |
| 3 | $\dfrac{10!}{3!7!}$ | $\dfrac{3\,628\,800}{6 \times 5\,040}$ | 120 |
| 4 | $\dfrac{10!}{4!6!}$ | $\dfrac{3\,628\,800}{24 \times 720}$ | 210 |
| 5 | $\dfrac{10!}{5!5!}$ | $\dfrac{3\,628\,800}{120 \times 120}$ | 252 |
| 6 | $\dfrac{10!}{6!4!}$ | $\dfrac{3\,628\,800}{720 \times 24}$ | 210 |
| 7 | $\dfrac{10!}{7!3!}$ | $\dfrac{3\,628\,800}{5\,040 \times 6}$ | 120 |
| 8 | $\dfrac{10!}{8!2!}$ | $\dfrac{3\,628\,800}{40\,320 \times 2}$ | 45 |
| 9 | $\dfrac{10!}{9!1!}$ | $\dfrac{3\,628\,800}{363\,880 \times 1}$ | 10 |
| 10 | $\dfrac{10!}{10!0!}$ | $\dfrac{3\,628\,800}{3\,628\,800 \times 1}$ | 1 |

The second stage is to calculate the relative probability factors of success and corresponding failure for each number of possible successes, $k$. In a binomial situation, there are only two possible outcomes for each individual toss of the coin. So, the probability for success or failure on a single toss equals 0.5 in both cases. Consequently, these probability factors are 0.5 raised to the power of $k$ or $n - k$.

*Experimental Design and Statistical Analysis for Pharmacology and the Biomedical Sciences*, First Edition. Paul J. Mitchell.
© 2022 John Wiley & Sons Ltd. Published 2022 by John Wiley & Sons Ltd.

| k success | $0.5^k$ | $0.5^{10-k}$ |
|---|---|---|
| 0 | $0.5^0 = 1$ | $0.5^{10} = 0.0009765625$ |
| 1 | $0.5^1 = 0.5$ | $0.5^9 = 0.001953125$ |
| 2 | $0.5^2 = 0.25$ | $0.5^8 = 0.00390625$ |
| 3 | $0.5^3 = 0.125$ | $0.5^7 = 0.0078125$ |
| 4 | $0.5^4 = 0.0625$ | $0.5^6 = 0.015625$ |
| 5 | $0.5^5 = 0.03125$ | $0.5^5 = 0.03125$ |
| 6 | $0.5^6 = 0.015625$ | $0.5^4 = 0.0625$ |
| 7 | $0.5^7 = 0.0078125$ | $0.5^3 = 0.125$ |
| 8 | $0.5^8 = 0.00390625$ | $0.5^2 = 0.25$ |
| 9 | $0.5^9 = 0.001953125$ | $0.5^1 = 0.5$ |
| 10 | $0.5^{10} = 0.0009765625$ | $0.5^0 = 1$ |

| k success | Probability mass function | Predicted number of successes | Actual number of successes |
|---|---|---|---|
| 0 | 0.000976 | 0.244 | 1 |
| 1 | 0.009765 | 2.44125 | 2 |
| 2 | 0.043945 | 10.98625 | 10 |
| 3 | 0.117188 | 29.297 | 29 |
| 4 | 0.205078 | 51.2695 | 53 |
| 5 | 0.246094 | 61.5235 | 62 |
| 6 | 0.205078 | 51.2695 | 51 |
| 7 | 0.117188 | 29.297 | 28 |
| 8 | 0.043945 | 10.98625 | 11 |
| 9 | 0.009765 | 2.44125 | 3 |
| 10 | 0.000976 | 0.244 | 0 |

The final table summarises the probability mass function for each level of success over 10 tosses of the coin according to the equation above, the total number of successes for 250 students predicted by the probability mass function for each number of possible successes, and the actual total number of success achieved for each level of $k$.

## A.2 Exponential distribution (Chapter 4. v1, Figure 4.5): Probability density function

The exponential distribution is used to model the time between independent events that occur at a constant rate (e.g. radioactive decay), $\lambda$. The probability density function of the exponential distribution is given by the formula;

$$\text{Pr} = \lambda e^{-\lambda x}$$

where $\lambda$ indicates the rate of change of the variable $x$. It is important to recognise that this distribution is infinitely divisible.

The example provided in Figure 4.5 shows the probability density curves of the exponential distribution for rate values ($\lambda$) of 0.5, 1.0, 1.5, and 2 for the stochastic variable, $x$. The probability values for the probability density function (Figure 4.5) were generated using the Excel function EXPON.DIST($x$, $\lambda$, FALSE), where $x$ = stochastic variable and $\lambda$ = rate factor.

Selected probability values are summarised in the table below.

| | Probability density values | | | | | Probability density values | | | |
|---|---|---|---|---|---|---|---|---|---|
| x | $\lambda = 0.5$ | $\lambda = 1.0$ | $\lambda = 1.5$ | $\lambda = 2.0$ | x | $\lambda = 0.5$ | $\lambda = 1.0$ | $\lambda = 1.5$ | $\lambda = 2.0$ |
| 0 | 0.5 | 1 | 1.5 | 2 | | | | | |
| 0.2 | 0.452419 | 0.818731 | 1.111227 | 1.34064 | 5.2 | 0.037137 | 0.005517 | 0.000615 | 6.09E-05 |
| 0.4 | 0.409365 | 0.67032 | 0.823217 | 0.898658 | 5.4 | 0.033603 | 0.004517 | 0.000455 | 4.08E-05 |
| 0.6 | 0.370409 | 0.548812 | 0.609854 | 0.602388 | 5.6 | 0.030405 | 0.003698 | 0.000337 | 2.73E-05 |
| 0.8 | 0.33516 | 0.449329 | 0.451791 | 0.403793 | 5.8 | 0.027512 | 0.003028 | 0.00025 | 1.83E-05 |
| 1.0 | 0.303265 | 0.367879 | 0.334695 | 0.270671 | 6 | 0.024894 | 0.002479 | 0.000185 | 1.23E-05 |
| 1.2 | 0.274406 | 0.301194 | 0.247948 | 0.181436 | 6.2 | 0.022525 | 0.002029 | 0.000137 | 8.24E-06 |
| 1.4 | 0.248293 | 0.246597 | 0.183685 | 0.12162 | 6.4 | 0.020381 | 0.001662 | 0.000102 | 5.52E-06 |
| 1.6 | 0.224664 | 0.201897 | 0.136077 | 0.081524 | 6.6 | 0.018442 | 0.00136 | 7.53E-05 | 3.7E-06 |
| 1.8 | 0.203285 | 0.165299 | 0.100808 | 0.054647 | 6.8 | 0.016687 | 0.001114 | 5.58E-05 | 2.48E-06 |
| 2.0 | 0.18394 | 0.135335 | 0.074681 | 0.036631 | 7 | 0.015099 | 0.000912 | 4.13E-05 | 1.66E-06 |
| 2.2 | 0.166436 | 0.110803 | 0.055325 | 0.024555 | 7.2 | 0.013662 | 0.000747 | 3.06E-05 | 1.11E-06 |
| 2.4 | 0.150597 | 0.090718 | 0.040986 | 0.016459 | 7.4 | 0.012362 | 0.000611 | 2.27E-05 | 7.47E-07 |
| 2.6 | 0.136266 | 0.074274 | 0.030363 | 0.011033 | 7.6 | 0.011185 | 0.0005 | 1.68E-05 | 5.01E-07 |
| 2.8 | 0.123298 | 0.06081 | 0.022493 | 0.007396 | 7.8 | 0.010121 | 0.00041 | 1.24E-05 | 3.36E-07 |
| 3.0 | 0.111565 | 0.049787 | 0.016663 | 0.004958 | 8 | 0.009158 | 0.000335 | 9.22E-06 | 2.25E-07 |
| 3.2 | 0.100948 | 0.040762 | 0.012345 | 0.003323 | 8.2 | 0.008286 | 0.000275 | 6.83E-06 | 1.51E-07 |
| 3.4 | 0.091342 | 0.033373 | 0.009145 | 0.002228 | 8.4 | 0.007498 | 0.000225 | 5.06E-06 | 1.01E-07 |
| 3.6 | 0.082649 | 0.027324 | 0.006775 | 0.001493 | 8.6 | 0.006784 | 0.000184 | 3.75E-06 | 6.78E-08 |
| 3.8 | 0.074784 | 0.022371 | 0.005019 | 0.001001 | 8.8 | 0.006139 | 0.000151 | 2.78E-06 | 4.54E-08 |
| 4.0 | 0.067668 | 0.018316 | 0.003718 | 0.000671 | 9 | 0.005554 | 0.000123 | 2.06E-06 | 3.05E-08 |
| 4.2 | 0.061228 | 0.014996 | 0.002754 | 0.00045 | 9.2 | 0.005026 | 0.000101 | 1.52E-06 | 2.04E-08 |
| 4.4 | 0.055402 | 0.012277 | 0.002041 | 0.000301 | 9.4 | 0.004548 | 8.27E-05 | 1.13E-06 | 1.37E-08 |
| 4.6 | 0.050129 | 0.010052 | 0.001512 | 0.000202 | 9.6 | 0.004115 | 6.77E-05 | 8.36E-07 | 9.17E-09 |
| 4.8 | 0.045359 | 0.00823 | 0.00112 | 0.000135 | 9.8 | 0.003723 | 5.55E-05 | 6.19E-07 | 6.15E-09 |
| 5.0 | 0.041042 | 0.006738 | 0.00083 | 9.08E-05 | 10 | 0.003369 | 4.54E-05 | 4.59E-07 | 4.12E-09 |

# A.3 Normal distribution (Chapter 4.vii, Figure 4.7): Probability density function

The probability density function of the normal distribution is given by the formula;

$$f\left(x \mid \mu, \sigma^2\right) = \frac{1}{\sqrt{2\pi\sigma^2}} e^{-\frac{(x-\mu)^2}{2\sigma^2}}$$

where

- $\mu$ is the mean of the data set,
- $\sigma$ is the standard deviation
- $\sigma^2$ is the variance

The example provided in Figure 4.7 shows the probability density curves of the normal distribution with mean = 30 and standard deviation = 2 (i.e., N(30, 2)). The probability values for the probability density function (Figure 4.7) were generated using the Excel function NORMDIST($x$, mean, standard deviation, FALSE), for $x$ values equal to four times the standard deviation below and above the mean (i.e. from $x = 22$ to 38, equivalent to $z$ scores = −4 to +4).

The example provided in Figure 5.1 also shows the probability density curves of the normal distribution with mean = 30 and standard deviations = 4 and 8 (i.e., N(30, 4) and N(30, 8), respectively). Likewise the Excel function was used to generate the probability densities for x values equal to four times the respective standard deviations below and above the mean (i.e. from $x = 14$ to 46 for N(30, 4) and x = −2 to +62 for N(30, 8), respectively, equivalent to $z$ scores = −4 to +4 in both cases).

Selected probability values are summarized in the table below.

| | Probability density | | | | Probability density | | |
|---|---|---|---|---|---|---|---|
| $z$ | N(30, 2) | N(30, 4) | N(30, 8) | $z$ | N(30, 2) | N(30, 4) | N(30, 8) |
| −4 | 6.69E-05 | 3.35E-05 | 1.67E-05 | | | | |
| −3.8 | 0.000146 | 7.3E-05 | 3.65E-05 | 0.2 | 0.195521 | 0.097761 | 0.04888 |
| −3.6 | 0.000306 | 0.000153 | 7.65E-05 | 0.4 | 0.184135 | 0.092068 | 0.046034 |
| −3.4 | 0.000616 | 0.000308 | 0.000154 | 0.6 | 0.166612 | 0.083306 | 0.041653 |
| −3.2 | 0.001192 | 0.000596 | 0.000298 | 0.8 | 0.144846 | 0.072423 | 0.036211 |
| −3 | 0.002216 | 0.001108 | 0.000554 | 1 | 0.120985 | 0.060493 | 0.030246 |
| −2.8 | 0.003958 | 0.001979 | 0.000989 | 1.2 | 0.097093 | 0.048547 | 0.024273 |
| −2.6 | 0.006791 | 0.003396 | 0.001698 | 1.4 | 0.074864 | 0.037432 | 0.018716 |
| −2.4 | 0.011197 | 0.005599 | 0.002799 | 1.6 | 0.05546 | 0.02773 | 0.013865 |
| −2.2 | 0.017737 | 0.008869 | 0.004434 | 1.8 | 0.039475 | 0.019738 | 0.009869 |
| −2 | 0.026995 | 0.013498 | 0.006749 | 2 | 0.026995 | 0.013498 | 0.006749 |
| −1.8 | 0.039475 | 0.019738 | 0.009869 | 2.2 | 0.017737 | 0.008869 | 0.004434 |
| −1.6 | 0.05546 | 0.02773 | 0.013865 | 2.4 | 0.011197 | 0.005599 | 0.002799 |
| −1.4 | 0.074864 | 0.037432 | 0.018716 | 2.6 | 0.006791 | 0.003396 | 0.001698 |
| −1.2 | 0.097093 | 0.048547 | 0.024273 | 2.8 | 0.003958 | 0.001979 | 0.000989 |
| −1 | 0.120985 | 0.060493 | 0.030246 | 3 | 0.002216 | 0.001108 | 0.000554 |
| −0.8 | 0.144846 | 0.072423 | 0.036211 | 3.2 | 0.001192 | 0.000596 | 0.000298 |
| −0.6 | 0.166612 | 0.083306 | 0.041653 | 3.4 | 0.000616 | 0.000308 | 0.000154 |
| −0.4 | 0.184135 | 0.092068 | 0.046034 | 3.6 | 0.000306 | 0.000153 | 7.65E-05 |
| −0.2 | 0.195521 | 0.097761 | 0.04888 | 3.8 | 0.000146 | 7.3E-05 | 3.65E-05 |
| 0 | 0.199471 | 0.099736 | 0.049868 | 4 | 6.69E-05 | 3.35E-05 | 1.67E-05 |

# A.4 Chi-square distribution (Chapter 4. viii, Figure 4.8): Probability density function

The probability density function of the chi-square distribution, with $k$ degrees of freedom, is given by the formula:

$$f(x;k) = \frac{1}{2^{k/2}\Gamma(k/2)} x^{k/2-1} e^{-x/2}$$

where $\Gamma(k/2)$ is the **gamma function** and $x$ are chi square values.

Factorials are used extensively in probability theory, and consequently most probability density functions in statistics use a **factorial function** in their calculation (see the Binomial distribution, above). The factorial function (denoted by N!) is the product of all positive integers less than or equal to N. By convention, 0! Is equal to 1. The factorial function may also be defined for non-integer values although this requires more advanced mathematics.

The Gamma function, denoted by $\Gamma(z)$, is one example that completes the values of the factorial defined for all complex numbers except non-positive integers. Thus,

$$\Gamma(z) = \int_0^\infty x^{z-1} e^{-x} dt$$

Where the relationship to factorials is that for any natural number, $n$, is

$$n! = \Gamma(n+1)$$

The probability values for the chi square probability density function (Figure 4.7) were generated using the Excel function CHISQ.DIST(x, df, FALSE), where $x$ = chi square and df = degrees of freedom for values 1, 2, 5, and 10. Selected probability values are summarised in the table below.

| Chi-square | Probability density values | | | | Chi-square | Probability density values | | | |
| | df = 1 | df = 2 | df = 5 | df = 10 | | df = 1 | df = 2 | df = 5 | df = 10 |
|---|---|---|---|---|---|---|---|---|---|
| 0.2 | 0.807171 | 0.452419 | 0.010762 | 1.89E-06 | 5.8 | 0.009115 | 0.027512 | 0.102206 | 0.081077 |
| 0.4 | 0.516442 | 0.409365 | 0.027544 | 2.73E-05 | 6.2 | 0.007218 | 0.022525 | 0.092483 | 0.086675 |
| 0.6 | 0.381545 | 0.370409 | 0.045785 | 0.000125 | 6.6 | 0.005728 | 0.018442 | 0.083164 | 0.091126 |
| 0.8 | 0.298984 | 0.33516 | 0.063783 | 0.000358 | 7.0 | 0.004553 | 0.015099 | 0.074371 | 0.094406 |
| 1.0 | 0.241971 | 0.303265 | 0.080657 | 0.00079 | 7.4 | 0.003626 | 0.012362 | 0.066183 | 0.096533 |
| 1.2 | 0.199868 | 0.274406 | 0.095937 | 0.001482 | 7.8 | 0.002891 | 0.010121 | 0.058638 | 0.097559 |
| 1.4 | 0.167433 | 0.248293 | 0.109389 | 0.002484 | 8.2 | 0.002309 | 0.008286 | 0.051749 | 0.097563 |
| 1.6 | 0.141715 | 0.224664 | 0.12093 | 0.003834 | 8.6 | 0.001846 | 0.006784 | 0.045506 | 0.096642 |
| 1.8 | 0.120895 | 0.203285 | 0.130567 | 0.005557 | 9.0 | 0.001477 | 0.005554 | 0.039887 | 0.094904 |
| 2.0 | 0.103777 | 0.18394 | 0.138369 | 0.007664 | 9.5 | 0.00112 | 0.004326 | 0.033688 | 0.091755987 |
| 2.2 | 0.089531 | 0.166436 | 0.144444 | 0.010153 | 10 | 0.00085 | 0.003369 | 0.028335 | 0.087733685 |
| 2.4 | 0.077562 | 0.150597 | 0.14892 | 0.013012 | 10.5 | 0.000646 | 0.002624 | 0.023743 | 0.083051971 |
| 2.6 | 0.067428 | 0.136266 | 0.151938 | 0.016216 | 11 | 0.000492 | 0.002043 | 0.019827 | 0.077909402 |
| 2.8 | 0.058792 | 0.123298 | 0.153643 | 0.019736 | 11.5 | 0.000374 | 0.001591 | 0.016506 | 0.072483119 |
| 3.0 | 0.051393 | 0.111565 | 0.15418 | 0.023533 | 12 | 0.000285 | 0.001239 | 0.013702 | 0.066926309 |
| 3.2 | 0.045026 | 0.100948 | 0.153689 | 0.027566 | 12.5 | 0.000218 | 0.000965 | 0.011345 | 0.061367484 |
| 3.4 | 0.039525 | 0.091342 | 0.152302 | 0.031787 | 13 | 0.000166 | 0.000752 | 0.009371 | 0.055911103 |
| 3.6 | 0.034756 | 0.082649 | 0.150146 | 0.036151 | 13.5 | 0.000127 | 0.000585 | 0.007723 | 0.050639114 |
| 3.8 | 0.03061 | 0.074784 | 0.147335 | 0.040608 | 14 | 9.72E-05 | 0.000456 | 0.006352 | 0.045613096 |
| 4.0 | 0.026995 | 0.067668 | 0.143976 | 0.045112 | 14.5 | 7.44E-05 | 0.000355 | 0.005214 | 0.040876697 |
| 4.2 | 0.023838 | 0.061228 | 0.140167 | 0.049616 | 15 | 5.7E-05 | 0.000277 | 0.004273 | 0.036458198 |
| 4.4 | 0.021073 | 0.055402 | 0.135994 | 0.054076 | 16 | 3.35E-05 | 0.000168 | 0.002855 | 0.028626144 |
| 4.6 | 0.018649 | 0.050129 | 0.131537 | 0.058451 | 17 | 1.97E-05 | 0.000102 | 0.001897 | 0.02212745 |
| 4.8 | 0.016519 | 0.045359 | 0.126866 | 0.062704 | 18 | 1.16E-05 | 6.17E-05 | 0.001253 | 0.016868578 |
| 5.0 | 0.014645 | 0.041042 | 0.122042 | 0.066801 | 19 | 6.85E-06 | 3.74E-05 | 0.000824 | 0.012701517 |
| 5.4 | 0.011538 | 0.033603 | 0.112146 | 0.074408 | 20 | 4.05E-06 | 2.27E-05 | 0.00054 | 0.009458319 |

# A.5 Student *t*-distribution (Chapter 4.ix, Figure 4.9): Probability density function

The probability density function of the Student *t*- distribution is a further extension of the Gamma function (see above) and is given by the formula:

$$f(t) = \frac{\Gamma\left(\dfrac{v+1}{2}\right)}{\sqrt{v\pi}\,\Gamma\left(\dfrac{v}{2}\right)} \left(1 + \frac{t^2}{v}\right)^{-\frac{v+1}{2}}$$

where *v* is the degrees of freedom and $\Gamma$ is the gamma function (see above). The probability density function is symmetric and the overall shape resembles the bell shape of the normal distribution with mean = 0 and standard deviation = 1 (i.e. N(0,1)), although it is slightly lower and wider with heavier tails. As the number of degrees of freedom (*v*) increases so the *t*-distribution approximates to the normal distribution (see Figure 4.8) and consequently *v* is known as the normality parameter.

The probability values for the probability density function for the *t*-distribution (Figure 4.8) were generated using the Excel function T.DIST(t, df, FALSE), where *t* = t value and df = degrees of freedom of 1, 2 and 4, respectively. Selected probability values are summarized in the table below.

| t value | df = 1 | df = 2 | df = 4 | t value | df = 1 | df = 2 | df = 4 |
|---|---|---|---|---|---|---|---|
| −4 | 0.018724 | 0.013095 | 0.006708 | 0.1 | 0.315158 | 0.350918 | 0.372666 |
| −3.9 | 0.019637 | 0.014006 | 0.007419 | 0.2 | 0.306067 | 0.343206 | 0.365787 |
| −3.8 | 0.020616 | 0.015002 | 0.008218 | 0.3 | 0.292027 | 0.330964 | 0.35471 |
| −3.7 | 0.021668 | 0.01609 | 0.009117 | 0.4 | 0.274405 | 0.315006 | 0.339976 |
| −3.6 | 0.022802 | 0.017282 | 0.01013 | 0.5 | 0.254648 | 0.296296 | 0.322262 |
| −3.5 | 0.024023 | 0.01859 | 0.011273 | 0.6 | 0.234051 | 0.275824 | 0.302319 |
| −3.4 | 0.025343 | 0.020027 | 0.012565 | 0.7 | 0.213631 | 0.254508 | 0.280909 |
| −3.3 | 0.026771 | 0.021608 | 0.014026 | 0.8 | 0.194091 | 0.233128 | 0.258754 |
| −3.2 | 0.028319 | 0.023352 | 0.015682 | 0.9 | 0.175862 | 0.212295 | 0.236493 |
| −3.1 | 0.030001 | 0.025279 | 0.01756 | 1 | 0.159155 | 0.19245 | 0.214663 |
| −3 | 0.031831 | 0.02741 | 0.019693 | 1.1 | 0.144032 | 0.173877 | 0.193681 |
| −2.9 | 0.033827 | 0.029773 | 0.022118 | 1.2 | 0.130455 | 0.156734 | 0.173854 |
| −2.8 | 0.036008 | 0.032397 | 0.024877 | 1.3 | 0.118331 | 0.141078 | 0.155382 |
| −2.7 | 0.038397 | 0.035316 | 0.028019 | 1.4 | 0.107537 | 0.126899 | 0.138378 |
| −2.6 | 0.041019 | 0.038569 | 0.031597 | 1.5 | 0.097942 | 0.114134 | 0.12288 |
| −2.5 | 0.043905 | 0.042201 | 0.035676 | 1.6 | 0.089413 | 0.102696 | 0.108873 |
| −2.4 | 0.047087 | 0.04626 | 0.040323 | 1.7 | 0.081828 | 0.092478 | 0.096302 |
| −2.3 | 0.050606 | 0.050805 | 0.045619 | 1.8 | 0.075073 | 0.083369 | 0.085081 |
| −2.2 | 0.054505 | 0.055901 | 0.051648 | 1.9 | 0.069048 | 0.075259 | 0.075114 |
| −2.1 | 0.058837 | 0.061619 | 0.058505 | 2 | 0.063662 | 0.068041 | 0.066291 |
| −2 | 0.063662 | 0.068041 | 0.066291 | 2.1 | 0.058837 | 0.061619 | 0.058505 |
| −1.9 | 0.069048 | 0.075259 | 0.075114 | 2.2 | 0.054505 | 0.055901 | 0.051648 |
| −1.8 | 0.075073 | 0.083369 | 0.085081 | 2.3 | 0.050606 | 0.050805 | 0.045619 |
| −1.7 | 0.081828 | 0.092478 | 0.096302 | 2.4 | 0.047087 | 0.04626 | 0.040323 |
| −1.6 | 0.089413 | 0.102696 | 0.108873 | 2.5 | 0.043905 | 0.042201 | 0.035676 |
| −1.5 | 0.097942 | 0.114134 | 0.12288 | 2.6 | 0.041019 | 0.038569 | 0.031597 |
| −1.4 | 0.107537 | 0.126899 | 0.138378 | 2.7 | 0.038397 | 0.035316 | 0.028019 |
| −1.3 | 0.118331 | 0.141078 | 0.155382 | 2.8 | 0.036008 | 0.032397 | 0.024877 |
| −1.2 | 0.130455 | 0.156734 | 0.173854 | 2.9 | 0.033827 | 0.029773 | 0.022118 |
| −1.1 | 0.144032 | 0.173877 | 0.193681 | 3 | 0.031831 | 0.02741 | 0.019693 |
| −1 | 0.159155 | 0.19245 | 0.214663 | 3.1 | 0.030001 | 0.025279 | 0.01756 |
| −0.9 | 0.175862 | 0.212295 | 0.236493 | 3.2 | 0.028319 | 0.023352 | 0.015682 |
| −0.8 | 0.194091 | 0.233128 | 0.258754 | 3.3 | 0.026771 | 0.021608 | 0.014026 |
| −0.7 | 0.213631 | 0.254508 | 0.280909 | 3.4 | 0.025343 | 0.020027 | 0.012565 |
| −0.6 | 0.234051 | 0.275824 | 0.302319 | 3.5 | 0.024023 | 0.01859 | 0.011273 |
| −0.5 | 0.254648 | 0.296296 | 0.322262 | 3.6 | 0.022802 | 0.017282 | 0.01013 |
| −0.4 | 0.274405 | 0.315006 | 0.339976 | 3.7 | 0.021668 | 0.01609 | 0.009117 |
| −0.3 | 0.292027 | 0.330964 | 0.35471 | 3.8 | 0.020616 | 0.015002 | 0.008218 |
| −0.2 | 0.306067 | 0.343206 | 0.365787 | 3.9 | 0.019637 | 0.014006 | 0.007419 |
| −0.1 | 0.315158 | 0.350918 | 0.372666 | 4 | 0.018724 | 0.013095 | 0.006708 |
| 0 | 0.31831 | 0.353553 | 0.375 | | | | |

# A.6 F distribution (Chapter 4.x, Figure 4.10): Probability density function

The F distribution is employed when the analysis of variance (ANOVA) test is used to examine the variability of values contained in more than two groups of data (see Chapters 15–17 and 20).

The probability density function of the F distribution is given by the formula:

$$f(x; d_1, d_2) = \frac{\sqrt{\dfrac{(d_1 x)^{d_1} d_2^{d_2}}{(d_1 x + d_2)^{d_1 + d_2}}}}{x B\left(\dfrac{d_1}{2}, \dfrac{d_2}{2}\right)}$$

where $x$ is a variable with an $F$ distribution and degrees of freedom $d_1$ and $d_2$, which are both positive integers, and B is the **beta function**.

The beta function is symmetrical and a key property of which is its relationship to the gamma function (see above). Thus,

$$B(x, y) = B(y, x) = \frac{\Gamma(x)\, \Gamma(y)}{\Gamma(x + y)}$$

Consequently, it follows from the definition of the gamma function that when both $x$ and $y$ are positive integers then,

$$B(x, y) = \frac{(x - 1)!\,(y - 1)!}{(x + y - 1)!}$$

The probability values for the probability density function of the F distribution (Figure 4.9) were generated using the Excel function F.DIST(F, df1, df2, FALSE), where $F$ = F ratio and df1 and df2 = degrees of freedom values, respectively. Selected probability values for df1 and df2 values of (1, 4), (2, 8), (4, 20), and (8, 32) are summarised in the table below.

| F ratio | Df (1, 4) | Df (2, 8) | Df (4,20) | Df 8, 32) | F ratio | Df (1, 4) | Df (2, 8) | Df (4,20) | Df 8, 32) |
|---|---|---|---|---|---|---|---|---|---|
| 0.2 | 0.742238 | 0.783526 | 0.549645 | 0.182603 | 5.2 | 0.020498 | 0.015537 | 0.004404 | 0.000496 |
| 0.4 | 0.467218 | 0.620921 | 0.69892 | 0.576143 | 5.4 | 0.019062 | 0.013953 | 0.003623 | 0.000361 |
| 0.6 | 0.341359 | 0.497177 | 0.677622 | 0.799283 | 5.6 | 0.017759 | 0.012559 | 0.00299 | 0.000265 |
| 0.8 | 0.265787 | 0.401878 | 0.592989 | 0.808814 | 5.8 | 0.016573 | 0.011328 | 0.002474 | 0.000195 |
| 1 | 0.214663 | 0.32768 | 0.493489 | 0.698238 | 6 | 0.015492 | 0.01024 | 0.002054 | 0.000144 |
| 1.2 | 0.177657 | 0.269329 | 0.399552 | 0.550656 | 6.2 | 0.014504 | 0.009275 | 0.001709 | 0.000107 |
| 1.4 | 0.149669 | 0.223014 | 0.318465 | 0.411067 | 6.4 | 0.013599 | 0.008417 | 0.001427 | 7.97E-05 |
| 1.6 | 0.127835 | 0.185934 | 0.251585 | 0.296485 | 6.6 | 0.012769 | 0.007652 | 0.001194 | 5.97E-05 |
| 1.8 | 0.110402 | 0.156013 | 0.197815 | 0.209248 | 6.8 | 0.012005 | 0.006969 | 0.001002 | 4.49E-05 |
| 2 | 0.096225 | 0.131687 | 0.155219 | 0.145703 | 7 | 0.011302 | 0.006358 | 0.000843 | 3.4E-05 |
| 2.2 | 0.084526 | 0.111774 | 0.121766 | 0.100656 | 7.2 | 0.010653 | 0.00581 | 0.000711 | 2.58E-05 |
| 2.4 | 0.074752 | 0.095367 | 0.095614 | 0.069253 | 7.4 | 0.010053 | 0.005318 | 0.000602 | 1.96E-05 |
| 2.6 | 0.066502 | 0.081767 | 0.075215 | 0.047582 | 7.6 | 0.009498 | 0.004875 | 0.00051 | 1.5E-05 |
| 2.8 | 0.059474 | 0.07043 | 0.059308 | 0.032711 | 7.8 | 0.008983 | 0.004476 | 0.000433 | 1.15E-05 |
| 3 | 0.053441 | 0.060927 | 0.046896 | 0.022532 | 8 | 0.008505 | 0.004115 | 0.000369 | 8.89E-06 |
| 3.2 | 0.048225 | 0.052922 | 0.037194 | 0.015567 | 8.2 | 0.008061 | 0.003789 | 0.000315 | 6.88E-06 |
| 3.4 | 0.043688 | 0.046147 | 0.029595 | 0.010795 | 8.4 | 0.007647 | 0.003493 | 0.000269 | 5.34E-06 |
| 3.6 | 0.039719 | 0.040386 | 0.023627 | 0.007517 | 8.6 | 0.007261 | 0.003224 | 0.000231 | 4.16E-06 |
| 3.8 | 0.036229 | 0.035467 | 0.018927 | 0.005259 | 8.8 | 0.006901 | 0.00298 | 0.000198 | 3.26E-06 |
| 4 | 0.033146 | 0.03125 | 0.015214 | 0.003696 | 9 | 0.006564 | 0.002758 | 0.000171 | 2.55E-06 |
| 4.2 | 0.03041 | 0.02762 | 0.012271 | 0.002611 | 9.2 | 0.00625 | 0.002555 | 0.000147 | 2.01E-06 |
| 4.4 | 0.027974 | 0.024485 | 0.009931 | 0.001854 | 9.4 | 0.005955 | 0.00237 | 0.000127 | 1.59E-06 |
| 4.6 | 0.025796 | 0.021767 | 0.008065 | 0.001323 | 9.6 | 0.005678 | 0.002201 | 0.00011 | 1.26E-06 |
| 4.8 | 0.023843 | 0.019404 | 0.006571 | 0.000949 | 9.8 | 0.005418 | 0.002046 | 9.53E-05 | 9.99E-07 |
| 5 | 0.022085 | 0.017342 | 0.005371 | 0.000685 | 10 | 0.005174 | 0.001904 | 8.28E-05 | 7.96E-07 |

# Write Your Own Notes

# Appendix B: Standard normal probabilities

Values in the following tables for $z$ indicate the area under the Standard Normal Distribution curve to the left of $z$. Area under the curve values to the right of the tabulated $z$ values may be calculated by 1 - (tabulated value for $z$). For example, if $z = -0.63$, then the corresponding area to the left of $z = 0.2643$ (i.e. 26.43%) while area to the right of $z = 1 - 0.2643 = 0.7357$ (i.e. 73.57%).

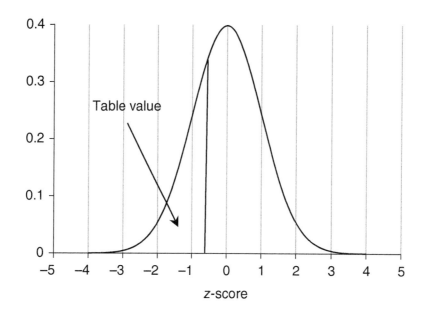

*Experimental Design and Statistical Analysis for Pharmacology and the Biomedical Sciences*, First Edition. Paul J. Mitchell.
© 2022 John Wiley & Sons Ltd. Published 2022 by John Wiley & Sons Ltd.

Table B.1 AUC values for z values below the mean (i.e. −z).

| z | .00 | .01 | .02 | .03 | .04 | .05 | .06 | .07 | .08 | .09 |
|---|-----|-----|-----|-----|-----|-----|-----|-----|-----|-----|
| −3.4 | 0.0003 | 0.0003 | 0.0003 | 0.0003 | 0.0003 | 0.0003 | 0.0003 | 0.0003 | 0.0003 | 0.0002 |
| −3.3 | 0.0005 | 0.0005 | 0.0005 | 0.0004 | 0.0004 | 0.0004 | 0.0004 | 0.0004 | 0.0004 | 0.0003 |
| −3.2 | 0.0007 | 0.0007 | 0.0006 | 0.0006 | 0.0006 | 0.0006 | 0.0006 | 0.0005 | 0.0005 | 0.0005 |
| −3.1 | 0.0010 | 0.0009 | 0.0009 | 0.0009 | 0.0008 | 0.0008 | 0.0008 | 0.0008 | 0.0007 | 0.0007 |
| −3.0 | 0.0013 | 0.0013 | 0.0013 | 0.0012 | 0.0012 | 0.0011 | 0.0011 | 0.0011 | 0.0010 | 0.0010 |
| −2.9 | 0.0019 | 0.0018 | 0.0018 | 0.00170 | 0.00160 | 0.0016 | 0.0015 | 0.0015 | 0.0014 | 0.0014 |
| −2.8 | 0.0026 | 0.0025 | 0.0024 | 0.0023 | 0.0023 | 0.0022 | 0.0021 | 0.0021 | 0.0020 | 0.0019 |
| −2.7 | 0.0037 | 0.0034 | 0.0033 | 0.0032 | 0.0031 | 0.0030 | 0.0029 | 0.0028 | 0.0027 | 0.0026 |
| −2.6 | 0.0047 | 0.0045 | 0.0044 | 0.0043 | 0.0041 | 0.0040 | 0.0039 | 0.0038 | 0.0037 | 0.0036 |
| −2.5 | 0.0062 | 0.0060 | 0.0059 | 0.0057 | 0.0055 | 0.0054 | 0.0052 | 0.0051 | 0.0049 | 0.0048 |
| −2.4 | 0.0082 | 0.0080 | 0.0078 | 0.0075 | 0.0073 | 0.0071 | 0.0069 | 0.0068 | 0.0066 | 0.0064 |
| −2.3 | 0.0107 | 0.0104 | 0.0102 | 0.0099 | 0.0096 | 0.0094 | 0.0091 | 0.0089 | 0.0087 | 0.0084 |
| −2.2 | 0.0139 | 0.0136 | 0.0132 | 0.0129 | 0.0125 | 0.0122 | 0.0119 | 0.0116 | 0.0113 | 0.0110 |
| −2.1 | 0.0179 | 0.0174 | 0.0170 | 0.0166 | 0.0162 | 0.0158 | 0.0154 | 0.0150 | 0.0146 | 0.0143 |
| −2.0 | 0.0228 | 0.0222 | 0.0217 | 0.0212 | 0.0207 | 0.0202 | 0.0197 | 0.0192 | 0.0188 | 0.0183 |
| −1.9 | 0.0287 | 0.0281 | 0.0274 | 0.0268 | 0.0262 | 0.0256 | 0.0250 | 0.0244 | 0.0239 | 0.0233 |
| −1.8 | 0.0359 | 0.0351 | 0.0344 | 0.0336 | 0.0329 | 0.0322 | 0.0314 | 0.0307 | 0.0301 | 0.0294 |
| −1.7 | 0.0446 | 0.0436 | 0.0427 | 0.0418 | 0.0409 | 0.0401 | 0.0392 | 0.0384 | 0.0375 | 0.0367 |
| −1.6 | 0.0548 | 0.0537 | 0.0526 | 0.0516 | 0.0505 | 0.0495 | 0.0485 | 0.0475 | 0.0465 | 0.0455 |
| −1.5 | 0.0668 | 0.0655 | 0.0643 | 0.0630 | 0.0618 | 0.0606 | 0.0594 | 0.0582 | 0.0571 | 0.0559 |
| −1.4 | 0.0808 | 0.0793 | 0.0778 | 0.0764 | 0.0749 | 0.0735 | 0.0721 | 0.0708 | 0.0694 | 0.0681 |
| −1.3 | 0.0968 | 0.0951 | 0.0934 | 0.0918 | 0.0901 | 0.0885 | 0.0869 | 0.0853 | 0.0838 | 0.0823 |
| −1.2 | 0.1151 | 0.1131 | 0.1112 | 0.1093 | 0.1075 | 0.1056 | 0.1038 | 0.1020 | 0.1003 | 0.0985 |
| −1.1 | 0.1357 | 0.1335 | 0.1314 | 0.1292 | 0.1271 | 0.1251 | 0.1230 | 0.1210 | 0.1190 | 0.1170 |
| −1.0 | 0.1587 | 0.1562 | 0.1539 | 0.1515 | 0.1492 | 0.1469 | 0.1446 | 0.1423 | 0.1401 | 0.1379 |
| −0.9 | 0.1841 | 0.1814 | 0.1788 | 0.1762 | 0.1736 | 0.1711 | 0.1685 | 0.1660 | 0.1635 | 0.1611 |
| −0.8 | 0.2119 | 0.2090 | 0.2061 | 0.2033 | 0.2005 | 0.1977 | 0.1949 | 0.1922 | 0.1894 | 0.1867 |
| −0.7 | 0.2420 | 0.2389 | 0.2358 | 0.2327 | 0.2296 | 0.2266 | 0.2236 | 0.2206 | 0.2177 | 0.2148 |
| −0.6 | 0.2743 | 0.2709 | 0.2676 | 0.2643 | 0.2611 | 0.2578 | 0.2546 | 0.2514 | 0.2483 | 0.2451 |
| −0.5 | 0.3085 | 0.3050 | 0.3015 | 0.2981 | 0.2946 | 0.2912 | 0.2877 | 0.2843 | 0.2810 | 0.2776 |
| −0.4 | 0.3446 | 0.3409 | 0.3372 | 0.3336 | 0.3300 | 0.3264 | 0.3228 | 0.3192 | 0.3156 | 0.3121 |
| −0.3 | 0.3821 | 0.3783 | 0.3745 | 0.3707 | 0.3669 | 0.3632 | 0.3594 | 0.3557 | 0.3520 | 0.3483 |
| −0.2 | 0.4207 | 0.4168 | 0.4129 | 0.4090 | 0.4052 | 0.4013 | 0.3974 | 0.3936 | 0.3897 | 0.3859 |
| −0.1 | 0.4602 | 0.4562 | 0.4522 | 0.4483 | 0.4443 | 0.4404 | 0.4364 | 0.4325 | 0.4286 | 0.4247 |
| −0.0 | 0.5000 | 0.4960 | 0.4920 | 0.4880 | 0.4840 | 0.4801 | 0.4761 | 0.4721 | 0.4681 | 0.4641 |

*Source:* Table values for B.1 were computed by the author.

Values in the following tables for $z$ indicate the area under the standard normal distribution curve to the left of $z$. Area under the curve values to the right of the tabulated $z$ values may be calculated by 1 - (tabulated value for $z$). For example, if $z = 0.63$, then the corresponding area to the left of $z = 0.7357$ (i.e. 73.57%), while area to the right of $z = 1 - 0.7357 = 0.2643$ (i.e. 26.43%).

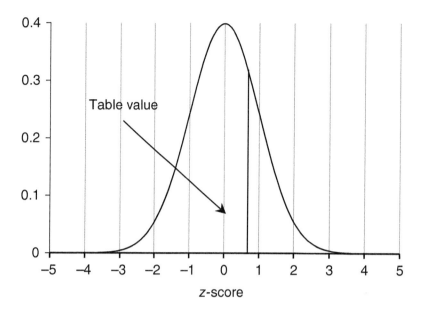

**Table B.2** AUC values for $z$ values above the mean (i.e. $+z$).

| $z$ | .00 | .01 | .02 | .03 | .04 | .05 | .06 | .07 | .08 | .09 |
|-----|-----|-----|-----|-----|-----|-----|-----|-----|-----|-----|
| 0.0 | 0.5000 | 0.5040 | 0.5080 | 0.5120 | 0.5160 | 0.5199 | 0.5239 | 0.5279 | 0.5319 | 0.5359 |
| 0.1 | 0.5398 | 0.5438 | 0.5478 | 0.5517 | 0.5557 | 0.5596 | 0.5636 | 0.5675 | 0.5714 | 0.5753 |
| 0.2 | 0.5793 | 0.5832 | 0.5871 | 0.5910 | 0.5948 | 0.5987 | 0.6026 | 0.6064 | 0.6103 | 0.6141 |
| 0.3 | 0.6179 | 0.6217 | 0.6255 | 0.6293 | 0.6331 | 0.6368 | 0.6406 | 0.6443 | 0.6480 | 0.6517 |
| 0.4 | 0.6554 | 0.6591 | 0.6628 | 0.6664 | 0.6700 | 0.6736 | 0.6772 | 0.6808 | 0.6844 | 0.6879 |
| 0.5 | 0.6915 | 0.6950 | 0.6985 | 0.7019 | 0.7054 | 0.7088 | 0.7123 | 0.7157 | 0.7190 | 0.7224 |
| 0.6 | 0.7257 | 0.7291 | 0.7324 | 0.7357 | 0.7389 | 0.7422 | 0.7454 | 0.7486 | 0.7517 | 0.7549 |
| 0.7 | 0.7580 | 0.7611 | 0.7642 | 0.7673 | 0.7704 | 0.7734 | 0.7764 | 0.7794 | 0.7823 | 0.7852 |
| 0.8 | 0.7881 | 0.7910 | 0.7939 | 0.7967 | 0.7995 | 0.8023 | 0.8051 | 0.8078 | 0.8106 | 0.8133 |
| 0.9 | 0.8159 | 0.8186 | 0.8212 | 0.8238 | 0.8264 | 0.8289 | 0.8315 | 0.8340 | 0.8365 | 0.8389 |
| 1.0 | 0.8413 | 0.8438 | 0.8461 | 0.8485 | 0.8508 | 0.8531 | 0.8554 | 0.8577 | 0.8599 | 0.8621 |
| 1.1 | 0.8643 | 0.8665 | 0.8686 | 0.8708 | 0.8729 | 0.8749 | 0.8770 | 0.8790 | 0.8810 | 0.8830 |
| 1.2 | 0.8849 | 0.8869 | 0.8888 | 0.8907 | 0.8925 | 0.8944 | 0.8962 | 0.8980 | 0.8997 | 0.9015 |
| 1.3 | 0.9032 | 0.9049 | 0.9066 | 0.9082 | 0.9099 | 0.9115 | 0.9131 | 0.9147 | 0.9162 | 0.9177 |
| 1.4 | 0.9192 | 0.9207 | 0.9222 | 0.9236 | 0.9251 | 0.9265 | 0.9279 | 0.9292 | 0.9306 | 0.9319 |
| 1.5 | 0.9332 | 0.9345 | 0.9357 | 0.9370 | 0.9382 | 0.9394 | 0.9406 | 0.9418 | 0.9429 | 0.9441 |
| 1.6 | 0.9452 | 0.9463 | 0.9474 | 0.9484 | 0.9495 | 0.9505 | 0.9515 | 0.9525 | 0.9535 | 0.9545 |
| 1.7 | 0.9554 | 0.9564 | 0.9573 | 0.9582 | 0.9591 | 0.9599 | 0.9608 | 0.9616 | 0.9625 | 0.9633 |
| 1.8 | 0.9641 | 0.9649 | 0.9656 | 0.9664 | 0.9671 | 0.9678 | 0.9686 | 0.9693 | 0.9699 | 0.9706 |
| 1.9 | 0.9713 | 0.9719 | 0.9726 | 0.9732 | 0.9738 | 0.9744 | 0.9750 | 0.9756 | 0.9761 | 0.9767 |
| 2.0 | 0.9772 | 0.9778 | 0.9783 | 0.9788 | 0.9793 | 0.9798 | 0.9803 | 0.9808 | 0.9812 | 0.9817 |
| 2.1 | 0.9821 | 0.9826 | 0.9830 | 0.9834 | 0.9838 | 0.9842 | 0.9846 | 0.9850 | 0.9854 | 0.9857 |
| 2.2 | 0.9861 | 0.9864 | 0.9868 | 0.9871 | 0.9875 | 0.9878 | 0.9881 | 0.9884 | 0.9887 | 0.9890 |
| 2.3 | 0.9893 | 0.9896 | 0.9898 | 0.9901 | 0.9904 | 0.9906 | 0.9909 | 0.9911 | 0.9913 | 0.9916 |
| 2.4 | 0.9918 | 0.9920 | 0.9922 | 0.9925 | 0.9927 | 0.9929 | 0.9931 | 0.9932 | 0.9934 | 0.9936 |
| 2.5 | 0.9938 | 0.9940 | 0.9941 | 0.9943 | 0.9945 | 0.9946 | 0.9948 | 0.9949 | 0.9951 | 0.9952 |
| 2.6 | 0.9953 | 0.9955 | 0.9956 | 0.9957 | 0.9959 | 0.9960 | 0.9961 | 0.9962 | 9.9963 | 0.9964 |
| 2.7 | 0.0065 | 0.9966 | 0.9967 | 0.9968 | 0.9969 | 0.9970 | 0.9971 | 0.9972 | 0.9973 | 0.9974 |
| 2.8 | 0.9974 | 0.9975 | 0.9976 | 0.9977 | 0.9977 | 0.9978 | 0.9979 | 0.9979 | 0.9980 | 0.9981 |
| 2.9 | 0.9981 | 0.9982 | 0.9982 | 0.9983 | 0.9984 | 0.9984 | 0.9985 | 0.9985 | 0.9986 | 0.9986 |
| 3.0 | 0.9987 | 0.9987 | 0.9987 | 0.9988 | 0.9988 | 0.9989 | 0.9989 | 0.9989 | 0.9990 | 0.9990 |
| 3.1 | 0.9990 | 0.9991 | 0.9991 | 0.9991 | 0.9992 | 0.9992 | 0.9992 | 0.9992 | 0.9993 | 0.9993 |
| 3.2 | 0.9993 | 0.9993 | 0.9994 | 0.9994 | 0.9994 | 0.9994 | 0.9994 | 0.9995 | 0.9995 | 0.9995 |
| 3.3 | 0.9995 | 0.9995 | 0.9995 | 0.9996 | 0.9996 | 0.9996 | 0.9996 | 0.9996 | 0.9996 | 0.9997 |
| 3.4 | 0.9997 | 0.9997 | 0.9997 | 0.9997 | 0.9997 | 0.9997 | 0.9997 | 0.9997 | 0.9997 | 0.9998 |

*Source:* Table values for B.2 were computed by the author.

# Appendix C: Critical values of the t-distribution

Values in the following table indicates the critical values of $t$ for $p = 0.05$ and $0.01$ for both one- and two-tailed tests according to the appropriate degrees of freedom.

| | $t_{crit}$ | | | | |
|---|---|---|---|---|---|
| | **Level of Significance for One-tailed test** | | | | |
| | 0.05 | 0.025 | 0.01 | 0.005 | 0.0005 |
| | **Level of Significance for Two-tailed test** | | | | |
| df | 0.10 | 0.05 | 0.02 | 0.01 | 0.001 |
| 1 | 6.314 | 12.706 | 31.821 | 63.657 | 636.620 |
| 2 | 2.920 | 4.303 | 6.965 | 9.925 | 31.599 |
| 3 | 2.353 | 3.182 | 4.541 | 5.841 | 12.924 |
| 4 | 2.132 | 2.776 | 3.747 | 4.604 | 8.610 |
| 5 | 2.015 | 2.571 | 3.365 | 4.032 | 6.869 |
| 6 | 1.943 | 2.447 | 3.143 | 3.707 | 5.959 |
| 7 | 1.895 | 2.365 | 2.998 | 3.499 | 5.408 |
| 8 | 1.860 | 2.306 | 2.896 | 3.355 | 5.041 |
| 9 | 1.833 | 2.262 | 2.821 | 3.250 | 4.781 |
| 10 | 1.812 | 2.228 | 2.764 | 3.169 | 4.587 |
| 11 | 1.796 | 2.201 | 2.718 | 3.106 | 4.437 |
| 12 | 1.782 | 2.179 | 2.681 | 3.055 | 4.318 |
| 13 | 1.771 | 2.160 | 2.650 | 3.012 | 4.221 |
| 14 | 1.761 | 2.145 | 2.624 | 2.977 | 4.140 |
| 15 | 1.753 | 2.131 | 2.602 | 2.947 | 4.073 |
| 16 | 1.746 | 2.120 | 2.583 | 2.921 | 4.015 |
| 17 | 1.740 | 2.110 | 2.567 | 2.898 | 3.965 |
| 18 | 1.734 | 2.101 | 2.552 | 2.878 | 3.922 |
| 19 | 1.729 | 2.093 | 2.539 | 2.861 | 3.883 |
| 20 | 1.725 | 2.086 | 2.528 | 2.845 | 3.850 |
| 21 | 1.721 | 2.080 | 2.518 | 2.831 | 3.819 |
| 22 | 1.717 | 2.074 | 2.508 | 2.819 | 3.792 |
| 23 | 1.714 | 2.069 | 2.500 | 2.807 | 3.768 |
| 24 | 1.711 | 2.064 | 2.492 | 2.797 | 3.745 |
| 25 | 1.708 | 2.060 | 2.485 | 2.787 | 3.725 |
| 26 | 1.706 | 2.056 | 2.479 | 2.779 | 3.707 |
| 27 | 1.703 | 2.052 | 2.473 | 2.771 | 3.690 |
| 28 | 1.701 | 2.048 | 2.467 | 2.763 | 3.674 |
| 29 | 1.699 | 2.045 | 2.462 | 2.756 | 3.659 |
| 30 | 1.697 | 2.042 | 2.457 | 2.750 | 3.646 |
| 35 | 1.690 | 2.030 | 2.438 | 2.724 | 3.592 |
| 40 | 1.684 | 2.021 | 2.423 | 2.704 | 3.551 |
| 45 | 1.679 | 2.014 | 2.412 | 2.690 | 3.521 |
| 50 | 1.676 | 2.009 | 2.403 | 2.678 | 3.496 |
| 100 | 1.660 | 1.984 | 2.364 | 2.626 | 3.390 |
| ∞(Z) | 1.645 | 1.960 | 2.326 | 2.576 | 3.291 |

*Source:* Table values were computed by the author.

*Experimental Design and Statistical Analysis for Pharmacology and the Biomedical Sciences*, First Edition. Paul J. Mitchell.
© 2022 John Wiley & Sons Ltd. Published 2022 by John Wiley & Sons Ltd.

# Write Your Own Notes

# Appendix D: Critical values of the Mann–Whitney *U*-statistic

Values in the following tables indicate the critical values for *U* for $p = 0.05$ and 0.01 for both one- (Tables D.1 and D.2, respectively) and two-tailed (Tables D.3 and D.4, respectively) tests.

If the observed value of *U* falls between the two values in the table for $n_1$ and $n_2$ then accept $H_0$. Otherwise reject $H_0$.

**Table D.1** Critical values for *U*; One-tailed test, $p = 0.05$.

| $n_1 \backslash n_2$ | 1 | 2 | 3 | 4 | 5 | 6 | 7 | 8 | 9 | 10 | 11 | 12 | 13 | 14 | 15 | 16 | 17 | 18 | 19 | 20 |
|---|---|---|---|---|---|---|---|---|---|---|---|---|---|---|---|---|---|---|---|---|
| 1 | | | | | | | | | | | | | | | | | | | 0 / 19 | 0 / 20 |
| 2 | | | | | 0 / 10 | 0 / 12 | 0 / 14 | 1 / 15 | 1 / 17 | 1 / 19 | 1 / 21 | 2 / 22 | 2 / 24 | 2 / 26 | 3 / 27 | 3 / 29 | 3 / 31 | 4 / 32 | 4 / 34 | 4 / 36 |
| 3 | | | 0 / 9 | 0 / 12 | 1 / 14 | 2 / 16 | 2 / 19 | 3 / 21 | 3 / 24 | 4 / 26 | 5 / 28 | 5 / 31 | 6 / 33 | 7 / 35 | 7 / 38 | 8 / 40 | 9 / 42 | 9 / 45 | 10 / 47 | 11 / 49 |
| 4 | | | 0 / 12 | 1 / 15 | 2 / 18 | 3 / 21 | 4 / 24 | 5 / 27 | 6 / 30 | 7 / 33 | 8 / 36 | 9 / 39 | 10 / 42 | 11 / 45 | 12 / 48 | 14 / 50 | 15 / 53 | 16 / 56 | 17 / 59 | 18 / 62 |
| 5 | | 0 / 10 | 1 / 14 | 2 / 18 | 4 / 21 | 5 / 25 | 6 / 29 | 8 / 32 | 9 / 36 | 11 / 39 | 12 / 43 | 13 / 47 | 15 / 50 | 16 / 54 | 18 / 57 | 19 / 61 | 20 / 65 | 22 / 68 | 23 / 72 | 25 / 75 |
| 6 | | 0 / 12 | 2 / 16 | 3 / 21 | 5 / 25 | 7 / 29 | 8 / 34 | 10 / 38 | 12 / 42 | 14 / 46 | 16 / 50 | 17 / 55 | 19 / 59 | 21 / 63 | 23 / 67 | 25 / 71 | 26 / 76 | 28 / 80 | 30 / 84 | 32 / 88 |
| 7 | | 0 / 14 | 2 / 19 | 4 / 24 | 6 / 29 | 8 / 34 | 11 / 38 | 13 / 43 | 15 / 48 | 17 / 53 | 19 / 58 | 21 / 63 | 24 / 67 | 26 / 72 | 28 / 77 | 30 / 82 | 33 / 86 | 35 / 91 | 37 / 96 | 39 / 101 |
| 8 | | 1 / 15 | 3 / 21 | 5 / 27 | 8 / 32 | 10 / 38 | 13 / 43 | 15 / 49 | 18 / 54 | 20 / 60 | 23 / 65 | 26 / 70 | 28 / 76 | 31 / 81 | 33 / 87 | 36 / 92 | 39 / 97 | 41 / 103 | 44 / 108 | 47 / 113 |
| 9 | | 1 / 17 | 3 / 24 | 6 / 30 | 9 / 36 | 12 / 42 | 15 / 48 | 18 / 54 | 21 / 60 | 24 / 66 | 27 / 72 | 30 / 78 | 33 / 84 | 36 / 90 | 39 / 96 | 42 / 102 | 45 / 108 | 48 / 114 | 51 / 120 | 54 / 126 |
| 10 | | 1 / 19 | 4 / 26 | 7 / 33 | 11 / 39 | 14 / 46 | 17 / 53 | 20 / 60 | 24 / 66 | 27 / 73 | 31 / 79 | 34 / 86 | 37 / 93 | 41 / 99 | 44 / 106 | 48 / 112 | 51 / 119 | 55 / 125 | 58 / 132 | 62 / 138 |
| 11 | | 1 / 21 | 5 / 28 | 8 / 36 | 12 / 43 | 16 / 50 | 19 / 58 | 23 / 65 | 27 / 72 | 31 / 79 | 34 / 87 | 38 / 94 | 42 / 101 | 46 / 108 | 50 / 115 | 54 / 122 | 57 / 130 | 61 / 137 | 65 / 144 | 69 / 151 |
| 12 | | 2 / 22 | 5 / 31 | 9 / 39 | 13 / 47 | 17 / 55 | 21 / 63 | 26 / 70 | 30 / 78 | 34 / 86 | 38 / 94 | 42 / 102 | 47 / 109 | 51 / 117 | 55 / 125 | 60 / 132 | 64 / 140 | 68 / 148 | 72 / 156 | 77 / 163 |
| 13 | | 2 / 24 | 6 / 33 | 10 / 42 | 15 / 50 | 19 / 59 | 24 / 67 | 28 / 76 | 33 / 84 | 37 / 93 | 42 / 101 | 47 / 109 | 51 / 118 | 56 / 126 | 61 / 134 | 65 / 143 | 70 / 151 | 75 / 159 | 80 / 167 | 84 / 176 |
| 14 | | 2 / 26 | 7 / 35 | 11 / 45 | 16 / 54 | 21 / 63 | 26 / 72 | 31 / 81 | 36 / 90 | 41 / 99 | 46 / 108 | 51 / 117 | 56 / 126 | 61 / 135 | 66 / 144 | 71 / 153 | 77 / 161 | 82 / 170 | 87 / 179 | 92 / 188 |
| 15 | | 3 / 27 | 7 / 38 | 12 / 48 | 18 / 57 | 23 / 67 | 28 / 77 | 33 / 87 | 39 / 96 | 44 / 106 | 50 / 115 | 55 / 125 | 61 / 134 | 66 / 144 | 72 / 153 | 77 / 163 | 83 / 172 | 88 / 182 | 94 / 191 | 100 / 200 |
| 16 | | 3 / 29 | 8 / 40 | 14 / 50 | 19 / 61 | 25 / 71 | 30 / 82 | 36 / 92 | 42 / 102 | 48 / 112 | 54 / 122 | 60 / 132 | 65 / 143 | 71 / 153 | 77 / 163 | 83 / 173 | 89 / 183 | 95 / 193 | 101 / 203 | 107 / 213 |
| 17 | | 3 / 31 | 9 / 42 | 15 / 53 | 20 / 65 | 26 / 76 | 33 / 86 | 39 / 97 | 45 / 108 | 51 / 119 | 57 / 130 | 64 / 140 | 70 / 151 | 77 / 161 | 83 / 172 | 89 / 183 | 96 / 193 | 102 / 204 | 109 / 214 | 115 / 225 |
| 18 | | 4 / 32 | 9 / 45 | 16 / 56 | 22 / 68 | 28 / 80 | 35 / 91 | 41 / 103 | 48 / 114 | 55 / 125 | 61 / 137 | 68 / 148 | 75 / 159 | 82 / 170 | 88 / 182 | 95 / 193 | 102 / 204 | 109 / 215 | 116 / 226 | 123 / 237 |
| 19 | 0 / 19 | 4 / 34 | 10 / 47 | 17 / 59 | 23 / 72 | 30 / 84 | 37 / 96 | 44 / 108 | 51 / 120 | 58 / 132 | 65 / 144 | 72 / 156 | 80 / 167 | 87 / 179 | 94 / 191 | 101 / 203 | 109 / 214 | 116 / 226 | 123 / 238 | 130 / 250 |
| 20 | 0 / 20 | 4 / 36 | 11 / 49 | 18 / 62 | 25 / 75 | 32 / 88 | 39 / 101 | 47 / 113 | 54 / 126 | 62 / 138 | 69 / 151 | 77 / 163 | 84 / 176 | 92 / 188 | 100 / 200 | 107 / 213 | 115 / 225 | 123 / 237 | 130 / 250 | 138 / 262 |

*Experimental Design and Statistical Analysis for Pharmacology and the Biomedical Sciences*, First Edition. Paul J. Mitchell.
© 2022 John Wiley & Sons Ltd. Published 2022 by John Wiley & Sons Ltd.

**Table D.2** Critical values for $U$; One-tailed test, $p = 0.01$.

| $n_1$ $n_2$ | 1 | 2 | 3 | 4 | 5 | 6 | 7 | 8 | 9 | 10 | 11 | 12 | 13 | 14 | 15 | 16 | 17 | 18 | 19 | 20 |
|---|---|---|---|---|---|---|---|---|---|---|---|---|---|---|---|---|---|---|---|---|
| **1** | | | | | | | | | | | | | | | | | | | | |
| **2** | | | | | | | | | | | | | 0 / 26 | 0 / 28 | 0 / 30 | 0 / 32 | 0 / 34 | 0 / 36 | 1 / 37 | 1 / 39 |
| **3** | | | | | | | 0 / 21 | 0 / 24 | 1 / 26 | 1 / 29 | 1 / 32 | 2 / 34 | 2 / 37 | 2 / 40 | 3 / 42 | 3 / 45 | 4 / 47 | 4 / 50 | 4 / 52 | 5 / 55 |
| **4** | | | | | 0 / 20 | 1 / 23 | 1 / 27 | 2 / 30 | 3 / 33 | 3 / 37 | 4 / 40 | 5 / 43 | 5 / 47 | 6 / 50 | 7 / 53 | 7 / 57 | 8 / 60 | 9 / 63 | 9 / 67 | 10 / 70 |
| **5** | | | | 0 / 20 | 1 / 24 | 2 / 28 | 3 / 32 | 4 / 36 | 5 / 40 | 6 / 44 | 7 / 48 | 8 / 52 | 9 / 56 | 10 / 60 | 11 / 64 | 12 / 68 | 13 / 72 | 14 / 76 | 15 / 80 | 16 / 84 |
| **6** | | | | 1 / 23 | 2 / 28 | 3 / 33 | 4 / 38 | 6 / 42 | 7 / 47 | 8 / 52 | 9 / 57 | 11 / 61 | 12 / 66 | 13 / 71 | 15 / 75 | 16 / 80 | 18 / 84 | 19 / 89 | 20 / 94 | 22 / 98 |
| **7** | | | 0 / 21 | 1 / 27 | 3 / 32 | 4 / 38 | 6 / 43 | 7 / 49 | 9 / 54 | 11 / 59 | 12 / 65 | 14 / 70 | 16 / 75 | 17 / 81 | 19 / 86 | 21 / 91 | 23 / 96 | 24 / 102 | 26 / 107 | 28 / 112 |
| **8** | | | 0 / 24 | 2 / 30 | 4 / 36 | 6 / 42 | 7 / 49 | 9 / 55 | 11 / 61 | 13 / 67 | 15 / 73 | 17 / 79 | 20 / 84 | 22 / 90 | 24 / 96 | 26 / 102 | 28 / 108 | 30 / 114 | 32 / 120 | 34 / 126 |
| **9** | | | 1 / 226 | 3 / 33 | 5 / 40 | 7 / 47 | 9 / 54 | 11 / 61 | 14 / 67 | 16 / 74 | 18 / 81 | 21 / 87 | 23 / 94 | 26 / 100 | 28 / 107 | 31 / 113 | 33 / 120 | 36 / 126 | 38 / 133 | 40 / 140 |
| **10** | | | 1 / 29 | 3 / 37 | 6 / 44 | 8 / 52 | 11 / 59 | 13 / 67 | 16 / 74 | 19 / 81 | 22 / 88 | 24 / 96 | 27 / 103 | 30 / 110 | 33 / 117 | 36 / 124 | 38 / 132 | 41 / 139 | 44 / 146 | 47 / 153 |
| **11** | | | 1 / 32 | 4 / 40 | 7 / 48 | 9 / 57 | 12 / 65 | 15 / 73 | 18 / 81 | 22 / 88 | 25 / 96 | 28 / 104 | 31 / 112 | 34 / 120 | 37 / 128 | 41 / 135 | 44 / 143 | 47 / 151 | 50 / 159 | 53 / 167 |
| **12** | | | 2 / 34 | 5 / 43 | 8 / 52 | 11 / 61 | 14 / 70 | 17 / 79 | 21 / 87 | 24 / 96 | 28 / 104 | 31 / 113 | 35 / 121 | 38 / 130 | 42 / 138 | 46 / 146 | 49 / 155 | 53 / 163 | 56 / 172 | 60 / 180 |
| **13** | | 0 / 26 | 2 / 37 | 5 / 47 | 9 / 56 | 12 / 66 | 16 / 76 | 20 / 84 | 23 / 94 | 27 / 103 | 31 / 112 | 35 / 121 | 39 / 130 | 43 / 139 | 47 / 148 | 51 / 157 | 55 / 166 | 59 / 175 | 63 / 184 | 67 / 193 |
| **14** | | 0 / 28 | 2 / 40 | 6 / 50 | 10 / 60 | 13 / 71 | 17 / 81 | 22 / 90 | 26 / 100 | 30 / 110 | 34 / 120 | 38 / 130 | 43 / 139 | 47 / 149 | 51 / 159 | 56 / 168 | 60 / 178 | 65 / 187 | 69 / 197 | 73 / 207 |
| **15** | | 0 / 30 | 3 / 42 | 7 / 53 | 11 / 64 | 15 / 75 | 19 / 86 | 24 / 96 | 28 / 107 | 33 / 117 | 37 / 128 | 42 / 138 | 47 / 148 | 51 / 159 | 56 / 169 | 61 / 179 | 66 / 189 | 70 / 200 | 75 / 210 | 80 / 220 |
| **16** | | 0 / 32 | 3 / 45 | 7 / 57 | 12 / 68 | 16 / 80 | 21 / 91 | 26 / 102 | 31 / 113 | 36 / 124 | 41 / 135 | 46 / 146 | 51 / 157 | 56 / 168 | 61 / 179 | 66 / 190 | 71 / 201 | 76 / 212 | 82 / 222 | 87 / 233 |
| **17** | | 0 / 34 | 4 / 47 | 8 / 60 | 13 / 72 | 18 / 84 | 23 / 96 | 28 / 108 | 33 / 120 | 38 / 132 | 44 / 143 | 49 / 155 | 55 / 166 | 60 / 178 | 66 / 189 | 71 / 201 | 77 / 212 | 82 / 224 | 88 / 234 | 93 / 247 |
| **18** | | 0 / 36 | 4 / 50 | 9 / 63 | 14 / 76 | 19 / 89 | 24 / 102 | 30 / 114 | 36 / 126 | 41 / 139 | 47 / 151 | 53 / 163 | 59 / 175 | 65 / 187 | 70 / 200 | 76 / 212 | 82 / 224 | 88 / 236 | 94 / 248 | 100 / 260 |
| **19** | | 1 / 37 | 4 / 53 | 9 / 67 | 15 / 80 | 20 / 94 | 26 / 107 | 32 / 120 | 38 / 133 | 44 / 146 | 50 / 159 | 56 / 172 | 63 / 184 | 69 / 197 | 75 / 210 | 82 / 222 | 88 / 235 | 94 / 248 | 101 / 260 | 107 / 273 |
| **20** | | 1 / 39 | 5 / 55 | 10 / 70 | 16 / 84 | 22 / 98 | 28 / 112 | 34 / 126 | 40 / 140 | 47 / 153 | 53 / 167 | 60 / 180 | 67 / 193 | 73 / 207 | 80 / 220 | 87 / 233 | 93 / 247 | 100 / 260 | 107 / 273 | 114 / 286 |

## Table D.3 Critical values for $U$; Two-tailed test, $p = 0.05$.

| $n_1$ \ $n_2$ | 1 | 2 | 3 | 4 | 5 | 6 | 7 | 8 | 9 | 10 | 11 | 12 | 13 | 14 | 15 | 16 | 17 | 18 | 19 | 20 |
|---|---|---|---|---|---|---|---|---|---|---|---|---|---|---|---|---|---|---|---|---|
| **1** | | | | | | | | | | | | | | | | | | | | |
| **2** | | | | | | | | 0<br>16 | 0<br>18 | 0<br>20 | 0<br>22 | 1<br>23 | 1<br>25 | 1<br>27 | 1<br>29 | 1<br>31 | 2<br>32 | 2<br>34 | 2<br>36 | 2<br>38 |
| **3** | | | | | 0<br>15 | 1<br>17 | 1<br>20 | 2<br>22 | 2<br>25 | 3<br>27 | 3<br>30 | 4<br>32 | 4<br>35 | 5<br>37 | 5<br>40 | 6<br>42 | 6<br>45 | 7<br>47 | 7<br>50 | 8<br>52 |
| **4** | | | | 0<br>16 | 1<br>19 | 2<br>22 | 3<br>25 | 4<br>28 | 4<br>32 | 5<br>35 | 6<br>38 | 7<br>41 | 8<br>44 | 9<br>47 | 10<br>50 | 11<br>53 | 11<br>57 | 12<br>60 | 13<br>63 | 13<br>67 |
| **5** | | | 0<br>15 | 1<br>19 | 2<br>23 | 3<br>27 | 5<br>30 | 6<br>34 | 7<br>38 | 8<br>42 | 9<br>46 | 11<br>49 | 12<br>53 | 13<br>57 | 14<br>61 | 15<br>65 | 17<br>68 | 18<br>72 | 19<br>76 | 20<br>80 |
| **6** | | | 1<br>17 | 2<br>22 | 3<br>27 | 5<br>31 | 6<br>36 | 8<br>40 | 10<br>44 | 11<br>49 | 13<br>53 | 14<br>58 | 16<br>62 | 17<br>67 | 19<br>71 | 21<br>75 | 22<br>80 | 24<br>84 | 25<br>89 | 27<br>93 |
| **7** | | | 1<br>20 | 3<br>25 | 5<br>30 | 6<br>36 | 8<br>41 | 10<br>46 | 12<br>51 | 14<br>56 | 16<br>61 | 18<br>66 | 20<br>71 | 22<br>76 | 24<br>81 | 26<br>86 | 28<br>91 | 30<br>96 | 32<br>101 | 34<br>106 |
| **8** | | 0<br>16 | 2<br>22 | 4<br>28 | 6<br>34 | 8<br>40 | 10<br>46 | 13<br>51 | 15<br>57 | 17<br>63 | 19<br>69 | 22<br>74 | 24<br>80 | 26<br>86 | 29<br>91 | 31<br>97 | 34<br>102 | 36<br>108 | 38<br>114 | 41<br>119 |
| **9** | | 0<br>18 | 2<br>25 | 4<br>32 | 7<br>38 | 10<br>44 | 12<br>51 | 15<br>57 | 17<br>64 | 20<br>70 | 23<br>76 | 26<br>82 | 28<br>89 | 31<br>95 | 34<br>101 | 37<br>107 | 39<br>114 | 42<br>120 | 45<br>126 | 48<br>132 |
| **10** | | 0<br>20 | 3<br>27 | 5<br>35 | 8<br>42 | 11<br>49 | 14<br>56 | 17<br>63 | 20<br>70 | 23<br>77 | 26<br>84 | 29<br>91 | 33<br>97 | 36<br>104 | 39<br>111 | 42<br>118 | 45<br>125 | 48<br>132 | 52<br>138 | 55<br>145 |
| **11** | | 0<br>22 | 3<br>30 | 6<br>38 | 9<br>46 | 13<br>53 | 16<br>61 | 19<br>69 | 23<br>76 | 26<br>84 | 30<br>91 | 33<br>99 | 37<br>106 | 40<br>114 | 44<br>121 | 47<br>129 | 51<br>136 | 55<br>143 | 58<br>151 | 62<br>158 |
| **12** | | 1<br>23 | 4<br>32 | 7<br>41 | 11<br>49 | 14<br>58 | 18<br>66 | 22<br>74 | 26<br>82 | 29<br>91 | 33<br>99 | 37<br>107 | 41<br>115 | 45<br>123 | 49<br>131 | 53<br>139 | 57<br>147 | 61<br>155 | 65<br>163 | 69<br>171 |
| **13** | | 1<br>25 | 4<br>35 | 8<br>44 | 12<br>53 | 16<br>62 | 20<br>71 | 24<br>80 | 28<br>89 | 33<br>97 | 37<br>106 | 41<br>115 | 45<br>124 | 50<br>132 | 54<br>141 | 59<br>149 | 63<br>158 | 67<br>167 | 72<br>175 | 76<br>184 |
| **14** | | 1<br>27 | 5<br>37 | 9<br>47 | 13<br>57 | 17<br>67 | 22<br>76 | 26<br>86 | 31<br>95 | 36<br>104 | 40<br>114 | 45<br>123 | 50<br>132 | 55<br>141 | 59<br>151 | 64<br>160 | 67<br>171 | 74<br>178 | 78<br>188 | 83<br>197 |
| **15** | | 1<br>29 | 5<br>40 | 10<br>50 | 14<br>61 | 19<br>71 | 24<br>81 | 29<br>91 | 34<br>101 | 39<br>111 | 44<br>121 | 49<br>131 | 54<br>141 | 59<br>151 | 64<br>161 | 70<br>170 | 75<br>180 | 80<br>190 | 85<br>200 | 90<br>210 |
| **16** | | 1<br>31 | 6<br>42 | 11<br>53 | 15<br>65 | 21<br>75 | 26<br>86 | 31<br>97 | 37<br>107 | 42<br>118 | 47<br>129 | 53<br>139 | 59<br>149 | 64<br>160 | 70<br>170 | 75<br>181 | 81<br>191 | 86<br>202 | 92<br>212 | 98<br>222 |
| **17** | | 2<br>32 | 6<br>45 | 11<br>57 | 17<br>68 | 22<br>80 | 28<br>91 | 34<br>102 | 39<br>114 | 45<br>125 | 51<br>136 | 57<br>147 | 63<br>158 | 67<br>171 | 75<br>180 | 81<br>191 | 87<br>202 | 93<br>213 | 99<br>224 | 105<br>235 |
| **18** | | 2<br>34 | 7<br>47 | 12<br>60 | 18<br>72 | 24<br>84 | 30<br>96 | 36<br>108 | 42<br>120 | 48<br>132 | 55<br>143 | 61<br>155 | 67<br>167 | 74<br>178 | 80<br>190 | 86<br>202 | 93<br>213 | 99<br>225 | 106<br>236 | 112<br>248 |
| **19** | | 2<br>36 | 7<br>50 | 13<br>63 | 19<br>76 | 25<br>89 | 32<br>101 | 38<br>114 | 45<br>126 | 52<br>138 | 58<br>151 | 65<br>163 | 72<br>175 | 78<br>188 | 85<br>200 | 92<br>212 | 99<br>224 | 106<br>236 | 113<br>248 | 119<br>261 |
| **20** | | 2<br>38 | 8<br>52 | 13<br>67 | 20<br>80 | 27<br>93 | 34<br>106 | 41<br>119 | 48<br>132 | 55<br>145 | 62<br>158 | 69<br>171 | 76<br>184 | 83<br>197 | 90<br>210 | 98<br>222 | 105<br>235 | 112<br>248 | 119<br>261 | 127<br>273 |

Table D.4  Critical values for $U$; Two-tailed test, $p = 0.01$.

| $n_1$ \ $n_2$ | 1 | 2 | 3 | 4 | 5 | 6 | 7 | 8 | 9 | 10 | 11 | 12 | 13 | 14 | 15 | 16 | 17 | 18 | 19 | 20 |
|---|---|---|---|---|---|---|---|---|---|---|---|---|---|---|---|---|---|---|---|---|
| 1 | | | | | | | | | | | | | | | | | | | | |
| 2 | | | | | | | | | | | | | | | | | | | 0/38 | 0/40 |
| 3 | | | | | | | | | 0/27 | 0/30 | 0/33 | 1/35 | 1/38 | 1/41 | 2/43 | 2/46 | 2/49 | 2/52 | 3/54 | 3/57 |
| 4 | | | | | | 0/24 | 0/28 | 1/31 | 1/35 | 2/38 | 2/42 | 3/45 | 3/49 | 4/52 | 5/55 | 5/59 | 6/62 | 6/66 | 7/69 | 8/72 |
| 5 | | | | | 0/25 | 1/29 | 1/34 | 2/38 | 3/42 | 4/46 | 5/50 | 6/54 | 7/58 | 7/63 | 8/67 | 9/71 | 10/75 | 11/79 | 12/83 | 13/87 |
| 6 | | | | 0/24 | 1/29 | 2/34 | 3/39 | 4/44 | 5/49 | 6/54 | 7/59 | 9/63 | 10/68 | 11/73 | 12/78 | 13/83 | 15/87 | 16/92 | 17/97 | 18/102 |
| 7 | | | | 0/28 | 1/34 | 3/39 | 4/45 | 6/50 | 7/56 | 9/61 | 10/67 | 12/72 | 13/78 | 15/83 | 16/89 | 18/94 | 19/100 | 2/105 | 22/111 | 24/116 |
| 8 | | | | 1/31 | 2/38 | 4/44 | 6/50 | 7/57 | 9/63 | 11/69 | 13/75 | 15/81 | 17/87 | 18/94 | 20/100 | 22/106 | 24/112 | 26/118 | 28/124 | 30/130 |
| 9 | | | 0/27 | 1/35 | 3/42 | 5/49 | 7/56 | 9/63 | 11/70 | 13/77 | 16/83 | 18/90 | 20/97 | 22/104 | 24/111 | 27/117 | 29/124 | 31/131 | 33/138 | 36/144 |
| 10 | | | 0/30 | 2/38 | 4/46 | 6/54 | 9/61 | 11/69 | 13/77 | 16/84 | 18/92 | 21/99 | 24/106 | 26/114 | 29/121 | 31/129 | 34/136 | 37/143 | 39/151 | 42/158 |
| 11 | | | 0/33 | 2/42 | 5/50 | 7/59 | 10/67 | 13/75 | 16/83 | 18/92 | 21/100 | 24/108 | 27/116 | 30/124 | 33/132 | 36/140 | 39/148 | 42/156 | 45/164 | 48/172 |
| 12 | | | 1/35 | 3/45 | 6/54 | 9/63 | 12/72 | 15/81 | 18/90 | 21/99 | 24/108 | 27/117 | 31/125 | 34/134 | 37/143 | 41/151 | 44/160 | 47/169 | 51/177 | 54/186 |
| 13 | | | 1/38 | 3/49 | 7/58 | 10/68 | 13/78 | 17/87 | 20/97 | 24/106 | 27/116 | 31/125 | 34/135 | 38/144 | 42/153 | 45/163 | 49/172 | 53/181 | 56/191 | 60/200 |
| 14 | | | 1/41 | 4/52 | 7/63 | 11/73 | 15/83 | 18/94 | 22/104 | 26/114 | 30/124 | 34/134 | 38/144 | 42/154 | 46/164 | 50/174 | 54/184 | 58/194 | 63/203 | 67/213 |
| 15 | | | 2/43 | 5/55 | 8/67 | 12/78 | 16/89 | 20/100 | 24/111 | 29/121 | 33/132 | 37/143 | 42/153 | 46/164 | 51/174 | 55/185 | 60/195 | 4/206 | 69/216 | 73/227 |
| 16 | | | 2/46 | 5/59 | 9/71 | 13/83 | 18/94 | 22/106 | 27/117 | 31/129 | 36/140 | 41/151 | 45/163 | 50/174 | 55/185 | 60/196 | 65/207 | 70/218 | 74/230 | 79/241 |
| 17 | | | 2/49 | 6/62 | 10/75 | 15/87 | 19/100 | 24/112 | 29/124 | 34/138 | 39/148 | 44/160 | 49/172 | 54/184 | 60/195 | 65/207 | 70/219 | 75/231 | 81/242 | 86/254 |
| 18 | | | 2/52 | 6/66 | 11/79 | 16/92 | 21/105 | 26/118 | 31/131 | 37/143 | 42/156 | 47/169 | 53/181 | 58/194 | 64/206 | 70/218 | 75/231 | 81/243 | 87/255 | 92/268 |
| 19 | | 0/38 | 3/54 | 7/69 | 12/83 | 17/97 | 22/111 | 28/124 | 33/138 | 39/151 | 45/164 | 51/177 | 56/191 | 63/203 | 69/216 | 74/230 | 81/242 | 87/255 | 93/268 | 99/281 |
| 20 | | 0/40 | 3/57 | 8/72 | 13/87 | 18/102 | 24/116 | 30/130 | 36/144 | 42/158 | 48/172 | 54/186 | 60/200 | 67/213 | 73/227 | 79/241 | 86/254 | 92/268 | 99/281 | 105/295 |

Source: From Mann, H.B. and Whitney, D.R. (1947). On a test of whether one of two random variables is stochastically larger than the other. *Annals of Mathematical Statistics* 18: 50–60 and Auble, D. (1958). Extended tables for the Mann-Whitney statistic. *Bulletin of the institute of Educational Research at Indianna University* 1 (2): 1–33.

# Appendix E: Critical values of the *F* distribution

V alues in the following tables indicate the critical values of *F* for $p = 0.05$, 0.01, and 0.001 (Tables E.1, E.2, and E.3, respectively).

**Table E.1**  Critical values of *F*, $p = 0.05$.

| $v_1$ $v_2$ | 1 | 2 | 3 | 4 | 5 | 6 | 7 | 8 | 10 | 12 | 24 | ∞ |
|---|---|---|---|---|---|---|---|---|---|---|---|---|
| 1 | 161.4 | 199.5 | 215.7 | 224.6 | 230.2 | 234.0 | 236.8 | 238.9 | 241.9 | 243.9 | 249.0 | 254.3 |
| 2 | 18.5 | 19.0 | 19.2 | 19.2 | 19.3 | 19.3 | 19.4 | 19.4 | 19.4 | 19.4 | 19.5 | 19.5 |
| 3 | 10.13 | 9.55 | 9.28 | 9.12 | 9.01 | 8.94 | 8.89 | 8.85 | 8.79 | 8.74 | 8.64 | 8.53 |
| 4 | 7.71 | 6.94 | 9.59 | 9.39 | 6.26 | 6.16 | 6.09 | 6.04 | 5.96 | 5.91 | 5.77 | 5.63 |
| 5 | 6.61 | 5.79 | 5.41 | 5.19 | 5.05 | 4.95 | 4.88 | 4.82 | 4.74 | 4.68 | 4.53 | 4.36 |
| 6 | 5.99 | 5.14 | 4.76 | 4.53 | 4.39 | 4.28 | 4.21 | 4.15 | 4.06 | 4.00 | 3.84 | 3.67 |
| 7 | 5.59 | 4.74 | 4.35 | 4.12 | 3.97 | 3.87 | 3.79 | 3.73 | 3.64 | 3.57 | 3.41 | 3.23 |
| 8 | 5.32 | 4.46 | 4.07 | 3.84 | 3.69 | 3.58 | 3.50 | 3.44 | 3.35 | 3.28 | 3.12 | 2.93 |
| 9 | 5.12 | 4.26 | 3.86 | 3.63 | 3.48 | 3.37 | 3.29 | 3.23 | 3.14 | 3.07 | 2.90 | 2.71 |
| 10 | 4.96 | 4.10 | 3.71 | 3.48 | 3.33 | 3.22 | 3.14 | 3.07 | 2.98 | 2.97 | 2.74 | 2.54 |
| 11 | 4.84 | 3.98 | 3.59 | 3.36 | 3.20 | 3.09 | 3.01 | 2.95 | 2.85 | 2.79 | 2.61 | 2.40 |
| 12 | 4.75 | 3.89 | 3.49 | 3.26 | 3.11 | 3.00 | 2.91 | 2.85 | 2.75 | 2.69 | 2.51 | 2.30 |
| 13 | 4.67 | 3.81 | 3.41 | 3.18 | 3.03 | 2.92 | 2.83 | 2.77 | 2.67 | 2.60 | 2.42 | 2.21 |
| 14 | 4.60 | 3.74 | 3.34 | 3.11 | 2.96 | 2.85 | 2.76 | 2.70 | 2.60 | 2.53 | 2.35 | 2.13 |
| 15 | 4.54 | 3.68 | 3.29 | 3.06 | 2.90 | 2.79 | 2.71 | 2.64 | 2.54 | 2.48 | 2.29 | 2.07 |
| 16 | 4.49 | 3.63 | 3.24 | 3.01 | 2.85 | 2.74 | 2.66 | 2.59 | 2.49 | 2.42 | 2.24 | 2.01 |
| 17 | 4.45 | 3.59 | 3.20 | 2.96 | 2.81 | 2.70 | 2.61 | 2.55 | 2.45 | 2.38 | 2.19 | 1.96 |
| 18 | 4.41 | 3.55 | 3.16 | 2.93 | 2.77 | 2.66 | 2.58 | 2.51 | 2.41 | 2.34 | 2.15 | 1.92 |
| 19 | 4.38 | 3.52 | 3.13 | 2.90 | 2.74 | 2.63 | 2.54 | 2.48 | 2.38 | 2.31 | 2.11 | 1.88 |
| 20 | 4.35 | 3.49 | 3.10 | 2.87 | 2.71 | 2.60 | 2.51 | 2.45 | 2.35 | 2.28 | 2.08 | 1.84 |
| 21 | 4.32 | 3.47 | 3.07 | 2.84 | 2.68 | 2.57 | 2.49 | 2.42 | 2.32 | 2.25 | 2.05 | 1.81 |
| 22 | 4.30 | 3.44 | 3.05 | 2.82 | 2.66 | 2.55 | 2.46 | 2.40 | 2.30 | 2.23 | 2.03 | 1.78 |
| 23 | 4.28 | 3.42 | 3.03 | 2.80 | 2.64 | 2.53 | 2.44 | 2.37 | 2.27 | 2.20 | 2.00 | 1.76 |
| 24 | 4.26 | 3.40 | 3.01 | 2.78 | 2.62 | 2.51 | 2.42 | 2.36 | 2.25 | 2.18 | 1.98 | 1.73 |
| 25 | 4.24 | 3.39 | 2.99 | 2.76 | 2.60 | 2.49 | 2.40 | 2.34 | 2.24 | 2.16 | 1.96 | 1.71 |
| 26 | 4.23 | 3.37 | 2.98 | 2.74 | 2.59 | 2.47 | 2.39 | 2.32 | 2.22 | 2.15 | 1.95 | 1.69 |
| 27 | 4.21 | 3.35 | 2.96 | 2.73 | 2.57 | 2.46 | 2.37 | 2.31 | 2.20 | 2.13 | 1.93 | 1.67 |
| 28 | 4.20 | 3.34 | 2.95 | 2.71 | 2.56 | 2.45 | 2.36 | 2.29 | 2.19 | 2.12 | 1.91 | 1.65 |
| 29 | 4.18 | 3.33 | 2.93 | 2.70 | 2.55 | 2.43 | 2.35 | 2.28 | 2.18 | 2.10 | 1.90 | 1.64 |
| 30 | 4.17 | 3.32 | 2.92 | 2.69 | 2.53 | 2.42 | 2.33 | 2.27 | 2.16 | 2.09 | 1.89 | 1.62 |
| 32 | 4.15 | 3.29 | 2.90 | 2.67 | 2.51 | 2.40 | 2.31 | 2.24 | 2.14 | 2.07 | 1.86 | 1.59 |
| 34 | 4.13 | 3.28 | 2.88 | 2.65 | 2.49 | 2.38 | 2.29 | 2.23 | 2.12 | 2.05 | 1.84 | 1.57 |
| 36 | 4.11 | 3.26 | 2.87 | 2.63 | 2.48 | 2.36 | 2.28 | 2.21 | 2.11 | 2.03 | 1.82 | 1.55 |
| 38 | 4.10 | 3.24 | 2.85 | 2.62 | 2.46 | 2.35 | 2.26 | 2.19 | 2.09 | 2.02 | 1.81 | 1.53 |
| 40 | 4.08 | 3.23 | 2.84 | 2.61 | 2.45 | 2.34 | 2.25 | 2.18 | 2.08 | 2.00 | 1.79 | 1.51 |
| 60 | 4.00 | 3.15 | 2.76 | 2.53 | 2.37 | 2.25 | 2.17 | 2.10 | 1.99 | 1.92 | 1.70 | 1.39 |
| 120 | 3.92 | 3.07 | 2.68 | 2.45 | 2.29 | 2.18 | 2.09 | 2.02 | 1.91 | 1.83 | 1.61 | 1.25 |
| ∞ | 3.84 | 3.00 | 2.60 | 2.37 | 2.21 | 2.10 | 2.01 | 1.94 | 1.83 | 1.75 | 1.52 | 1.00 |

*Experimental Design and Statistical Analysis for Pharmacology and the Biomedical Sciences*, First Edition. Paul J. Mitchell.
© 2022 John Wiley & Sons Ltd. Published 2022 by John Wiley & Sons Ltd.

Table E.2 Critical values of $F$, $p = 0.01$.

| $v_1$ $v_2$ | 1 | 2 | 3 | 4 | 5 | 6 | 7 | 8 | 10 | 12 | 24 | ∞ |
|---|---|---|---|---|---|---|---|---|---|---|---|---|
| 1 | 4052 | 5000 | ∞5403 | 5625 | 5764 | 5859 | 5928 | 5981 | 6056 | 6106 | 6235 | 6366 |
| 2 | 98.5 | 99.0 | 99.2 | 99.2 | 99.3 | 99.3 | 99.4 | 99.4 | 99.4 | 99.4 | 99.5 | 99.5 |
| 3 | 34.1 | 30.8 | 29.5 | 28.7 | 28.2 | 27.9 | 27.7 | 27.5 | 27.2 | 27.1 | 26.6 | 26.1 |
| 4 | 21.2 | 18.0 | 16.7 | 16.0 | 15.5 | 15.2 | 15.0 | 14.8 | 14.5 | 14.4 | 13.9 | 13.5 |
| 5 | 16.26 | 13.27 | 12.06 | 11.39 | 10.97 | 10.67 | 10.46 | 10.29 | 10.05 | 9.89 | 9.47 | 9.02 |
| 6 | 13.74 | 10.92 | 9.78 | 9.15 | 8.75 | 8.47 | 8.26 | 8.10 | 7.87 | 7.72 | 7.31 | 6.88 |
| 7 | 12.25 | 9.55 | 8.45 | 7.85 | 7.46 | 7.19 | 6.99 | 6.84 | 6.62 | 6.47 | 6.07 | 5.65 |
| 8 | 11.26 | 8.65 | 7.59 | 7.01 | 6.63 | 6.37 | 6.18 | 6.03 | 5.81 | 5.67 | 5.28 | 4.86 |
| 9 | 10.56 | 8.02 | 6.99 | 6.42 | 6.06 | 5.80 | 5.61 | 5.47 | 5.26 | 5.11 | 4.73 | 4.31 |
| 10 | 10.04 | 7.56 | 6.55 | 5.99 | 5.64 | 5.39 | 5.20 | 5.06 | 4.85 | 4.71 | 4.33 | 3.91 |
| 11 | 9.65 | 7.21 | 6.22 | 5.67 | 5.32 | 5.07 | 4.89 | 4.74 | 4.54 | 4.40 | 4.02 | 3.60 |
| 12 | 9.33 | 6.93 | 5.95 | 5.41 | 5.06 | 4.82 | 4.64 | 4.50 | 4.30 | 4.16 | 3.78 | 3.36 |
| 13 | 9.07 | 6.70 | 5.74 | 5.21 | 4.86 | 4.62 | 4.44 | 4.30 | 4.10 | 3.96 | 3.59 | 3.17 |
| 14 | 8.86 | 6.51 | 5.56 | 5.04 | 4.70 | 4.46 | 4.28 | 4.14 | 3.94 | 3.80 | 3.43 | 3.00 |
| 15 | 8.68 | 6.36 | 5.42 | 4.89 | 4.56 | 4.32 | 4.14 | 4.00 | 3.80 | 3.67 | 3.29 | 2.87 |
| 16 | 8.53 | 6.23 | 5.29 | 4.77 | 4.44 | 4.20 | 4.03 | 3.89 | 3.69 | 3.55 | 3.18 | 2.75 |
| 17 | 8.40 | 6.11 | 5.18 | 4.67 | 4.34 | 4.10 | 3.93 | 3.79 | 3.59 | 3.46 | 3.08 | 2.65 |
| 18 | 8.29 | 6.01 | 5.09 | 4.58 | 4.25 | 4.01 | 3.84 | 3.71 | 3.51 | 3.37 | 3.00 | 2.57 |
| 19 | 8.18 | 5.93 | 5.01 | 4.50 | 4.17 | 3.94 | 3.77 | 3.63 | 3.43 | 3.30 | 2.92 | 2.49 |
| 20 | 8.10 | 5.85 | 4.94 | 4.43 | 4.10 | 3.87 | 3.70 | 3.56 | 3.37 | 3.23 | 2.86 | 2.42 |
| 21 | 8.02 | 5.78 | 4.87 | 4.37 | 4.04 | 3.81 | 3.64 | 3.51 | 3.31 | 3.17 | 2.80 | 2.36 |
| 22 | 7.95 | 5.72 | 4.82 | 4.31 | 3.99 | 3.76 | 3.59 | 3.45 | 3.26 | 3.12 | 2.75 | 2.31 |
| 23 | 7.88 | 5.66 | 4.76 | 4.26 | 3.94 | 3.71 | 3.54 | 3.41 | 3.21 | 3.07 | 2.70 | 2.26 |
| 24 | 7.82 | 5.61 | 4.72 | 4.22 | 3.90 | 3.67 | 3.50 | 3.36 | 3.17 | 3.03 | 2.66 | 2.21 |
| 25 | 7.77 | 5.57 | 4.68 | 4.18 | 3.86 | 3.63 | 3.46 | 3.32 | 3.13 | 2.99 | 2.62 | 2.17 |
| 26 | 7.72 | 5.53 | 4.64 | 4.14 | 3.82 | 3.59 | 3.42 | 3.29 | 3.09 | 2.96 | 2.58 | 2.13 |
| 27 | 7.68 | 5.49 | 4.60 | 4.11 | 3.78 | 3.56 | 3.36 | 3.26 | 3.06 | 2.93 | 2.55 | 2.10 |
| 28 | 7.64 | 5.45 | 4.57 | 4.07 | 3.75 | 3.53 | 3.36 | 3.23 | 3.03 | 2.90 | 2.52 | 2.06 |
| 29 | 7.60 | 5.42 | 4.54 | 4.04 | 3.73 | 3.50 | 3.33 | 3.20 | 3.00 | 2.87 | 2.49 | 2.03 |
| 30 | 7.56 | 5.39 | 4.51 | 4.02 | 3.70 | 3.47 | 3.30 | 3.17 | 2.98 | 2.84 | 2.47 | 2.01 |
| 32 | 7.50 | 5.34 | 4.46 | 3.97 | 3.65 | 3.43 | 3.26 | 3.13 | 2.93 | 2.80 | 2.42 | 1.96 |
| 34 | 7.45 | 5.29 | 4.42 | 3.93 | 3.61 | 3.39 | 3.22 | 3.09 | 2.90 | 2.76 | 2.38 | 1.91 |
| 36 | 7.40 | 5.25 | 4.38 | 3.89 | 3.58 | 3.35 | 3.18 | 3.05 | 2.86 | 2.72 | 2.35 | 1.87 |
| 38 | 7.35 | 5.21 | 4.34 | 3.86 | 3.54 | 3.32 | 3.15 | 3.02 | 2.83 | 2.69 | 2.32 | 1.84 |
| 40 | 7.31 | 5.18 | 4.31 | 3.83 | 3.51 | 3.29 | 3.12 | 2.99 | 2.80 | 2.66 | 2.29 | 1.80 |
| 60 | 7.08 | 4.98 | 4.13 | 3.65 | 3.34 | 3.12 | 2.95 | 2.82 | 2.63 | 2.50 | 2.12 | 1.60 |
| 120 | 6.85 | 4.79 | 3.95 | 3.48 | 3.17 | 2.96 | 2.79 | 2.66 | 2.47 | 2.34 | 1.95 | 1.38 |
| ∞ | 6.63 | 4.61 | 3.78 | 3.32 | 3.02 | 2.80 | 2.64 | 2.51 | 2.32 | 2.18 | 1.79 | 1.00 |

**Table E.3** Critical values of $F$, $p = 0.001$.

| $v_1$ $v_2$ | 1 | 2 | 3 | 4 | 5 | 6 | 7 | 8 | 10 | 12 | 24 | ∞ |
|---|---|---|---|---|---|---|---|---|---|---|---|---|
| 1 | 405300 | 500000 | 540400 | 562500 | 576400 | 585900 | 592900 | 598100 | 605600 | 610700 | 623500 | 636600 |
| 2 | 998.5 | 999.0 | 999.2 | 999.2 | 999.3 | 999.3 | 999.4 | 999.4 | 999.4 | 999.4 | 999.5 | 999.5 |
| 3 | 167.0 | 148.5 | 141.1 | 137.1 | 134.6 | 132.8 | 131.5 | 130.6 | 129.2 | 128.3 | 125.9 | 123.5 |
| 4 | 74.14 | 61.25 | 56.18 | 53.44 | 51.71 | 50.53 | 49.66 | 49.00 | 48.05 | 47.41 | 45.77 | 44.05 |
| 5 | 47.18 | 37.12 | 33.20 | 31.09 | 29.75 | 28.83 | 28.16 | 27.65 | 26.92 | 26.42 | 25.14 | 23.79 |
| 6 | 35.51 | 27.00 | 23.70 | 21.92 | 20.80 | 20.03 | 19.46 | 19.03 | 18.41 | 17.99 | 16.90 | 15.75 |
| 7 | 29.25 | 21.69 | 18.77 | 17.20 | 16.21 | 15.52 | 15.02 | 14.63 | 14.08 | 13.71 | 12.73 | 11.70 |
| 8 | 25.42 | 18.49 | 15.83 | 14.39 | 13.48 | 12.86 | 12.40 | 12.05 | 11.54 | 11.19 | 10.30 | 9.34 |
| 9 | 22.76 | 16.39 | 13.90 | 12.56 | 11.71 | 11.13 | 10.69 | 10.37 | 9.87 | 9.57 | 8.72 | 7.81 |
| 10 | 21.04 | 14.91 | 12.55 | 11.28 | 10.48 | 9.93 | 9.52 | 9.20 | 8.74 | 8.44 | 7.64 | 6.76 |
| 11 | 19.69 | 13.81 | 11.56 | 10.35 | 9.58 | 9.05 | 8.66 | 8.35 | 7.92 | 7.63 | 6.85 | 6.00 |
| 12 | 18.64 | 12.97 | 10.80 | 9.63 | 8.89 | 8.38 | 8.0 | 7.71 | 7.29 | 7.00 | 6.25 | 5.42 |
| 13 | 17.82 | 12.31 | 10.21 | 9.07 | 8.35 | 7.86 | 7.49 | 7.21 | 6.80 | 6.52 | 5.78 | 4.97 |
| 14 | 17.14 | 11.78 | 9.73 | 8.62 | 7.92 | 7.44 | 7.08 | 6.80 | 6.40 | 6.13 | 5.41 | 4.60 |
| 15 | 16.59 | 11.34 | 9.34 | 8.25 | 7.57 | 7.09 | 6.74 | 6.47 | 6.08 | 5.81 | 5.10 | 4.31 |
| 16 | 16.12 | 10.97 | 9.01 | 7.94 | 7.27 | 6.80 | 6.46 | 6.19 | 5.81 | 5.55 | 4.85 | 4.06 |
| 17 | 15.72 | 10.66 | 8.73 | 7.68 | 7.02 | 6.56 | 6.22 | 5.96 | 5.58 | 5.32 | 4.63 | 3.85 |
| 18 | 15.38 | 10.39 | 8.49 | 7.46 | 6.81 | 6.35 | 6.02 | 5.76 | 5.39 | 5.13 | 4.45 | 3.67 |
| 19 | 15.08 | 10.16 | 8.28 | 7.27 | 6.62 | 6.18 | 5.85 | 5.59 | 5.22 | 4.97 | 4.29 | 3.51 |
| 20 | 14.82 | 9.95 | 8.10 | 7.10 | 6.46 | 6.02 | 5.69 | 5.44 | 5.08 | 4.82 | 4.15 | 3.38 |
| 21 | 14.59 | 9.77 | 7.94 | 6.95 | 6.32 | 5.88 | 5.56 | 5.31 | 4.95 | 4.70 | 4.03 | 3.26 |
| 22 | 14.38 | 9.61 | 7.80 | 6.81 | 6.19 | 5.76 | 5.44 | 5.19 | 4.83 | 4.58 | 3.92 | 3.15 |
| 23 | 14.19 | 9.47 | 7.67 | 6.70 | 6.08 | 5.65 | 5.33 | 5.09 | 4.73 | 4.48 | 3.82 | 3.05 |
| 24 | 14.03 | 9.34 | 7.55 | 6.59 | 5.98 | 5.55 | 5.23 | 4.99 | 4.64 | 4.39 | 3.74 | 2.97 |
| 25 | 13.88 | 9.22 | 7.45 | 6.49 | 5.89 | 5.46 | 5.15 | 4.91 | 4.56 | 4.31 | 3.66 | 2.89 |
| 26 | 13.74 | 9.12 | 7.36 | 6.41 | 5.80 | 5.38 | 5.07 | 4.83 | 4.48 | 4.24 | 3.59 | 2.82 |
| 27 | 13.61 | 9.02 | 7.27 | 6.33 | 5.73 | 5.31 | 5.00 | 4.76 | 4.41 | 4.17 | 3.52 | 2.75 |
| 28 | 13.50 | 8.93 | 7.19 | 6.25 | 5.66 | 5.24 | 4.93 | 4.69 | 4.35 | 4.11 | 3.46 | 2.69 |
| 29 | 13.39 | 8.85 | 7.12 | 6.19 | 5.59 | 5.18 | 4.87 | 4.64 | 4.29 | 4.05 | 3.41 | 2.64 |
| 30 | 13.29 | 8.77 | 7.05 | 6.12 | 5.53 | 5.12 | 4.82 | 4.58 | 4.24 | 4.0 | 3.36 | 2.59 |
| 32 | 13.12 | 8.64 | 6.94 | 6.01 | 5.43 | 5.02 | 4.72 | 4.48 | 4.14 | 3.91 | 3.27 | 2.50 |
| 34 | 12.97 | 8.52 | 6.83 | 5.92 | 5.34 | 4.93 | 4.63 | 4.40 | 4.06 | 3.83 | 3.19 | 2.42 |
| 36 | 12.83 | 8.42 | 6.74 | 5.84 | 5.26 | 4.86 | 4.56 | 4.33 | 3.99 | 3.76 | 3.12 | 2.35 |
| 38 | 12.71 | 8.33 | 6.66 | 5.76 | 5.19 | 4.79 | 4.49 | 4.26 | 3.93 | 3.70 | 3.06 | 2.29 |
| 40 | 12.61 | 8.25 | 6.59 | 5.70 | 5.13 | 4.73 | 4.44 | 4.21 | 3.87 | 3.64 | 3.01 | 2.23 |
| 60 | 11.97 | 7.77 | 6.17 | 5.31 | 4.76 | 4.37 | 4.09 | 3.86 | 3.54 | 3.32 | 2.69 | 1.89 |
| 120 | 11.38 | 7.32 | 5.78 | 4.95 | 4.42 | 4.04 | 3.77 | 3.55 | 3.24 | 3.02 | 2.40 | 1.54 |
| ∞ | 10.83 | 6.91 | 5.42 | 4.62 | 4.10 | 3.74 | 3.47 | 3.27 | 2.96 | 2.74 | 2.13 | 1.00 |

*Source:* From Lindley, D.V. and Miller, J.C.P. (1952). *Cambridge Elementary Statistical Tables*, 8–11. Cambridge University Press.

Write Your Own Notes

# Appendix F: Critical values of chi-square distribution

Values in the following tables indicate the critical values of the chi-square distribution for $p = 0.05$, $0.01$, and $0.001$ according to the number of degrees of freedom.

| Degrees of Freedom | Probability | | | Degrees of Freedom | Probability | | |
|---|---|---|---|---|---|---|---|
| | 0.05 | 0.01 | 0.001 | | 0.05 | 0.01 | 0.001 |
| 1 | 3.84 | 6.63 | 10.83 | 20 | 31.41 | 37.57 | 45.31 |
| 2 | 5.99 | 9.21 | 13.81 | 21 | 32.67 | 38.93 | 46.80 |
| 3 | 7.81 | 11.34 | 16.27 | 22 | 33.92 | 40.29 | 48.27 |
| 4 | 9.49 | 13.28 | 18.47 | 23 | 35.17 | 41.64 | 49.73 |
| 5 | 11.07 | 15.09 | 20.52 | 24 | 36.42 | 42.98 | 51.18 |
| 6 | 12.59 | 16.81 | 22.46 | 25 | 37.65 | 44.31 | 52.62 |
| 7 | 14.07 | 18.48 | 24.32 | 26 | 38.89 | 45.64 | 54.05 |
| 8 | 15.51 | 20.09 | 26.12 | 27 | 40.11 | 46.96 | 55.48 |
| 9 | 16.92 | 21.67 | 27.88 | 28 | 41.34 | 48.28 | 56.89 |
| 10 | 18.31 | 23.21 | 29.59 | 29 | 42.56 | 49.59 | 58.30 |
| 11 | 19.68 | 24.73 | 31.26 | 30 | 43.77 | 50.89 | 59.70 |
| 12 | 21.03 | 26.22 | 32.91 | 40 | 55.76 | 63.69 | 73.40 |
| 13 | 22.36 | 27.69 | 34.53 | 50 | 67.5 | 76.15 | 86.66 |
| 14 | 23.68 | 29.14 | 36.12 | 60 | 79.08 | 88.38 | 99.61 |
| 15 | 25.00 | 30.58 | 37.70 | 70 | 9.053 | 100.4 | 112.3 |
| 16 | 26.30 | 32.00 | 39.25 | 80 | 101.9 | 112.3 | 124.8 |
| 17 | 27.90 | 33.41 | 40.79 | 90 | 113.1 | 124.1 | 137.2 |
| 18 | 28.87 | 34.81 | 42.31 | 100 | 124.3 | 135.8 | 149.4 |
| 19 | 30.14 | 36.198 | 43.82 | 200 | 233.99 | 249.45 | |

*Source:* From Lindley, D.V. and Miller J.C.P. (1952). *Cambridge Elementary Statistical Tables*, 7. Cambridge University Press.

*Experimental Design and Statistical Analysis for Pharmacology and the Biomedical Sciences*, First Edition. Paul J. Mitchell.
© 2022 John Wiley & Sons Ltd. Published 2022 by John Wiley & Sons Ltd.

# Write Your Own Notes

# Appendix G: Critical *z* values for multiple non-parametric pairwise comparisons

V alues in the following tables indicate the critical values of *z* for a given number of comparisons and level of significance α = 0.05 or α = 0.01 for one- and two-tailed tests.

**Table G.1** Critical values of *z* according to the number of comparisons.

| Number of comparisons | α = 0.05 One-tailed | α = 0.05 Two-tailed |
|---|---|---|
| 1 | 1.645 | 1.960 |
| 2 | 1.960 | 2.241 |
| 3 | 2.128 | 2.394 |
| 4 | 2.241 | 2.498 |
| 5 | 2.326 | 2.576 |
| 6 | 2.394 | 2.638 |
| 7 | 2.450 | 2.690 |
| 8 | 2.498 | 2.734 |
| 9 | 2.539 | 2.773 |
| 10 | 2.576 | 2.807 |
| 11 | 2.608 | 2.838 |
| 12 | 2.638 | 2.866 |
| 15 | 2.713 | 2.935 |
| 21 | 2.823 | 3.038 |
| 28 | 2.913 | 3.125 |

Table values indicate the point on the standard normal distribution abscissa where the upper-tail probability is equal to $\frac{1}{2}$ α /number of comparisons.

Values of *z* outside the range of the table may be found in Appendix B.

**Table G.2** Alternative critical values of *z* according to the number of comparisons when all groups have an equal number of subjects.

| Number of comparisons | One-tailed α = 0.05 | One-tailed α = 0.01 | Two-tailed α = 0.05 | Two-tailed α = 0.01 |
|---|---|---|---|---|
| 1 | 1.65 | 2.33 | 1.96 | 2.58 |
| 2 | 1.92 | 2.56 | 2.21 | 2.79 |
| 3 | 2.06 | 2.69 | 2.35 | 2.92 |
| 4 | 2.16 | 2.77 | 2.44 | 3.00 |
| 5 | 2.24 | 2.84 | 2.51 | 3.06 |
| 6 | 2.29 | 2.89 | 2.57 | 3.11 |
| 7 | 2.34 | 2.94 | 2.61 | 3.15 |
| 8 | 2.38 | 2.97 | 2.65 | 3.19 |
| 9 | 2.42 | 3.00 | 2.69 | 3.22 |
| 10 | 2.45 | 3.03 | 2.72 | 3.25 |
| 11 | 2.48 | 3.06 | 2.74 | 3.27 |
| 12 | 2.5 | 3.08 | 2.77 | 3.29 |
| 15 | 2.57 | 3.17 | 2.83 | 3.35 |
| 20 | 2.64 | 3.21 | 2.91 | 3.42 |

Table values are adjusted critical values of *z* for a given value of α, and the number of comparisons to be used when all groups have equal number of subjects.
One tailed: Adapted from Gupta, S.S. (1963). Probability integrals of multivariate normal and multivariate t. *Annals of Mathematical Statistics* 34: 792–823.
Two tailed: Adapted from Dunnett, C.W. (1964). New tables for multiple comparisons with a control. *Biometrics* 20: 482–491.
N.B. From Siegel, S. and Castellan, N.J. Jr. (1988). *Nonparametric Statistics for the Behavioral Sciences*, 2e. Singapore: McGraw-Hill Book Co.

*Experimental Design and Statistical Analysis for Pharmacology and the Biomedical Sciences*, First Edition. Paul J. Mitchell.
© 2022 John Wiley & Sons Ltd. Published 2022 by John Wiley & Sons Ltd.

# Write Your Own Notes

# Appendix H: Critical values of correlation coefficients

Values in the following tables indicate the critical values of the Pearson product moment correlation coefficient, $r$, for $p = 0.05$, 0.01, and 0.001 according to the degrees of freedom, df, i.e. $(N - 2)$.

Table H.1 Pearson product moment correlation.

| df | Probability (two-tailed) | | | df | Probability (two-tailed) | | |
|---|---|---|---|---|---|---|---|
| | 0.05 | 0.01 | 0.001 | | 0.05 | 0.01 | 0.001 |
| 1 | 0.997 | 0.999 | 1.000 | 20 | 0.423 | 0.537 | 0.652 |
| 2 | 0.950 | 0.990 | 0.999 | 21 | 0.413 | 0.526 | 0.640 |
| 3 | 0.878 | 0.959 | 0.991 | 22 | 0.404 | 0.515 | 0.629 |
| 4 | 0.811 | 0.917 | 0.974 | 23 | 0.396 | 0.505 | 0.618 |
| 5 | 0.754 | 0.875 | 0.951 | 24 | 0.388 | 0.496 | 0.607 |
| 6 | 0.707 | 0.834 | 0.925 | 25 | 0.381 | 0.487 | 0.597 |
| 7 | 0.666 | 0.798 | 0.898 | 26 | 0.374 | 0.479 | 0.588 |
| 8 | 0.632 | 0.765 | 0.872 | 27 | 0.367 | 0.471 | 0.579 |
| 9 | 0.602 | 0.735 | 0.847 | 28 | 0.361 | 0.463 | 0.570 |
| 10 | 0.576 | 0.708 | 0.823 | 29 | 0.355 | 0.456 | 0.562 |
| 11 | 0.553 | 0.684 | 0.801 | 30 | 0.349 | 0.449 | 0.554 |
| 12 | 0.532 | 0.661 | 0.780 | 40 | 0.304 | 0.393 | 0.490 |
| 13 | 0.514 | 0.641 | 0.760 | 50 | 0.273 | 0.354 | 0.443 |
| 14 | 0.497 | 0.623 | 0.742 | 60 | 0.250 | 0.325 | 0.408 |
| 15 | 0.482 | 0.606 | 0.725 | 70 | 0.232 | 0.303 | 0.380 |
| 16 | 0.468 | 0.590 | 0.708 | 80 | 0.217 | 0.283 | 0.357 |
| 17 | 0.456 | 0.575 | 0.693 | 90 | 0.205 | 0.267 | 0.338 |
| 18 | 0.444 | 0.561 | 0.679 | 100 | 0.195 | 0.254 | 0.321 |
| 19 | 0.433 | 0.549 | 0.665 | 200 | 0.138 | 0.181 | 0.230 |

*Source:* Lentner, C. (ed.) (1984). *Geigy Scientific Tables*, 8e. Novartis.

*Experimental Design and Statistical Analysis for Pharmacology and the Biomedical Sciences*, First Edition. Paul J. Mitchell.
© 2022 John Wiley & Sons Ltd. Published 2022 by John Wiley & Sons Ltd.

Values in the following tables indicate the critical values of the Spearman Rank correlation coefficient, $r_s$, for $p = 0.05$, 0.01, and 0.001 according to the number of data pairs, $N$.

Table H.2 Spearman rank correlation.

| N | Probability (two-tailed) | | | N | Probability (two-tailed) | | |
|---|---|---|---|---|---|---|---|
|  | 0.05 | 0.01 | 0.001 |  | 0.05 | 0.01 | 0.001 |
| 3 |  |  |  | 20 | 0.447 | 0.570 | 0.693 |
| 4 |  |  |  | 21 | 0.436 | 0.556 | 0.678 |
| 5 | 1.000 |  |  | 22 | 0.425 | 0.544 | 0.665 |
| 6 | 0.886 | 1.000 |  | 23 | 0.416 | 0.532 | 0.652 |
| 7 | 0.786 | 0.929 | 1.000 | 24 | 0.407 | 0.521 | 0.640 |
| 8 | 0.738 | 0.881 | 0.976 | 25 | 0.398 | 0.511 | 0.628 |
| 9 | 0.700 | 0.833 | 0.933 | 26 | 0.390 | 0.501 | 0.618 |
| 10 | 0.648 | 0.794 | 0.903 | 27 | 0.383 | 0.492 | 0.607 |
| 11 | 0.618 | 0.755 | 0.873 | 28 | 0.375 | 0.483 | 0.597 |
| 12 | 0.587 | 0.727 | 0.846 | 29 | 0.368 | 0.475 | 0.588 |
| 13 | 0.560 | 0.703 | 0.824 | 30 | 0.362 | 0.467 | 0.579 |
| 14 | 0.538 | 0.679 | 0.802 | 40 | 0.313 | 0.405 | 0.506 |
| 15 | 0.521 | 0.654 | 0.779 | 50 | 0.279 | 0.363 | 0.456 |
| 16 | 0.503 | 0.635 | 0.762 | 60 | 0.255 | 0.331 | 0.417 |
| 17 | 0.488 | 0.618 | 0.743 | 70 | 0.235 | 0.307 | 0.387 |
| 18 | 0.472 | 0.600 | 0.725 | 80 | 0.220 | 0.287 | 0.363 |
| 19 | 0.460 | 0.584 | 0.709 | 90 | 0.207 | 0.271 | 0.343 |
|  |  |  |  | 100 | 0.197 | 0.257 | 0.326 |

Note: Tabulated critical values of $r_s$ are exact for $3 \leq N \leq 18$ and Edgeworth approximations for $N \geq 19$.
Source: Lentner, C. (ed.) (1984). Geigy Scientific Tables, 8e. Novartis.

Values in the following table indicate the critical values of the Kendall's tau, $\tau$, for $p = 0.05$ and 0.01 according to the number of data pairs, $N$.

Table H.3  Kendall's rank correlation (Kendall's tau).

| N | Probability (two-tailed) | |
|---|---|---|
| | 0.05 | 0.01 |
| 3 | | |
| 4 | | |
| 5 | 1.000 | |
| 6 | 0.867 | 1.000 |
| 7 | 0.714 | 0.905 |
| 8 | 0.643 | 0.786 |
| 9 | 0.556 | 0.722 |
| 10 | 0.551 | 0.644 |
| 11 | 0.491 | 0.600 |
| 12 | 0.455 | 0.576 |
| 13 | 0.436 | 0.564 |
| 14 | 0.407 | 0.516 |
| 15 | 0.390 | 0.505 |
| 16 | 0.383 | 0.483 |
| 17 | 0.368 | 0.471 |
| 18 | 0.346 | 0.451 |
| 19 | 0.333 | 0.439 |
| 20 | 0.326 | 0.421 |
| 21 | 0.314 | 0.410 |
| 22 | 0.307 | 0.378 |
| 23 | 0.296 | 0.391 |
| 24 | 0.290 | 0.377 |
| 25 | 0.287 | 0.367 |
| 26 | 0.280 | 0.360 |
| 27 | 0.271 | 0.356 |
| 28 | 0.265 | 0.344 |
| 29 | 0.261 | 0.340 |
| 30 | 0.255 | 0.333 |

*Source:* real-statistics.com.

# Summary Decision Flowchart

## Parametric chart

**If your data set meets the following criteria:**

| | |
|---|---|
| Data type: | Measurement |
| Form: | Continuos |
| Scale: | Interval / Ratio |
| Spread: | Homogeneity of variance: Levene's test: $p > 0.05$ |
| Distribution: | Approximately normally distributed K–S (D): $p > 0.05$ S–W (W): $p > 0.05$ |
| Skewness: | F–P skewness coefficient: F–P: $< \pm2$. z-score: $<1.96$, $p > 0.05$ |
| Kurtosis: | Kurtosis: $<5$ z-score: $<1.96$, $p > 0.05$ |

**Descriptive measures — Parametric data (raw or transformed)**

| | |
|---|---|
| Central tendency | Mean |
| Spread | Sum of squares |
| | Variance |
| | Standard deviation |
| | Standard error of the mean |

**Single or multiple pair-wise comparisons**

| Group type | Number of Groups = 2 ONLY! | Number of Groups > 2 — Grouping Factor(s) | ANOVA model | Post hoc multiple comparisons |
|---|---|---|---|---|
| Independent | Independent t-test (Chapter 11) | 1 Between Group | One-way ANOVA (Chapter 15) | • All Means comparisons or • Control group comparisons (Chapter 15: Table 15.13) |
| | | 2 Between Groups | Two-way ANOVA (Chapter 17) | As above or multiple independent t-tests with Bonferroni or Holme correction, as appropriate(Chapter 17) |
| | | 3 Between Groups | Three-way ANOVA (Chapter 17) | |
| Paired | Paired t-test (Chapter 12) | 1 Within Group | Repeated Measures ANOVA (Chapter 16) | • Turkey, Games-Howell. • Turkey with Bonferroni or Sidak correction • Multiple paired t-tests with Bonferroni or Holme correction (Chapter 16) |
| Mixed Independent and Paired | | 1 Between Group+ 1 Within Group | One-way ANOVA with Repeated Measures (Chapter 17) | Multiple Independent and Paired t-tests with Bonferroni correction as justified by each Main effect of the Grouping Factors and interaction(s) therein (Chapter 17) |
| | | 2 Between Groups + 1 Within Group | Two-way ANOVA with Repeated Measures (Chapter 17) | |

**Type of association**

| Group type | Type of association | Inferential test |
|---|---|---|
| Independent | Correlation | Pearson's product-moment correlation test (Chapter 19) |
| Independent and dependent | Regression | Linear regression (Chapter 20) |

## Non-parametric chart

**If your data set meets the following criteria:**

| | |
|---|---|
| Data type: | Nominal (Categories) Ordinal (Ranks) |
| Form: | Discrete |
| Scale: | Limited: defined maximum and minimum |
| Spread: | Homogeneity of variance: Levene's test: $p < 0.05$ |
| Distribution: | Non-normal distribution. K–S (D): $p < 0.05$ S–W (W): $p < 0.05$ |
| Skewness: | F–P skewness coefficient: F–P: $> \pm2$. z-score: $>1.96$, $p < 0.05$ |
| Kurtosis: | Kurtosis: $>5$ z-score: $>1.96$, $p < 0.05$ |

**Descriptive measures — Non-parametric data (or distribution unknown)**

| | |
|---|---|
| Central tendency | Nominal: Mode |
| | Ordinal: Median |
| Spread | Ordinal Lower quartile |
| | Upper quartile |
| | Interquartile range |
| | Range |

**Single or multiple pair-wise comparisons**

| Group type | Number of Groups = 2 ONLY! | Number of Groups > 2 — Grouping Factor(s) | ANOVA model | Post hoc multiple comparisons |
|---|---|---|---|---|
| Independent | Wilcoxon Rank Sum test or Mann-Whitney U-test (Chapter 13) | 1 Between Group | Kruskal-Wallis test (Chapter 18) | Multiple Mann-Whitney U-test with Bonferroni or Holme correction or independent variant of Dunn's test (Chapter 18) |
| | | 2 Between Group | Scheirer-Ray-Hare extension (Chapter 18) | |
| Paired | Wilcoxon Signed Rank test (Chapter 14) | 1 Within Group | Friedman test (Chapter 18) | Multiple Mann-Whitney U-test with Bonferroni or Holme correction or paired variant of Dunn's test (Chapter 18) |

**Type of association**

| Group type | Type of association | Inferential tests |
|---|---|---|
| Independent | Correlation | Spearman's test (tied or no tied ranks), Kendall's test (Chapter 19) |
| Independent | Categorical | Chi-square test (Chapter 21) |

# Index

*Experimental Design and Statistical Analysis for Pharmacology and the Biomedical Sciences*, First Edition. Paul J. Mitchell.
© 2022 John Wiley & Sons Ltd. Published 2022 by John Wiley & Sons Ltd.